ATLAS OF
Regional Anesthesia

ATLAS OF
Regional Anesthesia

Fourth Edition

David L. Brown, MD

Professor of Anesthesiology
Cleveland Clinic Learner College of Medicine
Chairman of Anesthesiology Institute
The Cleveland Clinic
Cleveland, Ohio

ILLUSTRATIONS BY
Jo Ann Clifford

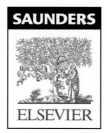

SAUNDERS
ELSEVIER

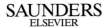

1600 John F. Kennedy Blvd.
Ste 1800
Philadelphia, PA 19103-2899

ATLAS OF REGIONAL ANESTHESIA   ISBN: 978-1-4160-6397-1
Copyright © 2010, 2006, 1999, 1992 by Saunders, an imprint of Elsevier Inc.

Library of Congress Cataloging-in-Publication Data
Brown, David L. (David Lee)
   Atlas of regional anesthesia / David L. Brown ; illustrations by Jo Ann Clifford and Joanna Wild King.—4th ed.
       p. ; cm.
   Includes bibliographical references and index.
   ISBN 978-1-4160-6397-1
   1. Conduction anesthesia—Atlases.   2. Local anesthesia—Atlases.   I. Title.
   [DNLM: 1. Anesthesia, Conduction—methods—Atlases. WO 517 B877a 2011]
   RD84.B76 2011
   617.9′64—dc22
                                                                       2010002699

Executive Publisher: Natasha Andjelkovic
Developmental Editor: Julie Goolsby
Publishing Services Manager: Tina Rebane
Project Manager: Amy Norwitz
Design Direction: Steven Stave

Printed in China

Last digit is the print number: 9 8 7 6 5 4 3 2 1

Dedicated to

Kathryn, Sarah, Eric, Noah, and Cody

And you who think to reveal the figure of a man in words, with his limbs arranged in all their different attitudes, banish the idea from you, for the more minute your description the more you will confuse the mind of the reader and the more you will lead him away from the knowledge of the thing described. It is necessary therefore for you to represent and describe.

LEONARDO DA VINCI

(1452–1519)

The Notebooks of Leonardo da Vinci, Vol. 1, Ch. III*

*Translator: Edward MacCurdy
Reynal & Hitchcock, New York, 1938

Contributors

André P. Boezaart, MD, PhD
Professor of Anesthesiology and Orthopaedic Surgery, University of Florida College of Medicine; Chief of Division of Acute Pain Medicine and Regional Anesthesia; Director of Acute Pain Medicine and Regional Anesthesia Fellowship Program, Department of Anesthesiology, University of Florida College of Medicine, Gainesville, Florida

Ursula A. Galway, MD
Assistant Professor, Cleveland Clinic Lerner College of Medicine of Case Western Reserve University; Staff Anesthesiologist, Department of General Anesthesiology, Cleveland Clinic Foundation, Cleveland, Ohio

James P. Rathmell, MD
Associate Professor of Anaesthesia, Harvard Medical School; Chief of Division of Pain Medicine, Department of Anesthesia, Critical Care and Pain Medicine, Massachusetts General Hospital, Boston, Massachusetts

Richard W. Rosenquist, MD
Professor of Anesthesia and Director of Pain Medicine Division, Department of Anesthesia, University of Iowa School of Medicine; Medical Director of Center for Pain Medicine and Regional Anesthesia, Department of Anesthesia, University of Iowa Hospitals and Clinics, Iowa City, Iowa

Brian D. Sites, MD
Associate Professor of Anesthesiology and Orthopedics, Dartmouth Medical School, Hanover; Director of Regional Anesthesiology and Orthopedics, Department of Anesthesiology, Dartmouth-Hitchcock Medical Center, Lebanon, New Hampshire

Brian C. Spence, MD
Assistant Professor of Anesthesiology, Dartmouth Medical School, Hanover; Director of Same-Day Surgery Program, Department of Anesthesiology, Dartmouth-Hitchcock Medical Center, Lebanon, New Hampshire

Preface to the Fourth Edition

Creating another edition of our *Atlas of Regional Anesthesia* demanded that we include the advances that are driving much of the change in regional anesthesia and pain practices, and we have wisely chosen experts in our specialty to contribute to this edition. The first two editions of the *Atlas* were based on my experience in my practice; thankfully, as my academic practice grew, others came alongside me to add their knowledge and practical experience. The goal with this fourth edition remains the same as with the first edition—to teach physicians needing to learn regional anesthesia and pain medicine technical procedures these techniques as they are practiced by physicians who use them daily, incorporating the pearls learned from this daily practice.

I remain indebted to my three outstanding physician contributors to the third edition, Drs. André Boezaart, James Rathmell, and Richard Rosenquist. Each has updated his contributions to this work. Additionally, two physicians helping to lead the revolution in ultrasound imaging in regional anesthesia have joined us, Drs. Brian Sites and Brian Spence. Their insights into the use of ultrasound will keep each of us focused on where our subspecialty is going. Finally, Dr. Ursula Galway has added her expertise in transversus abdominis plane block. Our artist for this edition remains Ms. Joanna Wild King; again she used her vision for simplification of images and concepts to improve on our technical messages.

I want to thank so many colleagues and patients across the country who share a belief that society as a whole benefits from physicians' becoming more adept at regional anesthesia and pain medicine techniques, as we are able to treat both acute and chronic pain more effectively.

David L. Brown

Introduction

The necessary, but somewhat artificial, separation of anesthetic care into regional or general anesthetic techniques often gives rise to the concept that these two techniques should not or cannot be mixed. Nothing could be farther from the truth. To provide comprehensive regional anesthesia care, it is absolutely essential that the anesthesiologist be skilled in all aspects of anesthesia. This concept is not original: John Lundy promoted this idea in the 1920s when he outlined his concept of "balanced anesthesia." Even before Lundy promoted this concept, George Crile had written extensively on the concept of anociassociation.

It is often tempting, and quite human, to trace the evolution of a discipline back through the discipline's developmental family tree. When such an investigation is carried out for regional anesthesia, Louis Gaston Labat, MD, often receives credit for being central in its development. Nevertheless, Labat's interest and expertise in regional anesthesia had been nurtured by Dr. Victor Pauchet of Paris, France, to whom Dr. Labat was an assistant. The real trunk of the developmental tree of regional anesthesia consists of the physicians willing to incorporate regional techniques into their early surgical practices. In Labat's original 1922 text *Regional Anesthesia: Its Technique and Clinical Application,* Dr. William Mayo in the foreword stated:

> The young surgeon should perfect himself in the use of regional anesthesia, which increases in value with the increase in the skill with which it is administered. The well equipped surgeon must be prepared to use the proper anesthesia, or the proper combination of anesthesias, in the individual case. I do not look forward to the day when regional anesthesia will wholly displace general anesthesia; but undoubtedly it will reach and hold a very high position in surgical practice.

Perhaps if the current generation of both surgeons and anesthesiologists keeps Mayo's concept in mind, our patients will be the beneficiaries.

It appears that these early surgeons were better able to incorporate regional techniques into their practices because they did not see the regional block as the "end all." Rather, they saw it as part of a comprehensive package that had benefit for their patients. Surgeons and anesthesiologists in that era were able to avoid the flawed logic that often seems to pervade application of regional anesthesia today. These individuals did not hesitate to supplement their blocks with sedatives or light general anesthetics; they did not expect each and every block to be "100%." The concept that a block has failed unless it provides complete anesthesia without supplementation seems to have occurred when anesthesiology developed as an independent specialty. To be successful in carrying out regional anesthesia, we must be willing to get back to our roots and embrace the concepts of these early workers who did not hesitate to supplement their regional blocks. Ironically, today some consider a regional block a failure if the initial dose does not produce complete anesthesia; yet these same individuals complement our "general anesthetists" who utilize the concept of anesthetic titration as a goal. Somehow, we need to meld these two views into one that allows comprehensive, titrated care to be provided for all our patients.

As Dr. Mayo emphasized in Labat's text, it is doubtful that regional anesthesia will "ever wholly displace general anesthesia." Likewise, it is equally clear that general anesthesia will probably never be able to replace the appropriate use of regional anesthesia. One of the principal rationales for avoiding the use of regional anesthesia through the years has been that it was "expensive" in terms of operating room and physician time. As is often the case, when examined in detail, some accepted truisms need rethinking. Thus, it is surprising that much of the renewed interest in regional anesthesia results from focusing on health care costs and the need to decrease the length and cost of hospitalization.

If regional anesthesia is to be incorporated successfully into a practice, there must be time for anesthesiologist and patient to discuss the upcoming operation and anesthetic prescription. Likewise, if regional anesthesia is to be effectively used, some area of an operating suite must be used to place the blocks prior to moving patients to the main operating room. Immediately at hand in this area must be both anesthetic and resuscitative equipment (such as regional trays), as well as a variety of local anesthetic drugs that span the timeline of anesthetic duration. Even after successful completion of the technical aspect of regional anesthesia, an anesthesiologist's work is really just beginning: it is as important to use appropriate sedation intraoperatively as it was preoperatively while the block was being administered.

Contents

SECTION I: INTRODUCTION

Chapter 1:
Local Anesthetics and Regional Anesthesia Equipment ... 3

David L. Brown with contributions from Richard W. Rosenquist, Brian D. Sites, and Brian C. Spence

Chapter 2:
Continuous Peripheral Nerve Blocks 17

André P. Boezaart

SECTION II: UPPER EXTREMITY BLOCKS

Chapter 3:
Upper Extremity Block Anatomy 31

Chapter 4:
Interscalene Block 41

David L. Brown with contributions from Brian D. Sites and Brian C. Spence

Chapter 5:
Supraclavicular Block 49

David L. Brown with contributions from Brian D. Sites and Brian C. Spence

Chapter 6:
Infraclavicular Block 59

Chapter 7:
Axillary Block 67

David L. Brown with contributions from Brian D. Sites and Brian C. Spence

Chapter 8:
Distal Upper Extremity Block 73

Chapter 9:
Intravenous Regional Block 81

SECTION III: LOWER EXTREMITY BLOCKS

Chapter 10:
Lower Extremity Block Anatomy 89

Chapter 11:
Lumbar Plexus Block 97

Chapter 12:
Sciatic Block 101

Chapter 13:
Femoral Block 111

David L. Brown with contributions from Brian D. Sites and Brian C. Spence

Chapter 14:
Lateral Femoral Cutaneous Block 121

Chapter 15:
Obturator Block 125

Chapter 16:
Popliteal and Saphenous Block 129

Chapter 17:
Ankle Block 135

SECTION IV: HEAD AND NECK BLOCKS

Chapter 18:
Head and Neck Block Anatomy 141

Chapter 19:
Occipital Block 147

Chapter 20:
Trigeminal (Gasserian) Ganglion Block 151

Chapter 21:
Maxillary Block 157

Chapter 22:
Mandibular Block 161

Chapter 23:
Distal Trigeminal Block 167

Chapter 24:
Retrobulbar (Peribulbar) Block 171

Chapter 25:
Cervical Plexus Block 177

Chapter 26:
Stellate Block 183

SECTION V: AIRWAY BLOCKS

Chapter 27:
Airway Block Anatomy 191

Chapter 28:
Glossopharyngeal Block 197

Chapter 29:
Superior Laryngeal Block 203

Chapter 30:
Translaryngeal Block 207

SECTION VI: TRUNCAL BLOCKS

Chapter 31:
Truncal Block Anatomy....................................213

Chapter 32:
Breast Block 217

Chapter 33:
Intercostal Block 221

Chapter 34:
Interpleural Anesthesia 227

Chapter 35:
Lumbar Somatic Block.....................231

Chapter 36:
Inguinal Block...................................239

Chapter 37:
Paravertebral Block...........................245

André P. Boezaart and Richard W. Rosenquist

Chapter 38:
Transversus Abdominis Plane Block 255

Ursula Galway

SECTION VII: NEURAXIAL BLOCKS

Chapter 39:
Neuraxial Block Anatomy 263

Chapter 40:
Spinal Block 271

Chapter 41:
Epidural Block 285

Chapter 42:
Caudal Block.....................................301

SECTION VIII: CHRONIC PAIN BLOCKS

Chapter 43:
Chronic and Cancer Pain Care: An Introduction
and Perspective................................311

Chapter 44:
Facet Block 315

Chapter 45:
Sacroiliac Block 327

Chapter 46:
Lumbar Sympathetic Block 335

Chapter 47:
Celiac Plexus Block 339

Chapter 48:
Superior Hypogastric Plexus Block.................................349

Chapter 49:
Selective Nerve Root Block 357

James P. Rathmell

Chapter 50:
Intrathecal Catheter Implantation 365

James P. Rathmell

Chapter 51:
Spinal Cord Stimulation....................375

James P. Rathmell

Bibliography......................................385

Index 391

SECTION I:
Introduction

Local Anesthetics and Regional Anesthesia Equipment

David L. Brown

with contributions from

Richard W. Rosenquist,
Brian D. Sites, and Brian C. Spence

1

Far too often, those unfamiliar with regional anesthesia regard it as complex because of the long list of local anesthetics available and the varied techniques described. Certainly, unfamiliarity with any subject will make it look complex; thus, the goal throughout this book is to simplify regional anesthesia rather than add to its complexity.

One of the first steps in simplifying regional anesthesia is to understand the two principal decisions necessary in prescribing a regional technique. First, the *appropriate technique* needs to be chosen for the patient, the surgical procedure, and the physicians involved. Second, the *appropriate local anesthetic and potential additives* must be matched to patient, procedure, regional technique, and physician. This book will detail how to integrate these concepts into your practice.

DRUGS

Not all procedures and physicians are created equal, at least regarding the amount of time needed to complete an operation. If anesthesiologists are to use regional techniques effectively, they must be able to choose a local anesthetic that lasts the right amount of time. To do this, they understand the local anesthetic timeline from the shorter-acting to the longer-acting agents (Fig. 1-1).

All local anesthetics share the basic structure of aromatic end, intermediate chain, and amine end (Fig. 1-2). This basic structure is subdivided clinically into two classes of drugs, the amino esters and the amino amides. The *amino esters* possess an ester linkage between the aromatic end and the intermediate chain. These drugs include cocaine, procaine, 2-chloroprocaine, and tetracaine (Figs. 1-3 and 1-4). The *amino amides* contain an amide link between the aromatic end and the intermediate chain. These drugs include lidocaine, prilocaine, etidocaine, mepivacaine, bupivacaine, and ropivacaine (see Figs. 1-3 and 1-4).

Amino Esters

Cocaine was the first local anesthetic used clinically, and it is used today primarily for topical airway anesthesia. It is unique among the local anesthetics in that it is a vasoconstrictor rather than a vasodilator. Some anesthesia departments have limited the availability of cocaine because of fears of its abuse potential. In those institutions, mixtures of lidocaine and phenylephrine rather than cocaine are used to anesthetize the airway mucosa and shrink the mucous membranes.

Procaine was synthesized in 1904 by Einhorn, who was looking for a drug that was superior to cocaine and other solutions in use. Currently, procaine is seldom used for peripheral nerve or epidural blocks because of its low potency, slow onset, short duration of action, and limited power of tissue penetration. It is an excellent local anesthetic for skin infiltration, and its 10% form can be used as a short-acting (i.e., lasting <1 hour) spinal anesthetic.

	Procaine	Chloroprocaine	Lidocaine	Mepivacaine	Tetracaine	Ropivacaine	Etidocaine	Bupivacaine
Infiltration	45–60		75–90					180–360
+ epi	60–90		90–180					200–400
Peripheral			90–120	100–150		360–480		480–780
+ epi			120–180	120–220		480–600		600–900
SAB*	60–75		60		70–90			90–110
+ epi	75–90		75–100		100–150			100–150
phenylephrine†	90–120				200–300			
Epidural		45–60	80–120	90–140		140–200	120–200	165–225
+ epi		60–90	120–180	140–200		160–220	150–225	180–240

Figure 1-1. Local anesthetic timeline (length in minutes of surgical anesthesia).

*Subarachnoid block.
†For lower extremity surgery.

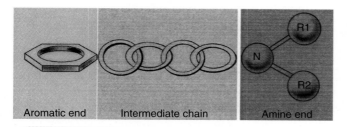

Figure 1-2. Basic local anesthetic structure.

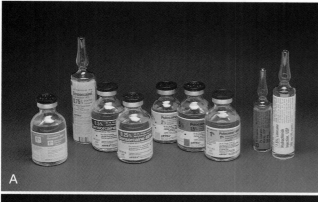

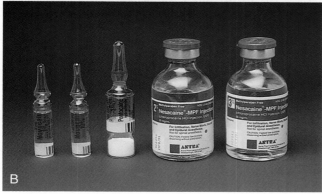

Figure 1-3. Local anesthetics commonly used in the United States. **A,** Amides. **B,** Esters.

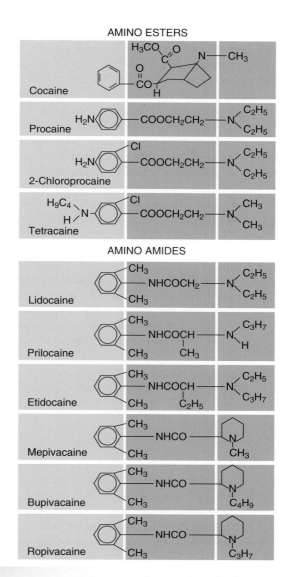

Figure 1-4. Chemical structure of commonly used amino ester and amino amide local anesthetics.

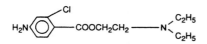

Chloroprocaine has a rapid onset and a short duration of action. Its principal use is in producing epidural anesthesia for short procedures (i.e., lasting <1 hour). Its use declined during the early 1980s after reports of prolonged sensory and motor deficits resulting from unintentional subarachnoid administration of an intended epidural dose. Since that time, the drug formulation has changed. Short-lived yet annoying back pain may develop after large (>30 mL) epidural doses of 3% chloroprocaine.

Tetracaine, first synthesized in 1931, has become widely used in the United States for spinal anesthesia. It may be used as an isobaric, hypobaric, or hyperbaric solution for spinal anesthesia. Without epinephrine it typically lasts 1.5 to 2.5 hours, and with the addition of epinephrine it may last up to 4 hours for lower extremity procedures. Tetracaine is also an effective topical airway anesthetic, although caution must be used because of the potential for systemic side effects. Tetracaine is available as a 1% solution for intrathecal use or as anhydrous crystals that are reconstituted as tetracaine solution by adding sterile water immediately before use. Tetracaine is not as stable as procaine or lidocaine in solution, and the crystals also undergo deterioration over time. Nevertheless, when a tetracaine spinal anesthetic is ineffective, one should question technique before "blaming" the drug.

Amino Amides

Lidocaine was the first clinically used amide local anesthetic, having been introduced by Lofgren in 1948.

Lidocaine has become the most widely used local anesthetic in the world because of its inherent potency, rapid onset, tissue penetration, and effectiveness during infiltration, peripheral nerve block, and both epidural and spinal blocks. During peripheral nerve block, a 1% to 1.5% solution is often effective in producing an acceptable motor blockade, whereas during epidural block, a 2% solution seems most effective. In spinal anesthesia, a 5% solution in dextrose is most commonly used, although it may also be used as a 0.5% hypobaric solution in a volume of 6 to 8 mL. Others use lidocaine as a short-acting 2% solution in a volume of 2 to 3 mL. The suggestion that lidocaine causes an unacceptable frequency of neurotoxicity with spinal use needs to be balanced against its long history of use. I believe that the basic science research may not completely reflect the typical clinical situation. In any event, I have reduced the total dose of subarachnoid lidocaine I administer to less than 75 mg per spinal procedure, inject it more rapidly than in the past, and no longer use it for continuous subarachnoid techniques. Patients often report that lidocaine causes the most common local anesthetic allergies. However, many of these reported allergies are simply epinephrine reactions resulting from intravascular injection of the local anesthetic epinephrine mixture, often during dental injection.

Prilocaine is structurally related to lidocaine, although it causes significantly less vasodilation than lidocaine and thus can be used without epinephrine. Prilocaine is formulated for infiltration, peripheral nerve block, and epidural anesthesia. Its anesthetic profile is similar to that of lidocaine, although in addition to producing less vasodilation, it has less potential for systemic toxicity in equal doses. This attribute makes it particularly useful for intravenous regional anesthesia. Prilocaine is not more widely used because, when metabolized, it can produce both orthotoluidine and nitrotoluidine, agents in methemoglobin formation.

Etidocaine is chemically related to lidocaine and is a long-acting amide local anesthetic. Etidocaine is associated with profound motor blockade and is best used when this attribute can be of clinical advantage. It has a more rapid onset of action than bupivacaine but is used less frequently. Those clinicians using etidocaine often use it for the initial epidural dose and then use bupivacaine for subsequent epidural injections.

Mepivacaine is structurally related to lidocaine and the two drugs have similar actions. Overall, mepivacaine is slightly longer acting than lidocaine, and this difference in duration is accentuated when epinephrine is added to the solutions.

Bupivacaine is a long-acting local anesthetic that can be used for infiltration, peripheral nerve block, and epidural and spinal anesthesia. Useful concentrations of the drug range from 0.125% to 0.75%. By altering the concentration of bupivacaine, sensory and motor blockade can be separated. Lower concentrations provide sensory blockade principally, and as the concentration is increased, the effectiveness of motor blockade increases with it. If an anesthesiologist had to select a single drug and a single drug concentration, 0.5% bupivacaine would be a logical choice because at that concentration it is useful for peripheral nerve block, subarachnoid block, and epidural block. Cardiotoxicity during systemic toxic reactions with bupivacaine became a concern in the 1980s. Although it is clear that bupivacaine alters myocardial conduction more dramatically than lidocaine, the need for appropriate and rapid resuscitation during any systemic toxic reaction cannot be overemphasized. Levobupivacaine is the single enantiomer (L-isomer) of bupivacaine and appears to have a systemic toxicity profile similar to that of ropivacaine, and clinically it has effects similar to those of racemic bupivacaine.

Ropivacaine is another long-acting local anesthetic, similar to bupivacaine; it was introduced in the United States in 1996. It may offer an advantage over bupivacaine because experimentally it appears to be less cardiotoxic. Whether that experimental advantage is borne out clinically remains to be seen. Initial studies also suggest that ropivacaine may produce less motor block than that produced by bupivacaine, with similar analgesia. Ropivacaine may also be slightly shorter acting than bupivacaine, with useful drug concentrations ranging from 0.25% to 1%. Many practitioners believe that ropivacaine may offer particular advantages for postoperative analgesic infusions and obstetric analgesia.

Vasoconstrictors

Vasoconstrictors are often added to local anesthetics to prolong the duration of action and improve the quality of the local anesthetic block. Although it is still unclear whether vasoconstrictors actually allow local anesthetics to have a longer duration of block or are effective because they produce additional antinociception through α-adrenergic action, their clinical effect is not in question.

Epinephrine is the most common vasoconstrictor used; overall, the most effective concentration, excluding spinal anesthesia, is a 1:200,000 concentration. When epinephrine is added to local anesthetic in the commercial production process, it is necessary to add stabilizing agents because epinephrine rapidly loses its potency on exposure to air and light. The added stabilizing agents lower the pH of the local anesthetic solution into the 3 to 4 range and, because of the higher pKas of local anesthetics, slow the onset of effective regional block. Thus, if epinephrine is to be used with local anesthetics, it should be added at the time the block is performed, at least for the initial block. In subsequent injections made during continuous epidural block, commercial preparations of local anesthetic–epinephrine solutions can be used effectively.

$$\text{(structure)} - CH - CH_2 - NH - CH_3$$

Phenylephrine also has been used as a vasoconstrictor, principally with spinal anesthesia; effective prolongation of block can be achieved by adding 2 to 5 mg of phenylephrine to the spinal anesthetic drug. Norepinephrine also has been used as a vasoconstrictor for spinal anesthesia, although it does not appear to be as long lasting as epinephrine, or to have any advantages over it. Because most local anesthetics are vasodilators, the addition of epinephrine often does not decrease blood flow as many fear it will; rather, the combination of local anesthetic and epinephrine results in tissue blood flow similar to that before injection.

NEEDLES, CATHETERS, AND SYRINGES

Effective regional anesthesia requires comprehensive knowledge of equipment—that is, the needles, syringes, and catheters that allow the anesthetic to be injected into the desired area. In early years, regional anesthesia found many variations in the method of joining needle to syringe. Around the turn of the century, Schneider developed the first all-glass syringe for Hermann Wolfing-Luer. Luer is credited with the innovation of a simple conical tip for easy exchange of needle to syringe, but the "Luer-Lok" found in use on most syringes today is thought to have been designed by Dickenson in the mid-1920s. The Luer fitting became virtually universal, and both the Luer slip tip and the Luer-Lok were standardized in 1955.

In almost all disposable and reusable needles used in regional anesthesia, the bevel is cut on three planes. The design theoretically creates less tissue laceration and discomfort than the earlier styles did, and it limits tissue coring. Many needles that are to be used for deep injection during regional block incorporate a security bead in the shaft so that the needle can be easily retrieved on the rare occasions when the needle hub separates from the needle shaft. Figure 1-5 contrasts a blunt-beveled, 25-gauge needle with a 25-gauge "hypodermic" needle. Traditional teach-

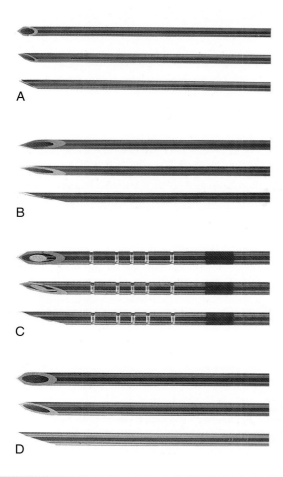

A

B

C

D

Figure 1-5. Frontal, oblique, and lateral views of regional block needles. **A,** Blunt-beveled, 25-gauge axillary block needle. **B,** Long-beveled, 25-gauge ("hypodermic") block needle. **C,** 22-gauge ultrasonography "imaging" needle. **D,** Short-beveled, 22-gauge regional block needle. (*A-D From Brown DL: Regional Anesthesia and Analgesia. Philadelphia, WB Saunders, 1996. By permission of the Mayo Foundation, Rochester, Minn.*)

ing holds that the short-beveled needle is less traumatic to neural structures. There is little clinical evidence that this is so, and experimental data about whether sharp or blunt needle tips minimize nerve injury are equivocal.

Figure 1-6 shows various spinal needles. The key to their successful use is to find the size and bevel tip that allow one to cannulate the subarachnoid space easily without causing repeated unrecognized puncture. For equivalent needle size, rounded needle tips that spread the dural fibers are associated with a lesser incidence of headache than are those that cut fibers. The past interest in very-small-gauge spinal catheters to reduce the incidence of spinal headache, with controllability of a continuous technique, faded during the controversy over lidocaine neurotoxicity.

Figure 1-7 depicts epidural needles. Needle tip design is often mandated by the decision to use a catheter with the epidural technique. Figure 1-8 shows two catheters available for either subarachnoid or epidural use. Although each has advantages and disadvantages, a single–end-hole catheter appears to provide the highest level of certainty of catheter tip location at the time of injection, whereas a multiple–side-hole catheter may be preferred for continuous analgesia techniques.

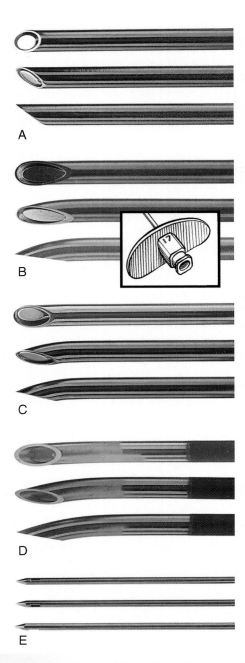

Figure 1-7. Frontal, oblique, and lateral views of common epidural needles. **A,** Crawford needle. **B,** Tuohy needle; the *inset* shows a winged hub assembly common to winged needles. **C,** Hustead needle. **D,** Curved, 18-gauge epidural needle. **E,** Whitacre, 27-gauge spinal needle. (*A-E From Brown DL: Regional Anesthesia and Analgesia. Philadelphia, WB Saunders, 1996. By permission of the Mayo Foundation, Rochester, Minn.*)

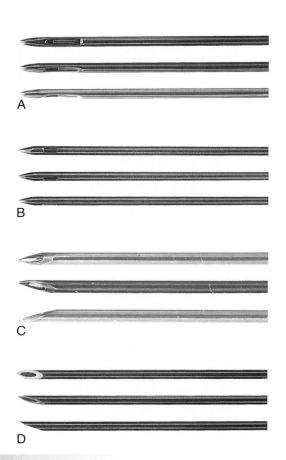

Figure 1-6. Frontal, oblique, and lateral views of common spinal needles. **A,** Sprotte needle. **B,** Whitacre needle. **C,** Greene needle. **D,** Quincke needle. (*A-D From Brown DL: Regional Anesthesia and Analgesia. Philadelphia, WB Saunders, 1996. By permission of the Mayo Foundation, Rochester, Minn.*)

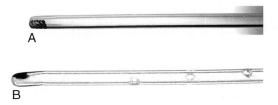

Figure 1-8. Epidural catheter designs. **A,** Single distal orifice. **B,** Closed tip with multiple side orifices. (*A and B From Brown DL: Regional Anesthesia and Analgesia. Philadelphia, WB Saunders, 1996. By permission of the Mayo Foundation, Rochester, Minn.*)

NERVE STIMULATORS

In recent years, use of nerve stimulators has increased from occasional use to common use and often critical importance. The growing emphasis on techniques that use either multiple injections near individual nerves or placement of stimulating catheters has provided impetus for this change. The primary impediment to successful use of a nerve stimulator in a clinical practice is that it is at least a three-handed or two-individual technique (Fig. 1-9), although there are devices allowing control of the stimulator current using a foot control, eliminating the need for a third hand or a second individual. In those situations requiring a second set of hands, correct operation of contemporary peripheral nerve stimulators is straightforward and easily taught during the course of the block. There are a variety of circumstances in which a nerve stimulator is helpful, such as in children and adults who are already anesthetized when a decision is made that regional block is an appropriate technique; in individuals who are unable to report paresthesias accurately; in performing local anesthetic administration on specific nerves; and in placement of stimulating catheters for anesthesia or postoperative analgesia. Another group that may benefit from the use of a nerve stimulator is patients with chronic pain, in whom accurate needle placement and reproduction of pain with electrical stimulation or elimination of pain with accurate administration of small volumes of local anesthetic may improve diagnosis and treatment.

When nerve stimulation is used during regional block, insulated needles are most appropriate because the current from such needles results in a current sphere around the needle tip, whereas uninsulated needles emit current at the tip as well as along the shaft, potentially resulting in less precise needle location. A peripheral nerve stimulator should allow between 0.1 and 10 milliamperes (mA) of current in pulses lasting approximately 200 msec at a frequency of 1 or 2 pulses per second. The peripheral nerve stimulator should have a readily apparent readout of when a complete circuit is present, a consistent and accurate

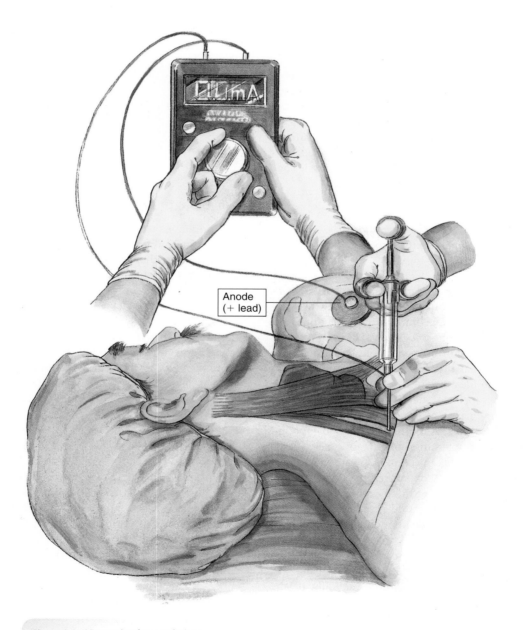

Anode
(+ lead)

Figure 1-9. Nerve stimulator technique.

current output over its entire range, and a digital display of the current delivered with each pulse. This facilitates generalized location of the nerve while stimulating at 2 mA and allows refinement of needle positioning as the current pulse is reduced to 0.5 to 0.1 mA. The nerve stimulator should have the polarity of the terminals clearly identified because peripheral nerves are most effectively stimulated by using the needle as the cathode (negative terminal). Alternatively, if the circuit is established with the needle as anode (positive terminal), approximately four times as much current is necessary to produce equivalent stimulation. The positive lead of the stimulator should be placed in a site remote from the site of stimulation by connecting the lead to a common electrocardiographic electrode (see Fig. 1-9).

The use of a nerve stimulator is not a substitute for a complete knowledge of anatomy and careful site selection for needle insertion; in fact, as much attention should be paid to the anatomy and technique when using a nerve stimulator as when not using it. Large myelinated motor fibers are stimulated by less current than are smaller unmyelinated fibers, and muscle contraction is most often produced before patient discomfort. The needle should be carefully positioned to a point where muscle contraction can be elicited with 0.5 to 0.1 mA. If a pure sensory nerve is to be blocked, a similar procedure is followed; however, correct needle localization will require the patient to report a sense of pulsed "tingling or burning" over the cutaneous distribution of the sensory nerve. Once the needle is in the final position and stimulation is achieved with 0.5 to 0.1 mA, 1 mL of local anesthetic should be injected through the needle. If the needle is accurately positioned, this amount of solution should rapidly abolish the muscle contraction or the sensation with pulsed current.

ULTRASONOGRAPHY (see *Video 1: Introduction to Ultrasound* on the Expert Consult Website)

In the last decade, image-guided peripheral nerve blocks have become the norm for anesthesiologists at the forefront of regional anesthesia innovation. The dominant method of imaging is ultrasonography. Ultrasonographic imaging devices are noninvasive, portable, and moderately priced. Most work has been done using scanning probes with frequencies in the range of 5 to 10 megahertz (MHz). These devices are capable of identifying vascular and bony structures but not nerves. Contemporary devices using high-resolution probes (12 to 15 MHz) and compound imaging allow clear visualization of nerves, vessels, catheters, and local anesthetic injection and can potentially improve the techniques of ultrasonography-assisted peripheral nerve block. Use of these devices is limited by their cost, the need for training in their use and familiarity with ultrasonographic image anatomy, and the extra set of hands required. They work best with superficial nerve plexuses and can be limited by excessive obesity or anatomically distant structures. One of the keys to using this technology effectively is a sound understanding of the physics behind ultrasonography. A corollary to understanding the physics is the need for study and appreciation of the relevant human anatomy.

Wavelength and Frequency

Ultrasound is a form of acoustic energy defined as the longitudinal progression of pressure changes (Fig. 1-10). These pressure changes consist of areas of compression and relaxation of particles in a given medium. For simplicity, an ultrasound wave is often modeled as a sine wave. Each ultrasound wave is defined by a specific wavelength (λ) measured in units of distance, amplitude (h) measured in decibels (dB), and frequency (f) measured in hertz (Hz) or cycles per second. Ultrasound is defined as a frequency of more than 20,000 Hz. Current transducers used for ultrasonography-guided regional anesthesia generate waves in the 3- to 13-MHz range (or 30,000 to 130,000 Hz).

Ultrasound Generation

Ultrasound is generated when multiple piezoelectric crystals inside a transducer rapidly vibrate in response to an alternating electric current. Ultrasound then travels into the body where, on contact with various tissues, it can be reflected, refracted, and scattered (Fig. 1-11).

To generate a clinically useful image, ultrasound waves must reflect off tissues and return to the transducer. The transducer, after emitting the wave, switches to a receive mode. When ultrasound waves return to the transducer, the piezoelectric crystals will vibrate once again, this time transforming the sound energy back into electrical energy. This process of transmission and reception can be repeated

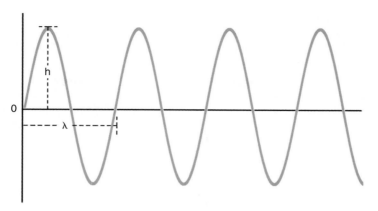

h = height of the wave, or amplitude
λ = wavelength

$$f = \frac{\text{velocity of ultrasound}}{\lambda}$$

Figure 1-10. Ultrasound wave basics.

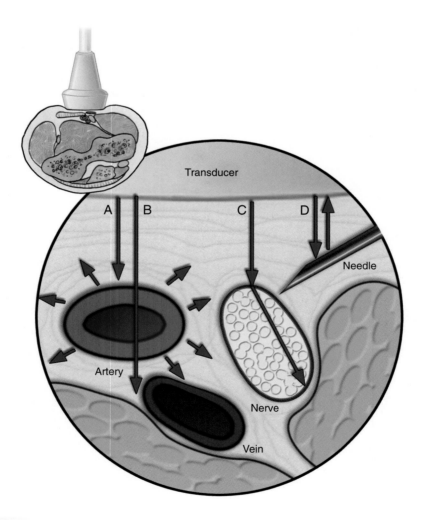

Figure 1-11. Production of an ultrasonographic image. This figure demonstrates the many responses that an ultrasound wave produces when traveling through tissue. A, Scatter reflection: the ultrasound wave is deflected in several random directions both toward and away from the probe. Scattering occurs with small or irregular objects. B, Transmission: the ultrasound wave continues through the tissue away from the probe. C, Refraction: when an ultrasound wave contacts the interface between two media with different propagation velocities, the wave is refracted (bent) to an extent depending on the difference in velocities. D, Specular reflection: a large, smooth object (e.g., the needle) returns (reflects) the ultrasound wave toward the probe when it is perpendicular to the ultrasound beam.

over 7000 times per second and, when coupled with computer processing, results in the generation of a real-time two-dimensional image that appears seamless. By convention, whiter (hyperechoic) objects represent a larger degree of reflection and higher signal intensities, whereas darker (hypoechoic) images represent less reflection and weaker signal intensities.

Clinical Issues Related to Physics

Resolution. Resolution refers to the ability to clearly distinguish two structures lying beside one another. Although there are several different types of resolution, anesthesiologists are mostly concerned with lateral resolution (left–right distinction) and axial resolution (front–back distinction). Ultrasonography systems with higher frequencies have better resolution and can effectively discriminate closely spaced peripheral neural structures. However, because of a process known as *attenuation*, high-frequency ultrasound cannot penetrate into deep tissue (Fig. 1-12). Attenuation is the loss of ultrasound energy into the surrounding tissue, primarily as heat. For superficial blocks between 1 and 4 cm in depth, frequencies greater than 10 MHz are preferred. For blocks at depths greater than 4 cm, frequencies less than 8 MHz should result in adequate tissue penetration, with a predictable degradation in resolution.

Focus. Although axial resolution is related simply to the frequency of ultrasound, lateral resolution also depends on beam thickness. Any maneuver that generates a narrow beam will increase the lateral resolution. Most ultrasonography machines have an electronic focus that generates a focal point (narrowest part of the beam) that can be placed directly over the target of interest. However, this increases the divergence of the beam beyond the region of the focus point (far field), resulting in image degradation of structures beyond this focal point. Thus, the beam focus should be placed at the level of the object that is being assessed to provide the clearest possible picture of the object (Fig. 1-13).

Gain. The overall gain and time gain compensation (TGC) controls allow the operator to increase or decrease the signal intensity. In clinical terms, the gain controls the "brightness" of the ultrasonographic image. The TGC control allows the operator to adjust gain at specific depths of the image. By increasing the overall gain or the TGC, one can compensate for the darker aspects of the ultrasonographic image, which are simply the result of ultrasound attenuation. Inappropriately low gain settings may result in the apparent absence of an existing structure (i.e., "missing structure" artifact), whereas inappropriately high gain settings can easily obscure existing structures.

Color Doppler

Color-flow Doppler ultrasonography relies on the fact that if an ultrasound pulse is sent out and strikes moving red blood cells, the ultrasound that is reflected back to the transducer will have a frequency that is different from the original emitted frequency. This change in frequency is known as the *Doppler shift*. It is this frequency change that

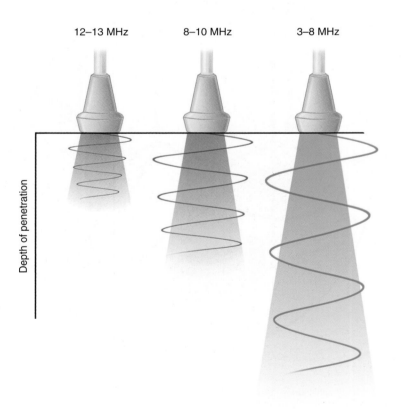

Figure 1-12. Probe frequency and depth of tissue penetration. Higher-frequency ultrasound attenuates to a larger degree at more superficial depths, although it provides more image detail.

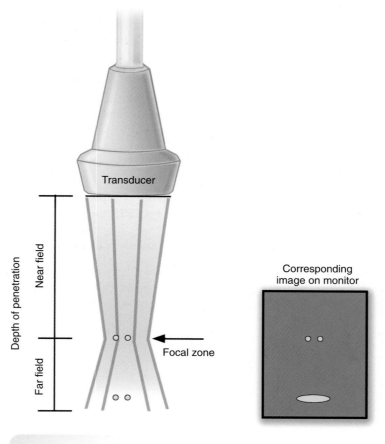

Figure 1-13. Basics of ultrasonographic probe focusing.

can be used in cardiac and vascular applications to calculate both blood flow velocity and blood flow direction. The Doppler equation states that

$$\text{Frequency shift} = 2 \times V \times Ft \times \text{cosine } \Phi / c$$

where V is velocity of the moving object, Ft is the transmitted frequency, Φ is the angle of incidence of the ultrasound beam and the direction of blood flow, and c is the speed of ultrasound in the medium. The direction of blood flow is not as crucial for regional anesthesia as it is for cardiovascular anesthesia. What is most important is being able to positively identify blood vessels by visualizing color flow. This is especially important when interrogating a projected trajectory of the needle when placing a block. By placing color-flow Doppler over the expected needle path, the clinician should be able to screen for and avoid any unanticipated vasculature.

General Principles of an Ultrasonography-Guided Nerve Block

During ultrasonographic needle guidance, most nerves are imaged in cross-section (short axis). Alternatively, if the transducer is moved 90 degrees from the short-axis view, the long-axis view is generated. The short-axis view is generally preferred because it allows the operator to assess the lateromedial perspective of the target nerve, which is lost in the long-axis view (Fig. 1-14).

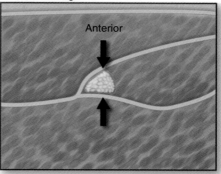

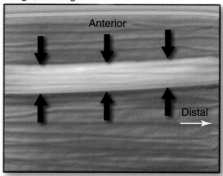

Figure 1-14. Short-axis *(top)* and long-axis *(bottom)* imaging of the median nerve.

Two techniques have emerged regarding the orientation of the needle with respect to the ultrasound beam (Fig. 1-15). The in-plane approach generates a long-axis view of the needle, allowing full visualization of the shaft and tip of the needle. The out-of-plane view generates a short-axis view of the needle. One disadvantage of the in-plane approach is the challenge of maintaining needle imaging with a very thin ultrasound beam. A limitation of the out-of-plane view is that it generates a short-axis view of the block needle, which may be very hard to visualize. With the out-of-plane view, the operator cannot confirm that the needle tip (rather than part of the shaft) is being imaged, and therefore the needle location is often inferred from tissue movement or small injections of solution.

In the pertinent images in this text, we provide a key for the recommended starting setup for each block used with ultrasonographic guidance in a corner of the image (Fig. 1-16). (Remember that because of anatomic variability among patients, these base settings may have to be adjusted based on clinical and patient variables.)

Regardless of the machine or transducer selected, there are four basic transducer manipulation techniques, which can be described as the "PART" of scanning:

Pressure (P): Various degrees of pressure are applied to the transducer that are translated onto the skin.

Alignment (A): Sliding the transducer defines the lengthwise course of the nerve and reference structures.

Rotation (R): The transducer is turned in either a clockwise or counterclockwise direction to optimize the image (either long- or short-axis) of the nerve and needle.

Tilting (T): The transducer is tilted in both directions to maximize the angle of incidence of the ultrasound beam to the target nerve, thereby maximizing reflection and optimizing image quality.

The primary objective of PART maneuvers is to optimize the amount of ultrasound that reflects off an object and returns to the transducer (Fig. 1-17).

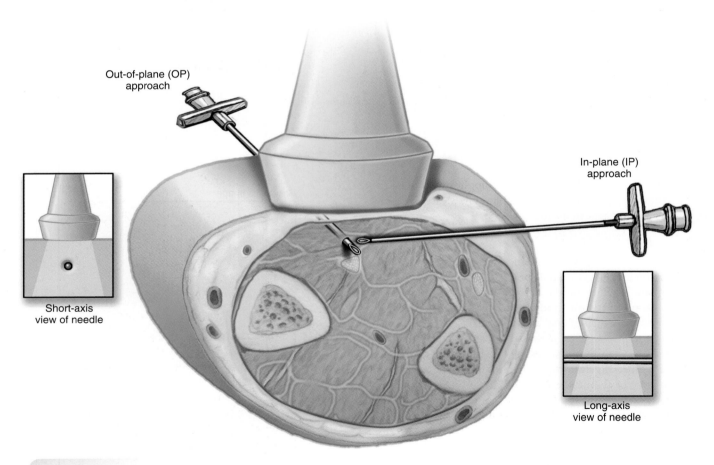

Out-of-plane (OP) approach

Short-axis view of needle

In-plane (IP) approach

Long-axis view of needle

Figure 1-15. The in-plane *(right)* and out-of-plane *(left)* needle approaches for needle insertion and ultrasonographic visualization.

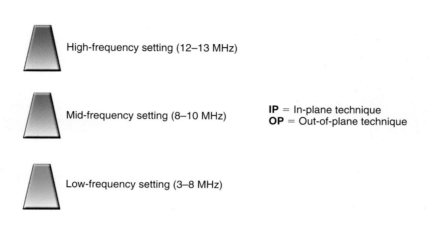

High-frequency setting (12–13 MHz)

Mid-frequency setting (8–10 MHz)

IP = In-plane technique
OP = Out-of-plane technique

Low-frequency setting (3–8 MHz)

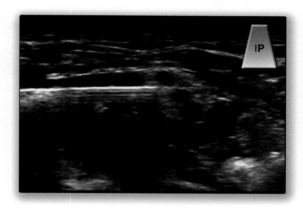

IP

Figure 1-16. Our system for ultrasonographic needle guidance recommendations. For a block for which we would recommend a high-frequency setting with the in-plane (IP) technique of needle visualization, a red scan plane with an "IP" inside the plane is shown. For a low-frequency setting with the out-of-plane (OP) technique for needle visualization, we show a green scan plane with an "OP" in the plane. The mid-frequency setting is indicated by a blue scan plane. An example is shown in the upper right of the figure. In this case, we recommend starting with a high-frequency probe setting and an in-plane technique for needle visualization.

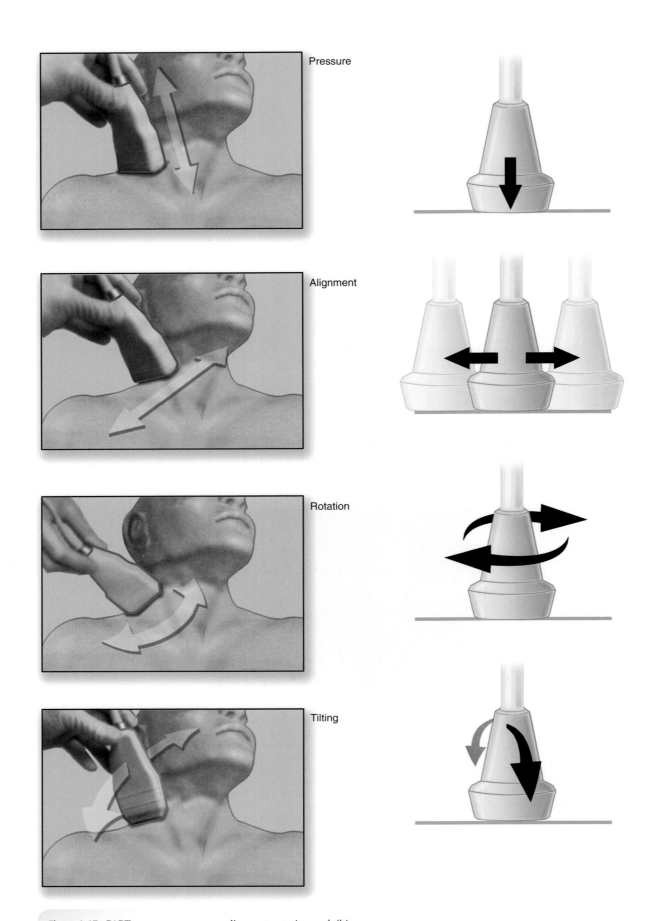

Figure 1-17. PART maneuvers: pressure, alignment, rotation, and tilting.

Continuous Peripheral Nerve Blocks

André P. Boezaart

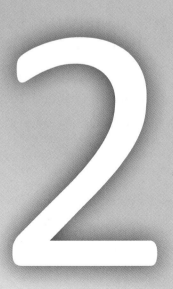

Acute pain medicine is a subspecialty of anesthesiology, and the capability to administer continuous nerve blocks (neuraxial, paraneuraxial, and peripheral) is a growing and essential skill of the acute pain specialist. Continuous nerve blocks provide analgesia over a continuum of hours to weeks and allow the clinician to control the spread, density, and duration of the nerve block, putting him or her firmly in control of the patient's analgesic requirements. These advances stimulated the ongoing development of continuous peripheral nerve blocks, the subject of this chapter. Research into reversible yet long-acting local anesthetics has been ongoing for many decades, but to date no effective long-acting drug is available—likely because long-lasting undesired side effects of the block will accompany the long-term desired effects of the block.

Advances in perineural techniques focus on improving catheter placement, thus reducing the diminishment of analgesia after the initial bolus injection. There are three primary techniques for placing perineural catheters: the nonstimulating catheter technique, the stimulating catheter technique, and the ultrasonography-guided technique. Most physicians use all three techniques in combinations that depend on the location of the block and the clinical situation; only a few use a single technique exclusively. The most popular and perhaps most effective way of placing a perineural catheter is under ultrasonographic guidance with or without nerve stimulation needle placement using a stimulating catheter.

GENERAL APPROACHES TO CONTINUOUS CATHETER PLACEMENT

Nonstimulating Catheter Technique

With the nonstimulating catheter technique, an insulated needle (usually a Tuohy needle) is advanced near a nerve with nerve stimulator or ultrasonographic guidance. Once the physician is satisfied with the position of the needle tip, saline or local anesthetic is injected through the needle to *expand* the potential perineural space, and a typical (usually multiorifice) epidural catheter is advanced through the needle. This technique is relatively easy to perform and usually provides an adequate initial or primary block, but the success rate of the secondary block—the block that develops as a result of the local anesthetic's infusing through the catheter after the initial local anesthetic bolus through the needle has worn off—is variable, depending on which nerve or plexus is being blocked.

Stimulating Catheter Technique

During stimulating catheter placement, an insulated needle (typically a Tuohy needle) is placed near the nerve to be blocked under nerve stimulator or ultrasonographic guidance; no bolus injection is made at the time of needle placement. The next step is to place a catheter with an electrically conductive tip through the needle; electrical stimulation is now performed through the catheter. If a bolus injection is made to expand the perineural space, 5% dextrose in water is used rather than saline or local anesthetic; the latter two will impair the nerve stimulation needed for correct catheter placement using this technique. This technique has more steps than a nonstimulating method. The primary success rate with this technique equals that of the nonstimulating technique, but in theory it has a higher secondary block success rate because of more precise catheter placement. Numerous formal outcome comparisons (nonstimulating vs. stimulating catheters) have been completed, and the findings show analgesic and even surgical outcomes significantly better with use of stimulating catheters. For optimum results, the stimulating catheter should be placed to block the entire region (limb) where the pain originates—for example, the brachial plexus in the case of shoulder surgery or the sciatic nerve in the case of ankle surgery (combined with a saphenous nerve block). Conversely, if only one of a number of nerves that innervate the area (limb) where the pain originates is blocked, such as the femoral nerve after major knee surgery, there seems to be no difference between the analgesic and surgical outcomes of stimulating and nonstimulating catheters. This is especially true if effective multimodal analgesia is also used.

TECHNIQUE DETAILS

Nonstimulating Catheter Technique

An insulated stimulating needle is directed near the peripheral nerve to be blocked with a stimulator current output of 1.5 mA, or under ultrasonographic guidance. The final needle position is confirmed by (1) observing an appropriate motor response with the nerve stimulator current output set at 0.3 to 0.5 mA, with a frequency of 1 to 2 Hz and a pulse width of 100 to 300 μsec; or (2) demonstrating the needle to be near the nerve by ultrasonography. When ultrasonography is used, it is customary to inject a small volume of fluid through the needle to demonstrate its spread around the nerve—so-called hydrodissection and doughnut sign formation. The needle

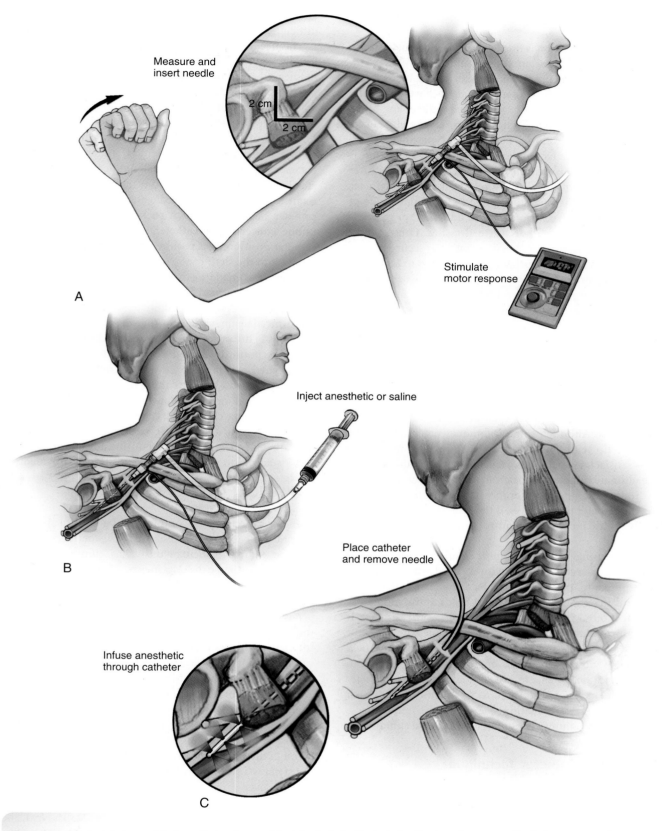

Measure and
insert needle

2 cm

2 cm

A

Stimulate
motor response

Inject anesthetic or saline

B

Place catheter
and remove needle

Infuse anesthetic
through catheter

C

Figure 2-1. Side-port device used during catheter placement for infraclavicular block. **A,** Localization of correct needle site by nerve stimulator guidance. **B,** Injection of local anesthetic to distend perineural space before catheter insertion. **C,** Insertion of catheter without additional guidance.

is often attached to a syringe by tubing from a side port (Fig. 2-1). This arrangement allows the physician to aspirate for blood or cerebrospinal fluid during needle placement and thus minimize unintentional intravascular or intrathecal injection; however, this can give potentially dangerous false-negative results because the suction produced by needle aspiration causes the surrounding tissue to obstruct the needle tip, thus allowing injection of local anesthetic into the intravascular or intrathecal space. Ultrasonography theoretically protects against missing the obstruction, although this depends on the operator's skill.

Once needle position is finalized the needle is held steady and the bolus of local anesthetic solution is injected in divided doses. Sometimes saline rather than a bolus injection of local anesthetic is used, as many believe that saline eases passage of the subsequently placed catheter and minimizes confusion of bolus local anesthetic effects with effects of the catheter injection. The catheter, typically an insulated 19- or 20-gauge epidural (multiorifice) catheter, is advanced 3 to 5 cm past the distal end of the needle. After catheter insertion the needle is removed and the catheter is secured with the operator's preferred technique, one of which is a combination of medical adhesive spray, Steri-Strips, and transparent occlusive dressing. Other physicians tunnel the catheter subcutaneously to secure it.

A variety of local anesthetic solutions are used for the block. Many prefer ropivacaine, but this choice depends on the clinical situation. More often than not during this method a bolus (20 to 40 mL) of the local anesthetic is injected through the needle before catheter insertion and provides the primary block. This is then followed by catheter placement and an infusion of local anesthetic solution through the catheter, producing what many call the secondary block (see Fig. 2-1C).

Unfortunately, catheters often curl when advanced, making it difficult to follow their eventual path with ultrasonography. Although some techniques of visualizing the catheter tip with color Doppler have been proposed, no fully satisfactory method is available to predictably identify the ultimate catheter tip location. After catheter placement, hydrodissection has been proposed as a means of identifying the catheter tip; however, if the catheter position proves faulty at this point the entire procedure needs to be repeated.

When using ultrasonographic guidance for catheter placement, a second person with a "third educated hand" is required to place the catheter: one hand holds and manipulates the needle, one hand holds and manipulates the ultrasound probe, and one hand places the catheter. If the "third educated hand" is not available, the operator removes the ultrasound transducer probe from the field and puts it down, leaving the operator with a free hand to place the catheter. This technical weakness—that catheter advancement is not observed directly (ultrasonography) or indirectly (nerve stimulation)—explains the frequent secondary block failures encountered with this technique.

Stimulating Catheter Technique

The insulated stimulating needle (Fig. 2-2A) is directed to the peripheral nerve to be blocked as in the nonstimulating technique approach described earlier, using either a nerve stimulator current output of 1.5 mA or ultrasonographic guidance. Adequate needle position is confirmed by observing an appropriate motor response with either (1) the nerve stimulator current output set at 0.3 to 0.5 mA, with a frequency of 1 to 2 Hz and a pulse width of 100 to 300 μsec or (2) the "doughnut sign" seen after hydrodissection when ultrasonography is used. Only 5% dextrose in water should be used for hydrodissection; saline or local anesthetic impairs the electrical stimulation of the nerve

and makes catheter placement with this technique difficult.

The needle is held steady in the desired position and, usually *without* injecting any solution through the needle, the negative lead off the nerve stimulator is clipped to the proximal end of the stimulating catheter, which is in turn advanced through the needle (Fig. 2-2B). The desired motor response with catheter advancement through the distal end of the needle should be similar to that elicited during initial needle placement. If the motor response decreases or disappears, it usually indicates that the catheter is being directed away from the nerve with advancement. Using this paired needle and catheter assembly, the catheter can be withdrawn back into the needle without undue concern over catheter shearing. If refinement in catheter positioning is required, the distal catheter is withdrawn into the shaft of the needle. Then, a small positioning change is made to the needle, typically by rotating it clockwise or counterclockwise or by advancing or withdrawing the needle a few millimeters, and then the catheter is advanced again, similar to the earlier catheter positioning steps. This process may be repeated until the desired motor response is elicited during catheter advancement. The desired motor response should continue as the catheter is advanced 3 to 5 cm along the neural structures.

The ultrasound transducer probe is normally also removed during catheter placement to leave the operator with a free hand to place the catheter. However, because the catheter is being stimulated during advancement, indirect visualization of the catheter's position is provided.

FIXATION OF THE CATHETER

Catheter dislodgement continues to be a problem during continuous catheter analgesia. In our experience, tunneling the catheter subcutaneously has eliminated a large number of catheter dislodgements. A variety of tunneling techniques are described. The first decision during catheter tunneling is whether a *skin bridge* will be used. A skin bridge allows easier catheter removal and is typically used during a short-term catheterization (1 to 7 days). Catheter tunneling without a skin bridge is often used for longer catheterizations (>7 days) and has the theoretic advantage of minimizing catheter infection.

For a skin bridge technique, the stylet of the Tuohy needle (Fig. 2-3A) is used as the needle guide and directed to enter the skin 2 to 3 cm from the catheter exit site. If a non–skin bridge technique is chosen, the stylet is placed through the skin at the catheter exit site. In each technique the stylet is advanced to the desired skin exit site subcutaneously over a distance of approximately 10 cm, or the length of the stylet. The Tuohy needle is then advanced in a retrograde fashion over the stylet (Fig. 2-3B). Next, the stylet is removed and the catheter is advanced through the needle (Fig. 2-3C) until it is secure and the needle can be withdrawn, leaving the catheter tunneled. If a skin bridge technique is used, a short length of plastic tubing is inserted to protect the skin under the skin bridge (Fig. 2-3D).

After the catheter tunneling has been completed, the catheter should be checked for stable distal catheter tip position. For this purpose, a device such as the SnapLock

Text continued on page 26

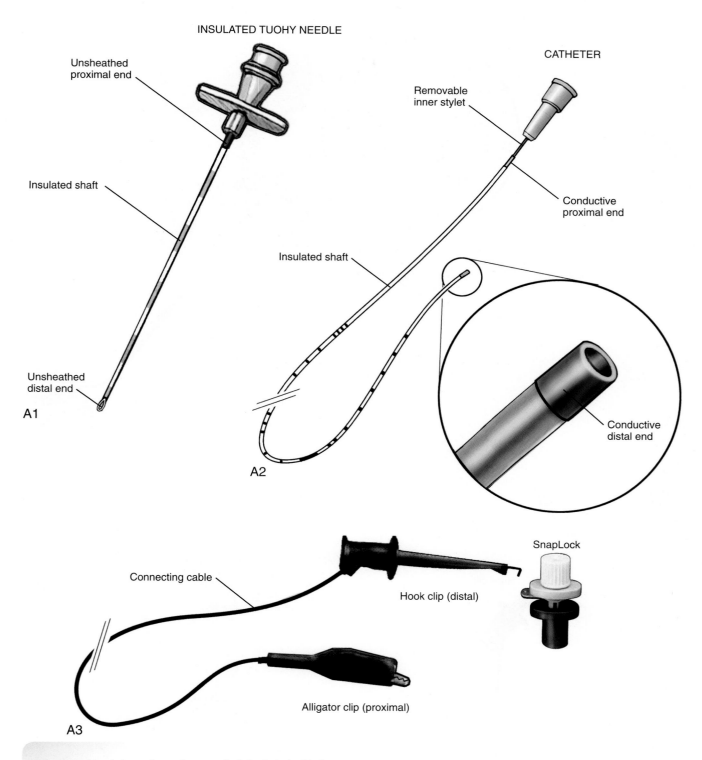

INSULATED TUOHY NEEDLE

Unsheathed proximal end

Insulated shaft

Unsheathed distal end

A1

CATHETER

Removable inner stylet

Conductive proximal end

Insulated shaft

Conductive distal end

A2

Connecting cable

Hook clip (distal)

Alligator clip (proximal)

SnapLock

A3

Figure 2-2. Stimulation catheter placement for infraclavicular block. **A,** Equipment used with StimuCath technique. **A1,** Insulated needle for initial insertion. **A2,** Electrically isolated catheter that allows stimulation by catheter tip. **A3,** Alligator extension adapter that allows stimulation by both needle and catheter. Catheter stimulation is possible with initial catheter insertion; after placement of a Tuohy-like end-adapter, stimulation and potential manipulation using the needle can be done if refined catheter positioning is desired.

Continued

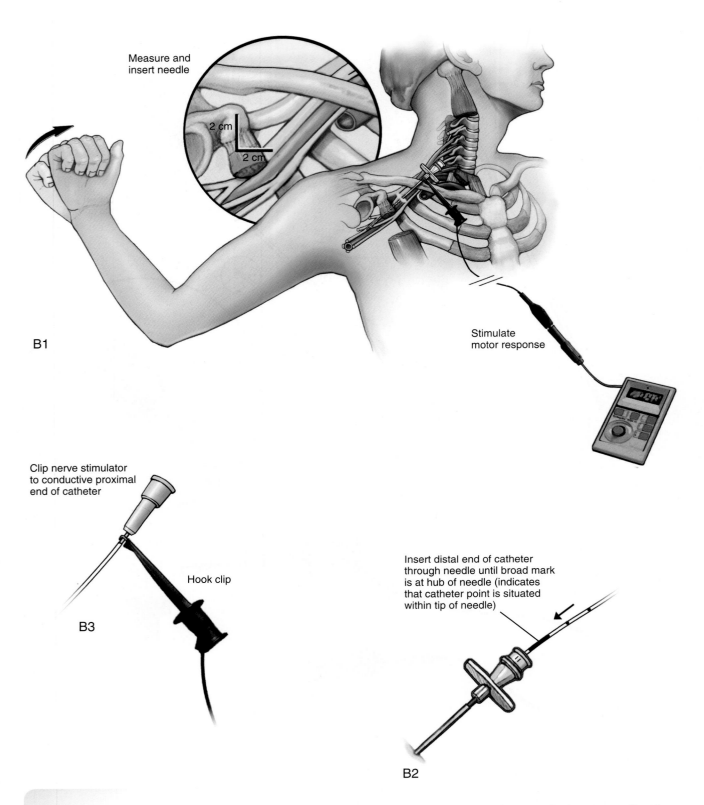

Measure and insert needle

2 cm

2 cm

B1

Stimulate motor response

Clip nerve stimulator to conductive proximal end of catheter

Hook clip

B3

Insert distal end of catheter through needle until broad mark is at hub of needle (indicates that catheter point is situated within tip of needle)

B2

Figure 2-2, cont'd. B, Block technique with StimuCath. **B1,** Initial needle placement with stimulation. **B2,** Placement of catheter into needle without passing needle tip. **B3,** Attachment of alligator extension adapter to catheter before catheter insertion.

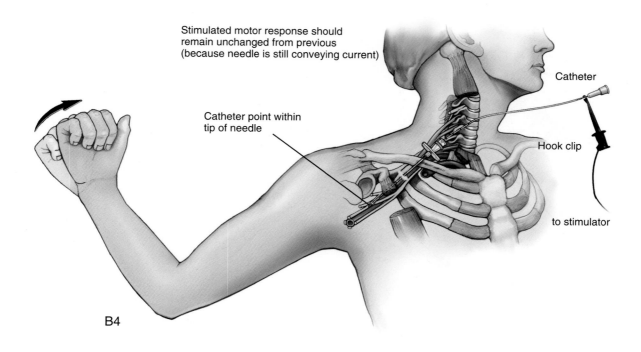

Stimulated motor response should remain unchanged from previous (because needle is still conveying current)

Catheter point within tip of needle

Catheter

Hook clip

to stimulator

B4

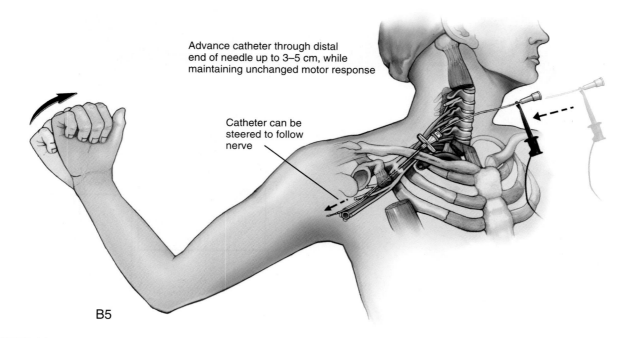

Advance catheter through distal end of needle up to 3–5 cm, while maintaining unchanged motor response

Catheter can be steered to follow nerve

B5

Figure 2-2, cont'd. **B4,** Advancement of catheter while using catheter stimulation. **B5,** Finalizing placement of catheter based on adequate stimulation pattern.

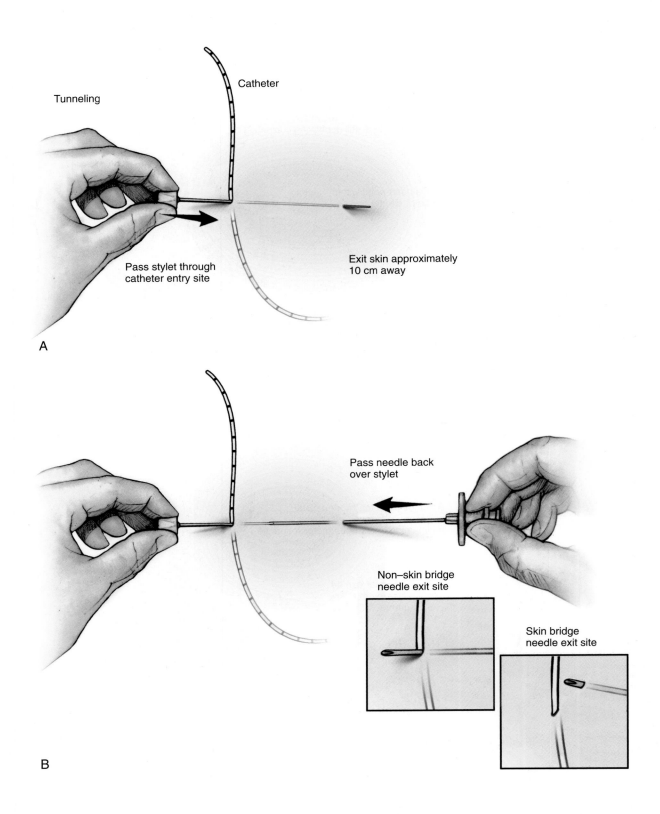

Tunneling

Catheter

Pass stylet through
catheter entry site

Exit skin approximately
10 cm away

A

Pass needle back
over stylet

Non–skin bridge
needle exit site

Skin bridge
needle exit site

B

Figure 2-3. Skin bridge and non–skin bridge techniques used in securing the catheters. **A,** Tuohy stylet is inserted. **B,** Tuohy needle is passed over stylet as a guide.

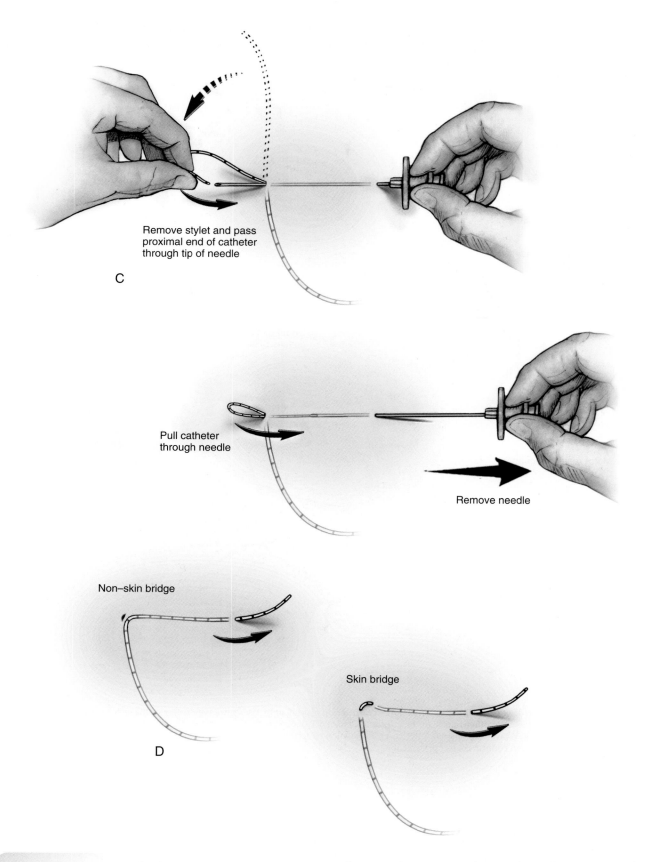

C, Remove stylet and pass proximal end of catheter through tip of needle

Pull catheter through needle

Remove needle

Non–skin bridge

Skin bridge

D

Figure 2-3, cont'd. C, Proximal catheter end is threaded into Tuohy lumen. **D,** Catheter and needle are withdrawn through final skin entry site.

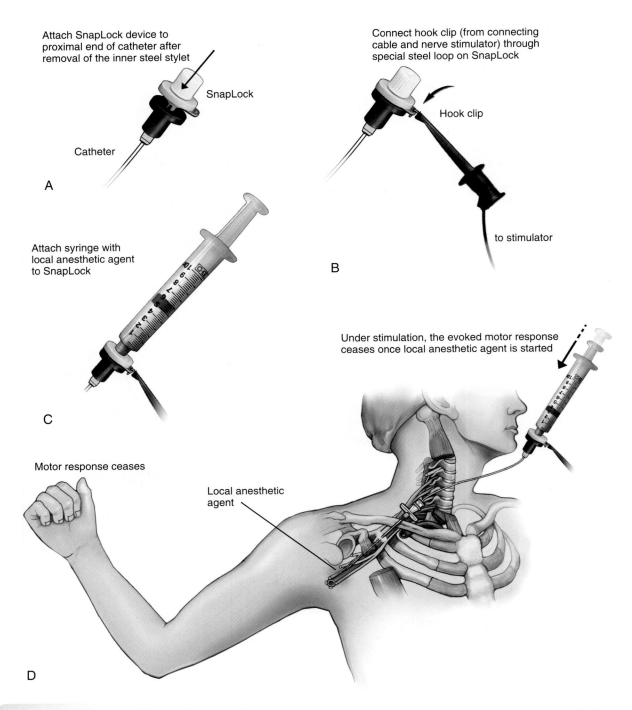

Attach SnapLock device to
proximal end of catheter after
removal of the inner steel stylet

SnapLock

Catheter

A

Connect hook clip (from connecting
cable and nerve stimulator) through
special steel loop on SnapLock

Hook clip

to stimulator

B

Attach syringe with
local anesthetic agent
to SnapLock

C

Under stimulation, the evoked motor response
ceases once local anesthetic agent is started

Motor response ceases

Local anesthetic
agent

D

Figure 2-4. The SnapLock device and confirmation of correct catheter tip placement by the appropriate fading of the catheter-stimulated motor response after injection of local anesthetic through the catheter. **A,** SnapLock device attached to catheter. **B,** Alligator extension adapter attached to SnapLock device. **C,** Syringe attached to SnapLock device. **D,** Stimulation pattern is sought through catheter stimulation, and this should fade with injection of local anesthetic to confirm correct placement.

(Arrow International, Reading, Penn), which allows continuous nerve stimulation through the catheter, is attached to the catheter. The syringe containing the local anesthetic is attached to the SnapLock (Fig. 2-4) and then, while stimulation of the catheter continues to elicit a motor response, the injection of local anesthetic is started. The evoked motor response should cease immediately on injection due to the dispersion of the current by the conductive fluid. Saline injected through the catheter will result in the same discontinuation of motor response, but plain sterile water will not. More current will therefore be required to produce a motor response.

PEARLS

Patient anxiety is the major cause of discomfort during continuous nerve block placement; hence, appropriate sedation or verbal reassurance through explanation of the procedure is important. A continuous block will typically take a slightly longer time to place than a single-injection block. Appropriate infiltration of local anesthetic at the site of the block and at the site of tunneling is important and should not be rushed. When making adjustments in needle position while establishing the initial optimum catheter position, ensure that the tip of the catheter is fully inside the shaft of the needle before needle manipulation. Continuous peripheral block catheters are often left in place for an extended time, so adherence to sterile technique is required. After catheter placement the site should be covered with a transparent dressing so that daily inspection of the catheter exit site and skin bridge area can be made for signs of inflammation.

The entire limb is usually insensitive for the duration of the continuous block. Blockaded nerves vulnerable to injury, external pressure, or traction should be specifically protected. These commonly include the ulnar nerve at the elbow, the radial nerve at the mid-humeral level, and the common peroneal nerve at the fibular head area. Ambulatory patients with a continuous brachial plexus block in place should always use a properly fitted arm sling to prevent traction injury to the brachial plexus or injury to the radial nerve by the sling. Pressure or undue traction to the ulnar nerve (hyperflexion at the elbow) should be avoided. When the block involves the quadriceps and hamstrings muscles, there is a possibility of falling with ambulation in the immediate postoperative period; leg splints should be routinely fitted and patients should not ambulate unassisted.

When removing the catheter it is ideal to withdraw it after full limb sensation has returned. Radiating pain experienced during catheter removal may indicate that the catheter is intertwined with a nerve or nerve root. Surgical removal of catheters after fluoroscopic examination may be indicated if the radiating pain persists with removal attempts. This is an extremely rare occurrence.

SECTION II:
Upper Extremity Blocks

Upper Extremity Block Anatomy

3

Man uses his arms and hands constantly ... as a result he exposes his arms and hands to injury constantly. ... Man also eats constantly. ... Man's stomach is never really empty. ... The combination of man's prehensibility and his unflagging appetite keeps a steady flow of patients with injured upper extremities and full stomachs streaming into hospital emergency rooms. This is why the brachial plexus is so frequently the anesthesiologist's favorite group of nerves.

Classical Anesthesia Files, David Little, 1963

The late David Little's appropriate observations do not always lead anesthesiologists to choose a regional anesthetic for upper extremity surgery. However, those selecting regional anesthesia recognize that there are multiple sites at which the brachial plexus block can be induced. If anesthesiologists are to deliver comprehensive anesthesia care, they should be familiar with brachial plexus blocks. Familiarity with these techniques demands an understanding of brachial plexus anatomy. One problem with understanding this anatomy is that the traditional wiring diagram for the brachial plexus is unnecessarily complex and intimidating.

Figure 3-1 illustrates that the plexus is formed by the ventral rami of the fifth to eighth cervical nerves and the greater part of the ramus of the first thoracic nerve. In addition, small contributions may be made by the fourth cervical and the second thoracic nerves. The intimidating part of this anatomy is what happens from the time these ventral rami emerge from between the middle and anterior scalene muscles until they end in the four terminal branches to the upper extremity: the musculocutaneous, median, ulnar, and radial nerves. Most of what happens to the roots on their way to becoming peripheral nerves is not clinically essential information for an anesthesiologist. There are some broad concepts that may help clinicians understand the brachial plexus anatomy; throughout, my goal in this chapter is to simplify this anatomy.

After the roots pass between the scalene muscles, they reorganize into trunks—superior, middle, and inferior. The trunks continue toward the first rib. At the lateral edge of the first rib, these trunks undergo a primary anatomic division, into ventral and dorsal divisions. This is also the point at which understanding of brachial plexus anatomy gives way to frustration and often unnecessary complexity. This anatomic division is significant because

nerves destined to supply the originally ventral part of the upper extremity separate from those that supply the dorsal part. As these divisions enter the axilla, the divisions give way to cords. The posterior divisions of all three trunks unite to form the posterior cord; the anterior divisions of the superior and middle trunks form the lateral cord; and the ununited, anterior division of the inferior trunk forms the medial cord. These cords are named according to their relationship to the second part of the axillary artery.

At the lateral border of the pectoralis minor muscle (which inserts onto the coracoid process), the three cords reorganize to give rise to the peripheral nerves of the upper extremity. Simplified, the branches of the lateral and medial cords are all "ventral" nerves to the upper extremity. The posterior cord, in contrast, provides all "dorsal" innervation to the upper extremity. Thus, the radial nerve supplies all the dorsal musculature in the upper extremity below the shoulder. The musculocutaneous nerve supplies muscular innervation in the arm, while providing cutaneous innervation to the forearm. In contrast, the median and ulnar nerves are nerves of passage in the arm, but in the forearm and hand they provide the ventral musculature with motor innervation. These nerves can be further categorized: the median nerve innervates more heavily in the forearm, whereas the ulnar nerve innervates more heavily in the hand.

Some writers have focused anesthesiologists' attention on the fascial investment of the brachial plexus. As the brachial plexus nerve roots leave the transverse processes, they do so between prevertebral fascia that divides to invest both the anterior and the middle scalene muscles. Many suggest that this prevertebral fascia surrounding the brachial plexus is tubular throughout its course, thus allowing needle placement within the "sheath" to produce brachial plexus block easily. There is no question that the brachial plexus is invested with prevertebral fascia; however, the fascial covering is discontinuous, with septa subdividing portions of the sheath into compartments that clinically may prevent adequate spread of local anesthetics. Ultrasonographic observation of injections near the brachial plexus confirms our earlier clinical impressions of fascial discontinuity. My clinical impression is that the discontinuity of the "sheath" increases as one moves from transverse process to axilla.

Most upper extremity surgery is performed with the patient resting supine on an operating table with the arm extended on an arm board. Thus, anesthesiologists must understand and clearly visualize the innervation of the upper extremity while the patient is in this position. Figures 3-2 through 3-7 illustrate these features with the

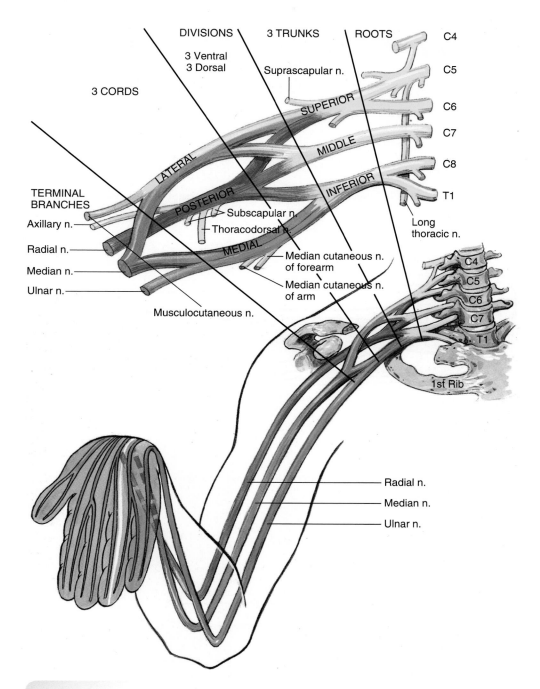

DIVISIONS
3 Ventral
3 Dorsal

3 TRUNKS

ROOTS

C4

C5

Suprascapular n.

C6

SUPERIOR

C7

3 CORDS

LATERAL

MIDDLE

C8

INFERIOR

T1

TERMINAL
BRANCHES

POSTERIOR

Subscapular n.

Long
thoracic n.

Axillary n.

Thoracodorsal n.

Radial n.

MEDIAL

Median cutaneous n.
of forearm

Median n.

Ulnar n.

Median cutaneous n.
of arm

Musculocutaneous n.

C4
C5
C6
C7
T1

1st Rib

Radial n.

Median n.

Ulnar n.

Figure 3-1. Brachial plexus anatomy.

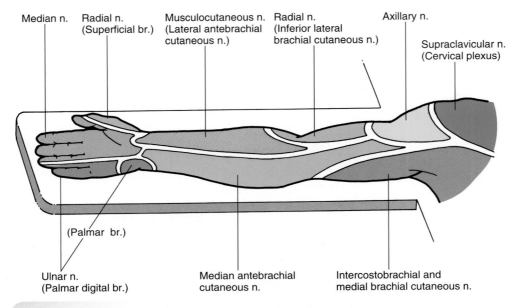

Median n.   Radial n.   Musculocutaneous n.   Radial n.   Axillary n.
(Superficial br.)   (Lateral antebrachial   (Inferior lateral
   cutaneous n.)   brachial cutaneous n.)

Supraclavicular n.
(Cervical plexus)

(Palmar br.)

Ulnar n.
(Palmar digital br.)

Median antebrachial
cutaneous n.

Intercostobrachial and
medial brachial cutaneous n.

Figure 3-2. Upper extremity peripheral nerve innervation with arm supinated on arm board.

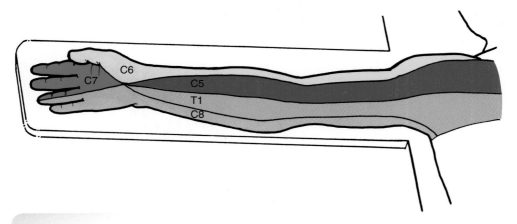

C6
C7
C5
T1
C8

Figure 3-3. Upper extremity dermatome innervation with arm supinated on arm board.

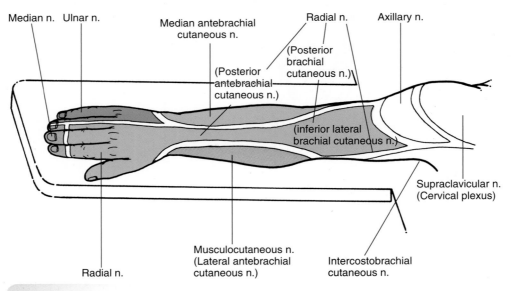

Median n.   Ulnar n.   Median antebrachial   Radial n.   Axillary n.
   cutaneous n.

(Posterior
brachial
cutaneous n.)

(Posterior
antebrachial
cutaneous n.)

(inferior lateral
brachial cutaneous n.)

Supraclavicular n.
(Cervical plexus)

Radial n.

Musculocutaneous n.
(Lateral antebrachial
cutaneous n.)

Intercostobrachial
cutaneous n.

Figure 3-4. Upper extremity peripheral nerve innervation with arm pronated on arm board.

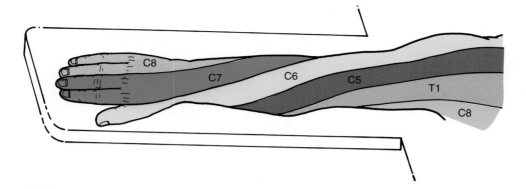

Figure 3-5. Upper extremity dermatome innervation with arm pronated on arm board.

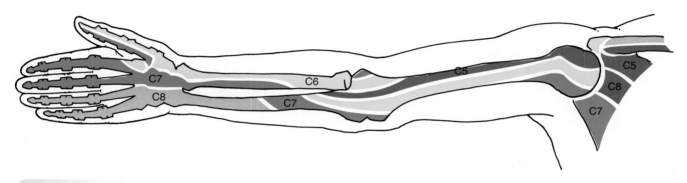

Figure 3-6. Upper extremity osteotomes with arm supinated.

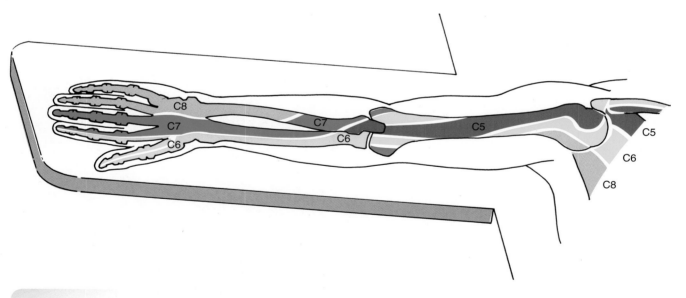

Figure 3-7. Upper extremity osteotomes with arm pronated on arm board.

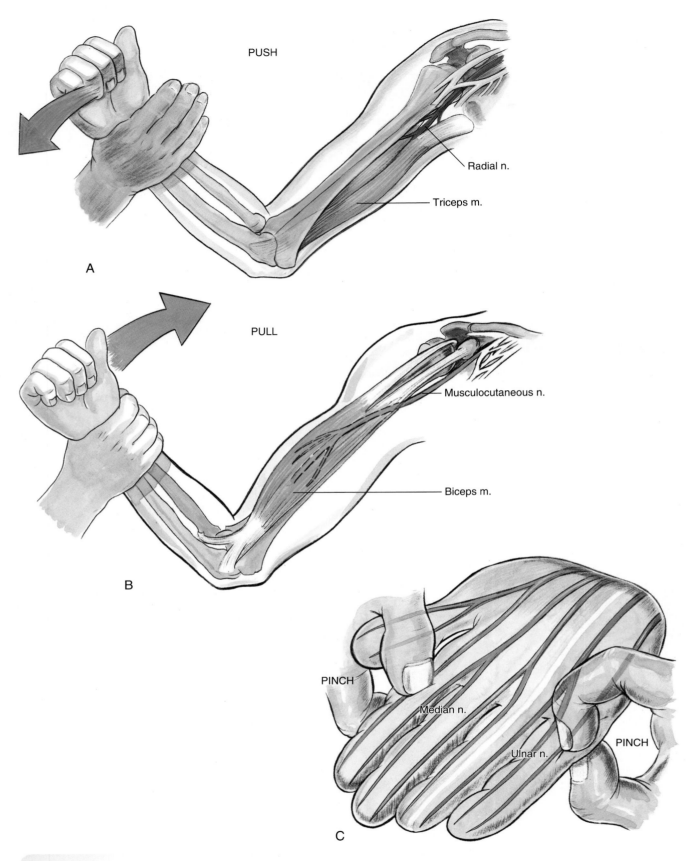

PUSH

Radial n.

Triceps m.

A

PULL

Musculocutaneous n.

Biceps m.

B

PINCH

Median n.

Ulnar n.

PINCH

C

Figure 3-8. Upper extremity peripheral nerve function mnemonic: "push (**A**), pull (**B**), pinch, pinch (**C**)."

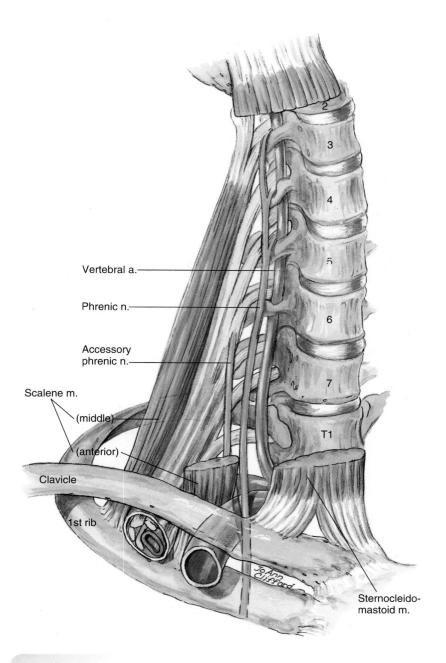

Vertebral a.

Phrenic n.

Accessory
phrenic n.

Scalene m.

(middle)

(anterior)

Clavicle

1st rib

Sternocleido-
mastoid m.

Figure 3-9. Supraclavicular regional block: functional anatomy.

arm in the supinated and pronated positions for the cutaneous nerves and dermatomal and osteotomal patterns, respectively.

An additional clinical "pearl" that will help anesthesiologists check brachial plexus block before initiation of the surgical procedure is the "four Ps." Figure 3-8 shows how the mnemonic "push, pull, pinch, pinch" can help an anesthesiologist remember how to check the four peripheral nerves of interest in the brachial plexus block. By having the patient resist the anesthesiologist's pulling the forearm away from the upper arm, motor innervation to the biceps muscle is assessed. If this muscle has been weakened, one can be certain that local anesthetic has reached the musculocutaneous nerve. Likewise, by asking the patient to attempt to extend the forearm by contracting the triceps muscle, one assesses the radial nerve. Finally, pinching the

fingers in the distribution of the ulnar or median nerve—that is, at the base of the fifth or second digit, respectively—helps the anesthesiologist develop a sense of the adequacy of block of both the ulnar and median nerves. Typically, if these maneuvers are performed shortly after brachial plexus block, motor weakness will be evident before sensory block. As a historical highlight, this technique for checking the upper extremity was developed during World War II to allow medics a method of quick analysis of injuries to the brachial plexus.

Although some of the brachial plexus neural anatomy of interest to anesthesiologists has been outlined, there are some anatomic details that should be highlighted (Fig. 3-9). As the cervical roots leave the transverse processes on their way to the brachial plexus, they exit in the gutter of the transverse process immediately posterior to the vertebral artery. The vertebral arteries leave the brachiocephalic and subclavian arteries on the right and left, respectively, and travel cephalad, normally entering a bony canal in the transverse process at the level of C6 and above. Thus, one must be constantly aware of needle tip location in relationship to the vertebral artery. It should be remembered that the vertebral artery lies anterior to the roots of the brachial plexus as they leave the cervical vertebrae.

Another structure of interest in the brachial plexus anatomy is the phrenic nerve. It is formed from branches of the third, fourth, and fifth cervical nerves and passes through the neck on its way to the thorax on the ventral surface of the anterior scalene muscle. It is almost always blocked during interscalene block and less frequently with supraclavicular techniques or with cervical paravertebral block. Avoidance of phrenic blockade is important in only a small percentage of patients, although phrenic nerve location should be kept in mind for those with significantly decreased pulmonary function—that is, those whose day-to-day activities are limited by their pulmonary impairment.

Another detail of the brachial plexus anatomy that needs amplification is the organization of the brachial plexus nerves (divisions) as they cross the first rib. Textbooks often depict the nerves in a stacked arrangement at this point. However, radiologic, clinical, ultrasonographic, and anatomic investigations demonstrate that the nerves are not discretely "stacked" at this point but rather assume a posterior and cranial relationship to the subclavian artery (Fig. 3-10). This is important when one is carrying out supraclavicular nerve block and is using the rib as an anatomic landmark. The relationship of the nerves to the artery means that if one simply walks the needle tip closely

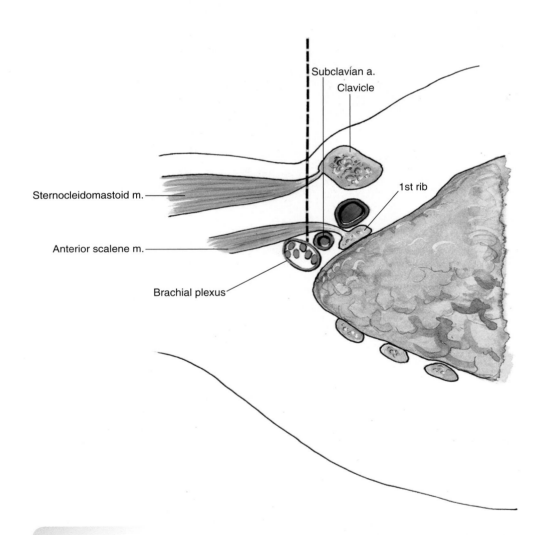

Figure 3-10. Supraclavicular block anatomy: functional anatomy of brachial plexus, subclavian artery, and first rib.

along the first rib, one may not as easily elicit paresthesias because the nerves are more cranial in relationship to the first rib.

Another anatomic detail needing highlighting is the proximal axillary anatomy at a parasagittal section through the coracoid process. At this transition site, the brachial plexus is changing from the brachial plexus cords to the peripheral nerves as it surrounds the subclavian and axillary arteries (Fig. 3-11). At the site of this parasagittal section the borders of the proximal axilla are formed by the following anatomic structures:

Anterior: posterior border of the pectoralis minor muscle and brachial head of the biceps

Posterior: scapula and subscapularis, latissimus dorsi, and teres major muscles

Medial: lateral aspect of chest wall, including the ribs and intercostal and serratus anterior muscles

Lateral: medial aspect of upper arm

These anatomic relationships are important during continuous techniques of infraclavicular block.

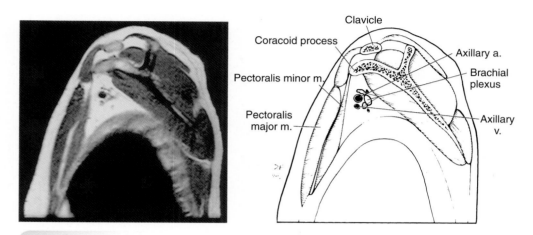

Figure 3-11. Parasagittal magnetic resonance image and line drawing of the important anatomy in the infraclavicular block. *(By permission of the Mayo Foundation, Rochester, Minn.)*

Interscalene Block

David L. Brown

with contributions from

Brian D. Sites and Brian C. Spence

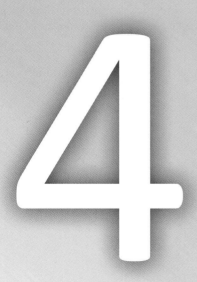

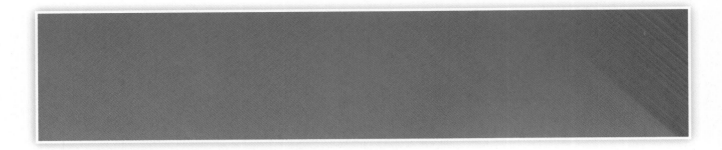

Interscalene block (classic anterior approach) is especially effective for surgery of the shoulder or upper arm because the roots of the brachial plexus are most easily blocked with this technique. Frequently the ulnar nerve and its more peripheral distribution in the hand can be spared, unless one makes a special effort to inject local anesthetic caudad to the site of the initial paresthesia. This block is ideal for reduction of a dislocated shoulder and often can be achieved with as little as 10 to 15 mL of local anesthetic. This block also can be performed with the arm in almost any position and thus can be useful when brachial plexus block needs to be repeated during a prolonged upper extremity procedure.

Patient Selection. Interscalene block is applicable to nearly all patients because even obese patients usually have identifiable scalene and vertebral body anatomy. However, interscalene block should be avoided in patients with significantly impaired pulmonary function. This point may be moot if one is planning to use a combined regional and general anesthetic technique, which allows intraoperative control of ventilation. Even when a long-acting local anesthetic is chosen for the interscalene technique, usually phrenic nerve, and thus pulmonary, function has returned to a level that patients can tolerate by the time the average-length surgical procedure is completed.

Pharmacologic Choice. Useful agents for interscalene block are primarily the amino amides. Lidocaine and mepivacaine provide surgical anesthesia for 2 to 3 hours without epinephrine and for 3 to 5 hours when epinephrine is added. These drugs can be useful for less complex or outpatient surgical procedures. For more extensive surgical procedures requiring hospital admission, longer-acting agents such as bupivacaine or ropivacaine can be chosen. The more complex surgical procedures on the shoulder often require muscle relaxation; thus, bupivacaine concentrations of at least 0.5% are needed. Plain bupivacaine produces surgical anesthesia lasting from 4 to 6 hours; the addition of epinephrine may prolong this to 8 to 12 hours. Ropivacaine's effects are slightly shorter in duration.

Traditional Block Technique

Anatomy. Surface anatomy of importance to anesthesiologists includes the larynx, sternocleidomastoid muscle, and external jugular vein. Interscalene block is most often performed at the level of the C6 vertebral body, which is at the level of the cricoid cartilage. Thus, by projecting a line laterally from the cricoid cartilage, one can identify the level at which one should roll the fingers off the sternocleidomastoid muscle onto the belly of the anterior scalene and then into the interscalene groove. When firm pressure is applied, in most individuals it is possible to feel the transverse process of C6, and in some people it is possible to elicit a paresthesia by deep palpation. The external jugular vein often overlies the interscalene groove at the level of C6, although this should not be relied on (Fig. 4-1).

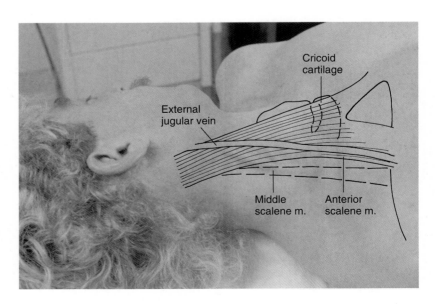

Figure 4-1. Interscalene block: surface anatomy.

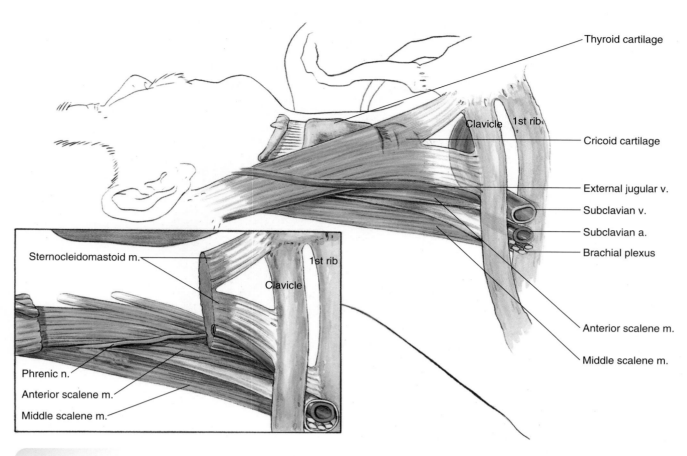

Figure 4-2. Interscalene block: functional anatomy of scalene muscles.

It is important to visualize what lies under the palpating fingers; again, the key to carrying out successful interscalene block is the identification of the interscalene groove. Figure 4-2 allows us to look beneath surface anatomy and develop a sense of how closely the lateral border of the anterior scalene muscle deviates from the border of the sternocleidomastoid muscle. This feature should be constantly kept in mind. The anterior scalene muscle and the interscalene groove are oriented at an oblique angle to the long axis of the sternocleidomastoid muscle. Figure 4-3 removes the anterior scalene and highlights the fact that at the level of C6, the vertebral artery begins its route to the base of the brain by traveling through the root of the transverse process in each of the more cephalad cervical vertebrae.

Position. The patient lies supine with the neck in the neutral position and the head turned slightly opposite the site to be blocked. The anesthesiologist then asks the patient to lift the head off the table to tense the sternocleidomastoid muscle and allow identification of its lateral border. The fingers then roll onto the belly of the anterior scalene and subsequently into the interscalene groove. This maneuver should be carried out in the horizontal plane through the cricoid cartilage—thus, at the level of C6. To roll the fingers effectively (Fig. 4-4), the operator should stand at the patient's side.

Needle Puncture. When the interscalene groove has been identified and the operator's fingers are firmly pressing in it, the needle is inserted, as shown in Figure 4-5, in a slightly caudal and slightly posterior direction. As a further directional help, if the needle for this block is imagined to be long and inserted deeply enough, it would exit the neck posteriorly in approximately the midline at the level of the C7 or T1 spinous process. If a paresthesia or motor response is not elicited on insertion, the needle is "walked," while maintaining the same needle angulation as shown in Figure 4-4, in a plane joining the cricoid cartilage to the C6 transverse process. Because the brachial plexus traverses the neck at virtually a right angle to this plane, a paresthesia or motor response is almost guaranteed if small enough steps of needle reinsertion are carried out. When undertaking the block for shoulder surgery, this is probably the one brachial plexus block in which a large volume of local anesthetic coupled with a single needle position allows effective anesthesia. For shoulder surgery, 25 to 35 mL of lidocaine, mepivacaine, bupivacaine, or ropivacaine can be used. If the interscalene block is being carried out for forearm or hand surgery, a second, more caudal needle position is desirable, in which 10 to 15 mL of additional local anesthetic is injected to allow spread along more caudal roots.

POTENTIAL PROBLEMS

Problems that can arise from interscalene block include subarachnoid injection, epidural block, intravascular injection (especially in the vertebral artery), pneumothorax, and phrenic block.

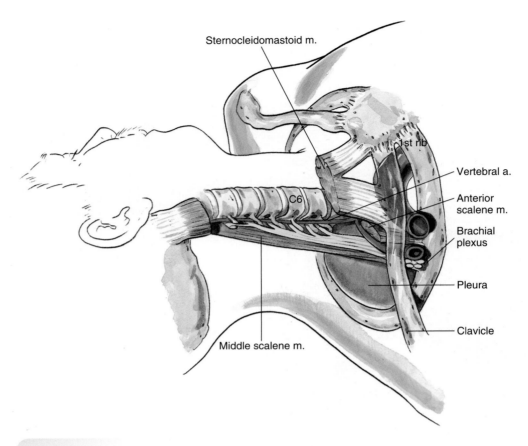

Figure 4-3. Interscalene block: functional anatomy of vertebral artery.

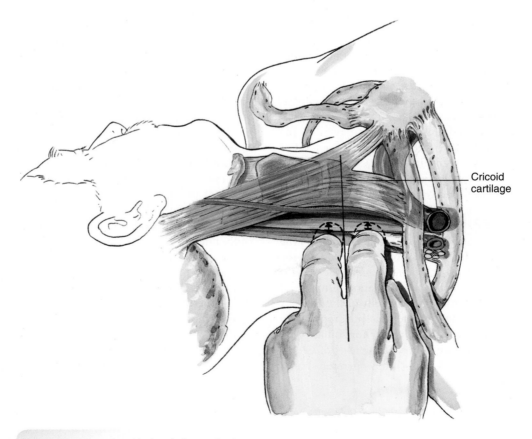

Figure 4-4. Interscalene block technique: palpation.

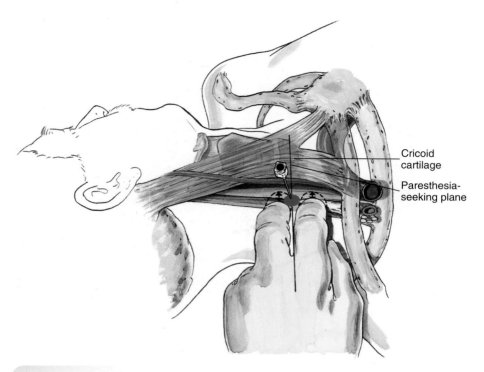

Figure 4-5. Interscalene block technique: "paresthesia-seeking" plane.

PEARLS

This block is most applicable to shoulder procedures, as opposed to forearm and hand surgical procedures, although some practitioners combine interscalene and axillary blocks to produce an approximation of a supraclavicular block. For shoulder surgery block that requires muscle relaxation, a local anesthetic concentration that provides adequate motor block should be chosen (i.e., mepivacaine and lidocaine at 1.5%, bupivacaine at 0.5%, and ropivacaine at 0.75% concentrations). Because this block is most often carried out through a single injection site and the operator relies on the spread of local anesthetic solution, one must allow sufficient "soak time" after the injection. This often means from 20 to 35 minutes.

If there is difficulty in identifying the anterior scalene muscle, one maneuver is to have the patient maximally inhale while the anesthesiologist palpates the neck. During this maneuver the scalene muscles should contract before the sternocleidomastoid muscle contracts, and this may allow clarification of the anterior scalene muscle in the difficult-to-palpate neck. Further, if the operator is finding it difficult to elicit a paresthesia or produce a motor response during nerve stimulation with this block, it is almost always because the needle entry site has been placed too far posteriorly. For example, Figure 4-6 shows that if the right side of the neck is divided into a 180-degree arc, the needle entry site should be approximately at 60 degrees from the sagittal plane to optimize production of the block.

Most of the injection difficulties that result in complications can be avoided if one remembers that this should be a very "superficial" block; if the palpating fingers apply sufficient pressure, no more than 1 to 1.5 cm of the needle should be necessary to reach the plexus. It is when the needle is inserted deeply that one must be cautious about subarachnoid, epidural, and intravascular injection. For an operation that requires ulnar nerve block, I would not choose the interscalene block. The ulnar nerve is difficult to block with the interscalene approach because it is derived from the eighth cervical nerve (this nerve is difficult to block after injection at a more cephalic injection site). Finally, one should be cautious about using this block in a patient with significant pulmonary impairment because phrenic block is almost guaranteed with the interscalene block.

Ultrasonography-Guided Technique

The goals of an ultrasonography-guided interscalene nerve block include defining normal anatomy, visualizing the brachial plexus, observing the advancing needle, and confirming correct intrasheath spread of local anesthetic. With the patient in the same position as for the surface landmark technique, the ultrasound transducer is placed in the midneck at the level of the cricoid cartilage. The operator should be at the head of the patient's bed, directing the transducer with his or her nondominant hand (Fig. 4-7). The first two structures identified are the carotid artery (a pulsatile, hypoechoic circle that resists compression) and internal jugular vein (a nonpulsatile and compressible hypoechoic circle). The probe is then moved in a latero-posterior direction approximately 1 to 2 cm. This should generate the sonogram depicted in Figure 4-7. The brachial plexus can be seen between the anterior and middle scalene muscles as distinct hypoechoic circles with hyperechoic rings. The scalene muscles appear as hypoechoic ovals or

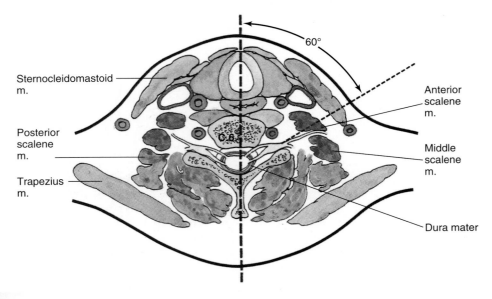

Figure 4-6. Interscalene block anatomy: an angle of approximately 60 degrees from the sagittal plane is the optimal needle angle for the block.

Sternocleidomastoid
m.

Posterior
scalene
m.

Trapezius
m.

60°

Anterior
scalene
m.

Middle
scalene
m.

Dura mater

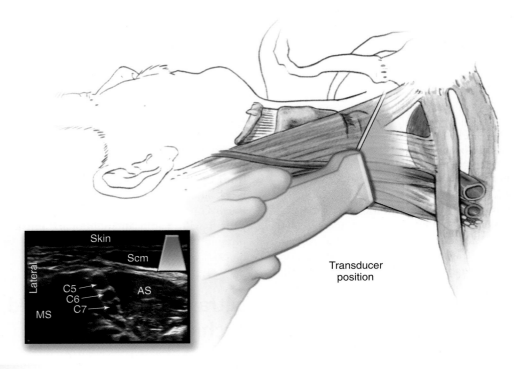

Figure 4-7. Interscalene block: transducer position and ultrasonographic anatomy. AS, anterior scalene muscle; MS, middle scalene muscle; Scm, sternocleidomastoid muscle.

circles lying deep to the overlying hypoechoic and triangle-shaped sternocleidomastoid muscle. Using the in-plane approach, the needle is inserted through either the middle scalene muscle (posterior approach) or the anterior scalene muscle (anterior approach); refer to Figure 4-8 for orientation. The needle is advanced until it enters into the brachial plexus sheath between the C5 and C6 ventral nerve roots. A distinct "popping" sensation is both felt and visualized (see *Video 2: Interscalene Nerve Block: In-Plane Technique* on the Expert Consult Website). After a test injection, the solution should be seen filling the brachial plexus sheath (see Fig. 4-8). If intramuscular spread is noted, the needle should be repositioned.

PEARLS

Given the superficial nature of this block, a high-frequency ultrasound transducer (>12 MHz) is preferred because it will provide the best axial and lateral image resolution. Of all of the PART maneuvers—pressure, alignment, rotation, and tilting—tilting has the largest impact on image quality in the interscalene region. Tilting the transducer 10 to 20 degrees cephalad often dramatically improves image quality. Good procedure ergonomics is critical to the effective performance of this nerve block. Operators are encouraged to rest their scanning arm and their needle arm on separate supporting structures (e.g., firm pillows) to help

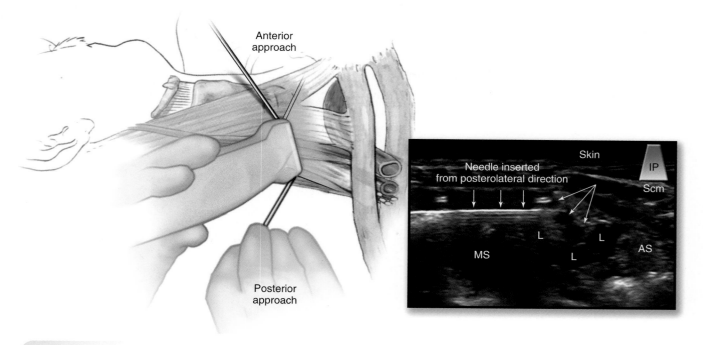

Figure 4-8. Interscalene block: anterior and posterior approaches. The sonogram shows a successful intrasheath injection from the posterior approach. AS, anterior scalene muscle; L, local anesthetic; MS, middle scalene muscle; Scm, sternocleidomastoid muscle; *arrows* identify nerve roots.

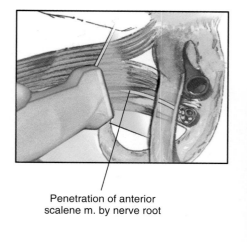

Penetration of anterior
scalene m. by nerve root

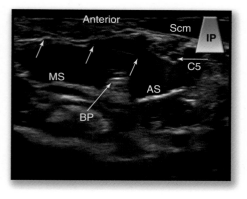

Figure 4-9. Interscalene block: anatomic anomaly injection. AS, anterior scalene muscle; BP, brachial plexus; MS, middle scalene muscle; Scm, sternocleidomastoid muscle; *arrows* identify needle course.

prevent fatigue and unintentional probe movement. The decision about which approach to perform (anterior vs. posterior) is usually based on patient characteristics, operator preferences, and individual bed-stretcher characteristics being used. It is often ergonomically and technically easier for a right-handed individual to perform an anterior approach for a right-sided interscalene block, especially when access is limited to the head of the bed. With the ultrasonographic image confirming the characteristic spread of local anesthetic within the brachial plexus sheath, no additional injections should be needed. Clinical experi-

ence has suggested that volumes as low as 10 to 15 mL can achieve effective blockade.

The operator should be on the lookout for common anatomic variants that can compromise the quality of the nerve block. Cadaver studies suggest that the "typical" situation of the brachial plexus lying between the anterior and middle scalene muscles exists in only 60% of situations. The most common variation (34%) is direct penetration of the anterior scalene muscle by the C5 or C6 ventral nerve roots (Fig. 4-9). Such anatomic variations explain failure of surface landmark–based approaches to the interscalene block in which the scalene muscle may serve as a barrier to the distribution of local anesthesia. In these special situations, several injections may be necessary given the anatomic separation of the nerve roots (see Fig. 4-9).

It can be helpful to scan the anticipated needled trajectory with color Doppler to identify unsuspected vascularity (see *Video 3: Interscalene Anatomy: Prescan Utility of Color Doppler* on the Expert Consult Website). Finally, the injection of local anesthetic should be made where the image of the ventral nerve roots is clearest. This ideal image is often found 1 to 3 cm caudal to the traditional entry point predicted by surface landmarks.

Supraclavicular Block

David L. Brown

with contributions from
Brian D. Sites and Brian C. Spence

5

PERSPECTIVE

Supraclavicular block provides anesthesia of the entire upper extremity in the most consistent, efficient manner of any brachial plexus technique. It is the most effective block for all portions of the upper extremity and is carried out at the division level of the brachial plexus; perhaps this is why there is often little or no sparing of peripheral nerves if an adequate paresthesia is obtained. If this block is to be used for shoulder surgery, it should be supplemented with a superficial cervical plexus block to anesthetize the skin overlying the shoulder.

Patient Selection. Almost all patients are candidates for this block, with the exception of those who are uncooperative. In addition, in less experienced hands it may be inappropriate for outpatients. Although pneumothorax is an infrequent complication of the block, such an event often becomes apparent only after a delay of several hours, when an outpatient may already be at home. Also, because the supraclavicular block relies principally on bony and muscular landmarks, very obese patients are not good candidates because they often have supraclavicular fat pads that interfere with easy application of this technique.

Pharmacologic Choice. As with other brachial plexus blocks, the prime consideration in drug selection should be the length of the procedure and the degree of motor blockade desired. Mepivacaine (1% to 1.5%), lidocaine (1% to 1.5%), bupivacaine (0.5%), and ropivacaine (0.5 to 0.75%) are all applicable to brachial plexus block. Lidocaine and mepivacaine will produce 2 to 3 hours of surgical anesthesia without epinephrine and 3 to 5 hours when epinephrine is added. These drugs can be useful for less involved or outpatient surgical procedures. For extensive surgical procedures requiring hospital admission, a longer-acting agent like bupivacaine can be chosen. Plain bupivacaine produces surgical anesthesia lasting from 4 to 6 hours, and the addition of epinephrine may prolong this time to 8 to 12 hours, whereas ropivacaine is slightly shorter acting.

Traditional Block Technique

PLACEMENT

Anatomy. The anatomy of interest for this block is the relationship between the brachial plexus and the first rib, the subclavian artery, and the cupola of the lung (Fig. 5-1).

My experience suggests that this block is more difficult to teach than many of the other regional blocks, and for that reason two approaches to the supraclavicular block are illustrated: the classic Kulenkampff approach and the vertical ("plumb bob") approach. The vertical approach has been developed in an attempt to overcome the difficulty and time necessary to become skilled in the classic supraclavicular block approach. Both techniques are clinically useful, once mastered. As the subclavian artery and brachial plexus pass over the first rib, they do so between the insertion of the anterior and middle scalene muscles onto the first rib (Fig. 5-2). The nerves lie in a cephaloposterior relationship to the artery; thus, a paresthesia may be elicited before the needle contacts the first rib. At the point where the artery and plexus cross the first rib, the rib is broad and flat, sloping caudad as it moves from posterior to anterior, and although the rib is a curved structure, there is a distance of 1 to 2 cm on which a needle can be "walked" in a parasagittal anteroposterior direction. Remember that immediately medial to the first rib is the cupola of the lung; when the needle angle is too medial, pneumothorax may result.

Position: Classic Supraclavicular Block. The patient lies supine without a pillow, with the head turned opposite the side to be blocked. The arms are at the sides, and the anesthesiologist can stand either at the head of the table or at the side of the patient, near the arm to be blocked.

Needle Puncture: Classic Supraclavicular Block. In the classic approach, the needle insertion site is approximately 1 cm superior to the clavicle at the clavicular midpoint (Fig. 5-3). This entry site is closer to the middle of the clavicle than to the junction of the middle and medial thirds (as often described in other regional anesthesia texts). In addition, if the artery is palpable in the supraclavicular fossa, it can be used as a landmark. From this point, the needle and syringe are inserted in a plane approximately parallel to the patient's neck and head, taking care that the axis of the syringe and needle does not aim medially toward the cupola of the lung. A 22-gauge, 5-cm needle typically will contact rib at a depth of 3 to 4 cm, although in a very large patient it is sometimes necessary to insert it to a depth of 6 cm. The initial needle insertion should not be carried out past 3 to 4 cm until a careful search in an anteroposterior plane does not identify the first rib. During the insertion of the needle and syringe, the assembly should be controlled with the hand, as illustrated in Figure 5-4. The hand can rest lightly against the patient's supraclavicular fossa because patients often move the shoulder with elicitation of a paresthesia.

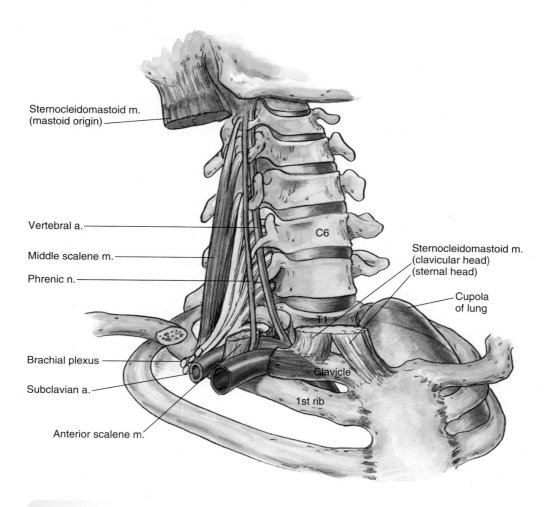

Sternocleidomastoid m.
(mastoid origin)

Vertebral a.

Middle scalene m.

Phrenic n.

C6

Sternocleidomastoid m.
(clavicular head)
(sternal head)

Cupola
of lung

T1

Brachial plexus

Subclavian a.

Clavicle

1st rib

Anterior scalene m.

Figure 5-1. Supraclavicular block: anatomy.

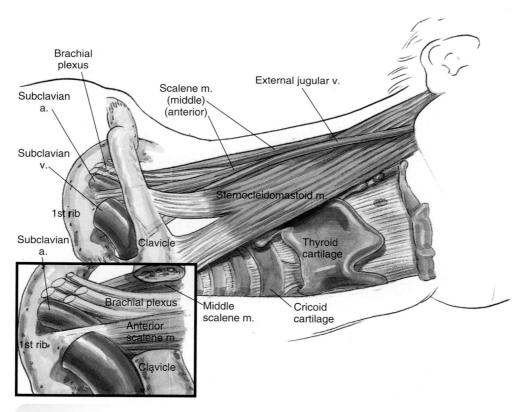

Brachial
plexus

Subclavian
a.

Scalene m.
(middle)
(anterior)

External jugular v.

Subclavian
v.

1st rib

Subclavian
a.

Clavicle

Sternocleidomastoid m.

Thyroid
cartilage

Brachial plexus

Middle
scalene m.

Cricoid
cartilage

Anterior
scalene m.

1st rib

Clavicle

Figure 5-2. Supraclavicular block: functional anatomy (with detail).

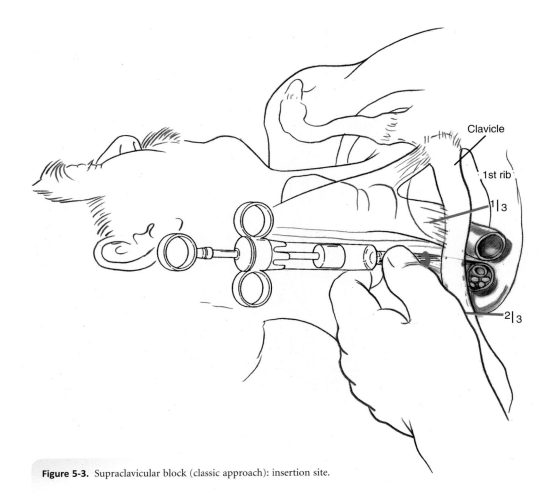

Figure 5-3. Supraclavicular block (classic approach): insertion site.

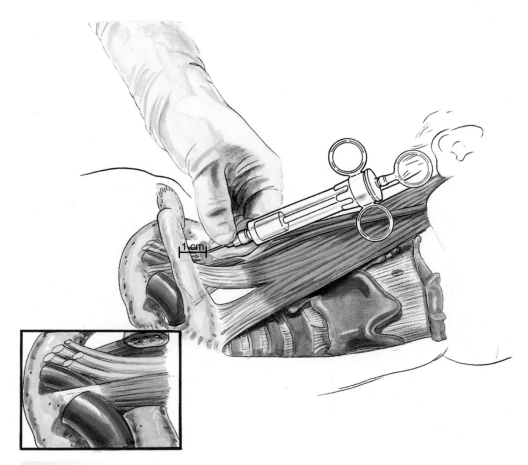

Figure 5-4. Supraclavicular block (classic approach): hand and syringe assembly positioning.

Figure 5-5. Supraclavicular block
(plumb bob): functional anatomy.

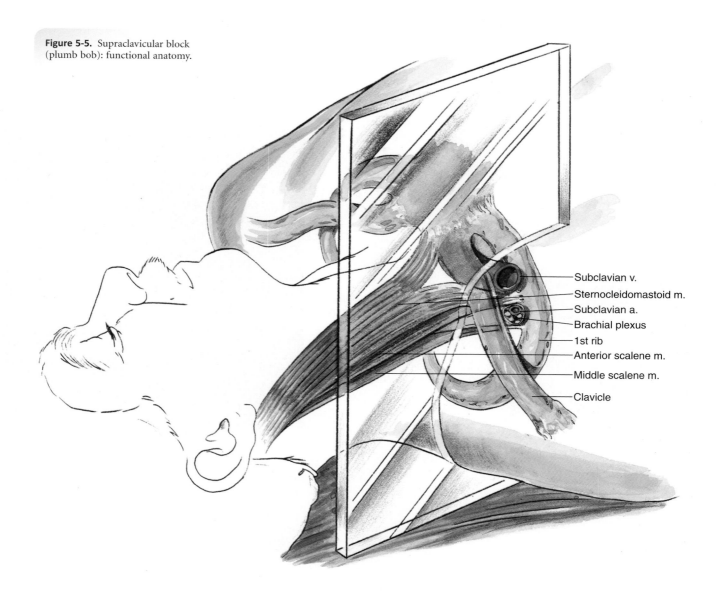

- Subclavian v.
- Sternocleidomastoid m.
- Subclavian a.
- Brachial plexus
- 1st rib
- Anterior scalene m.
- Middle scalene m.
- Clavicle

Position: Vertical (Plumb Bob) Supraclavicular Block. The vertical approach to the supraclavicular block was developed to simplify the anatomic projection necessary for the block. The patient should be positioned in a manner similar to that used for the classic approach, lying supine without a pillow, with the head turned slightly away from the side to be blocked. The anesthesiologist should stand lateral to the patient at the level of the patient's upper arm. This block involves inserting the needle and syringe assembly at approximately a 90-degree angle to that used in the classic approach.

Needle Puncture: Vertical (Plumb Bob) Supraclavicular Block. Patients are asked to raise the head slightly off the block table so that the lateral border of the sternocleidomastoid muscle can be marked as it inserts onto the clavicle. From that point, a plane is visualized running parasagittally through that site (Fig. 5-5). The name "plumb bob" was chosen for this block concept because if one were to suspend a plumb bob vertically over the entry site (Fig. 5-6), needle insertion through that point, along the continuation of the vertical line defined by the plumb bob, would result in contact with the brachial plexus in most

patients. Figure 5-6 also illustrates a parasagittal section obtained by magnetic resonance imaging in the sagittal plane necessary to carry out this block. As illustrated, the brachial plexus at the level of the first rib lies posterior and cephalad to the subclavian artery. Once this skin mark has been placed immediately superior to the clavicle at the lateral border of the sternocleidomastoid muscle as it inserts into the clavicle, the needle is inserted in the parasagittal plane at a 90-degree angle to the tabletop. If a paresthesia is not elicited on the first pass, the needle and syringe are redirected cephalad in small steps through an arc of approximately 20 degrees. If a paresthesia still has not been obtained, needle and syringe are reinserted at the starting position and then moved in small steps through an arc of approximately 20 degrees caudad (Fig. 5-7).

Because the brachial plexus lies cephaloposterior to the artery as it crosses the first rib, often a paresthesia can be elicited before either the artery or the first rib is contacted. If that occurs, approximately 30 mL of local anesthetic is inserted at this single site.

If a paresthesia is not elicited with the maneuvers described but the first rib is contacted, the block is carried out just as it is in the classic approach—by "walking" along

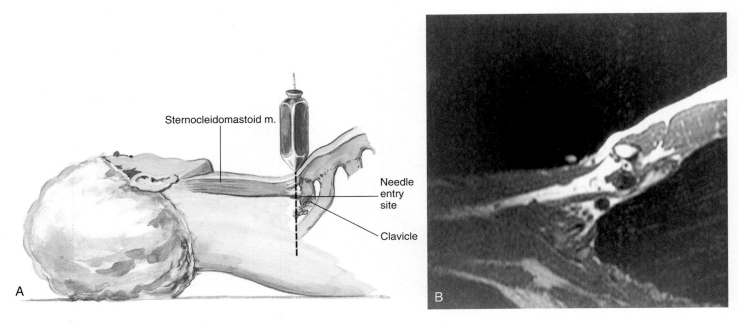

Sternocleidomastoid m.

Needle entry site

Clavicle

A

B

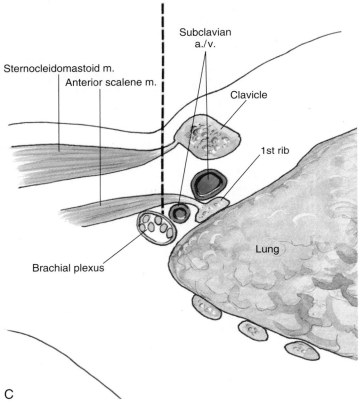

Subclavian a./v.

Sternocleidomastoid m.

Anterior scalene m.

Clavicle

1st rib

Brachial plexus

Lung

C

Figure 5-6. Supraclavicular block (plumb bob): parasagittal anatomy. **A,** Schematic, showing plumb bob and needle path. **B,** Magnetic resonance image. **C,** Needle path.

Figure 5-7. Supraclavicular block (plumb bob): paresthesia-seeking approach.

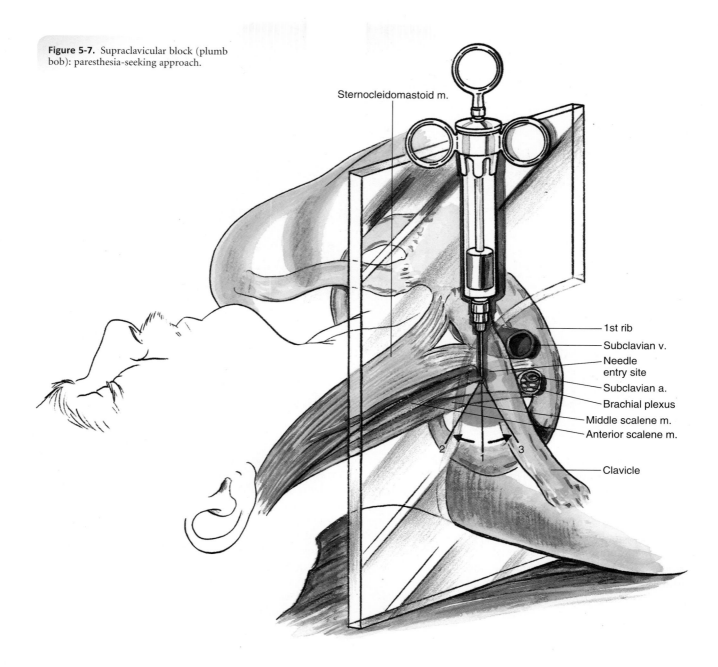

Sternocleidomastoid m.

1st rib
Subclavian v.
Needle entry site
Subclavian a.
Brachial plexus
Middle scalene m.
Anterior scalene m.
Clavicle

2   1   3

the first rib until a paresthesia is elicited. As in the classic approach, care should be taken not to allow the syringe and needle assembly to aim medially toward the cupola of the lung.

POTENTIAL PROBLEMS

The most feared complication of this block is pneumothorax, the principal cause of which is a needle/syringe angle that aims toward the cupola of the lung. Special attention should be directed to "walking" the needle in a strict anteroposterior direction. Pneumothorax incidence is between 0.5% and 5% and becomes less frequent as an anesthesiologist becomes skilled. The cupola of the lung rises proportionally higher in the neck in thin, asthenic individuals, and perhaps in these individuals the incidence of pneumothorax is higher. Pneumothorax most often develops over a number of hours as the result of impinge-

ment of the needle on the lung, rather than due to immediate entrance of air into the pleural space as the needle is inserted. Phrenic nerve block occurs, probably in the range of 30% to 50% of patients, and the block's use in patients with significantly impaired pulmonary function must be weighed. The development of hematoma after supraclavicular block, as a result of puncture of the subclavian artery, usually simply requires observation.

PEARLS

The predictability and rapid onset of this block allow the anesthesiologist to keep up with a fast orthopedic surgeon. Use of this block allows regional anesthesia to be used for hand surgery, even in a busy practice. Because this block requires a longer time for the anesthesiologist to attain proficiency than most other regional blocks, the anesthesiologist should develop a system for its use. "Wishful"

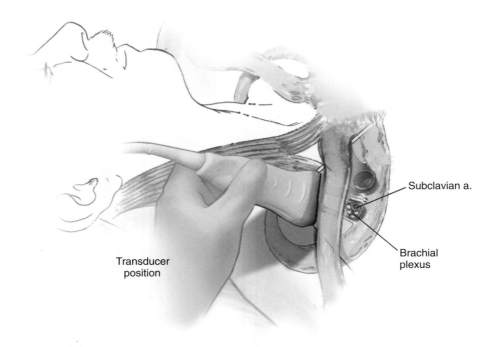

Figure 5-8. Supraclavicular block, ultrasonography-guided approach: transducer position.

probing at the root of the neck without a system is not the way to approach this block. Likewise, one should choose either the classic or the vertical approach and give each a fair trial before abandoning either.

If a pneumothorax occurs after supraclavicular block, it most often can be observed while the patient is reassured. If the pneumothorax is large enough to cause dyspnea or patient discomfort, aspiration of the pneumothorax through a small-gauge catheter is often all that is necessary for treatment. The patient should be admitted for observation; however, it is the exceptional patient who needs formal, large-bore chest tube placement for reexpansion of the lung. Obviously difficult patients should not be chosen as subjects while the anesthesiologist is developing expertise with this block.

Some anesthesiologists combine the axillary and interscalene blocks (in the so-called AXIS block) to approximate the results achieved from a more typical supraclavicular block. An AXIS block requires that the total doses of local anesthetic be increased; one must be willing to use almost 60 mL of whichever drug is injected. Time will tell whether this combined approach offers any advantages over the supraclavicular block. In the AXIS block, the axillary portion should be blocked first, with the interscalene block performed second to minimize the risk of injecting into an area already blocked by local anesthetic.

Ultrasonography-Guided Technique

Our team refers to the supraclavicular approach to the brachial plexus as the "spinal of the arm"; however, with traditional techniques there is a significant risk

of pneumothorax and subclavian artery puncture. With ultrasonographic guidance, this block becomes more efficient, and at-risk structures can be readily identified and avoided.

To start, the transducer should be placed in the supraclavicular fossa (Fig. 5-8). With this approach, the goal is to image the subclavian artery and brachial plexus in their short axis. If there is difficulty finding the subclavian artery, slide the transducer medially to first identify the distal carotid artery, then move the transducer laterally to image the subclavian artery. The subclavian artery will appear as a pulsatile, hypoechoic circular structure. Confirm the pulsation with color-flow Doppler. Once the subclavian artery has been located, the plexus will appear as several hypoechoic circles lateral and superior (cephaloposterior) to the artery (Fig. 5-9). The exact number of hypoechoic circles vary (three to six is common) because the image represents a variable portion of the brachial plexus from the trunks to divisions. Several other structures that are important to identify include the first rib and pleura. The first rib appears as a hyperechoic line with a characteristic acoustic dropout shadow posterior to it. The pleura appears as a hyperechoic line that moves with respiration (see *Video 4: Supraclavicular Anatomy: A Case of a Large Anomalous Branch of the Subclavian Artery* on the Expert Consult Website).

The transducer should be manipulated such that the subclavian artery and brachial plexus appear on the medial side of the ultrasonographic screen, which will allow an appropriate trajectory. Using the in-plane needle insertion technique, the needle is advanced from lateral to medial with the goal of having the tip enter the brachial plexus sheath at the most posterior imaged aspect (Fig. 5-10). This tends to be in an area previously described as the "corner pocket" for the needle using the aforementioned technique

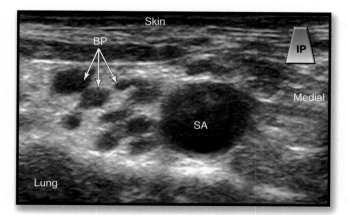

Figure 5-9. Supraclavicular block, ultrasonography-guided approach: image obtained with transducer placement as in Figure 5-8. BP, brachial plexus; SA, subclavian artery.

(see *Video 5: Supraclavicular Nerve Block* on the Expert Consult Website).

PEARLS

If there is difficulty locating the brachial plexus or the subclavian artery, the operator should identify the brachial plexus at the interscalene groove and then trace it down the neck to the subclavian fossa. (This can also be applied in reverse if you are having trouble identifying the brachial plexus in the interscalene groove.) There is usually (although not always) a visual and tactile "pop" once the needle punctures the sheath structures surrounding the brachial plexus. For rapid generation of surgical anesthesia, the goal is to have local anesthetic spread around the various imaged neural components adjacent to the subclavian artery. This objective is often facilitated by several injections near the brachial plexus structures.

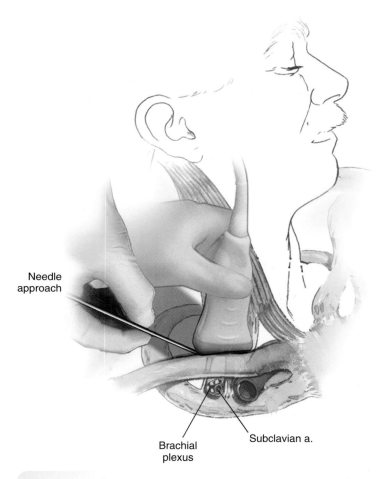

Figure 5-10. Supraclavicular block, ultrasonography-guided approach: needle placement for "corner pocket."

Infraclavicular Block

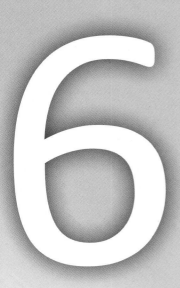

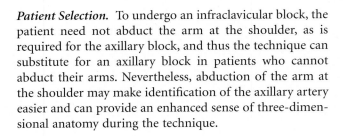

PERSPECTIVE

Infraclavicular brachial plexus block is often used for patients requiring prolonged brachial plexus analgesia and is increasingly used for surgical anesthesia by modifying it into a single-injection technique. Anesthesia or analgesia with this technique results in a "high" axillary block. Thus, it is most useful for patients undergoing procedures on the elbow, forearm, or hand. Like the axillary block, this technique is carried out distant from both the neuraxial structures and the lung, thus minimizing complications associated with those areas (see *Video 6: Infraclavicular Nerve Block* on the Expert Consult Website).

Patient Selection. To undergo an infraclavicular block, the patient need not abduct the arm at the shoulder, as is required for the axillary block, and thus the technique can substitute for an axillary block in patients who cannot abduct their arms. Nevertheless, abduction of the arm at the shoulder may make identification of the axillary artery easier and can provide an enhanced sense of three-dimensional anatomy during the technique.

Pharmacologic Choice. Because prolonged brachial plexus analgesia requires less motor blockade than is needed for surgical anesthesia, the concentration of local anesthetic can be decreased during postoperative analgesia regimens. An appropriate drug is bupivacaine 0.25% or ropivacaine 0.2%, both administered at initial rates of approximately 8 to 12 mL/hr. If a single-injection technique is used, appropriate drugs are lidocaine (1% to 1.5%), mepivacaine (1% to 1.5%), bupivacaine (0.5%), or ropivacaine (0.5% to 0.75%). Lidocaine and mepivacaine produce 2 to 3 hours of surgical anesthesia without epinephrine and 3 to 5 hours with the addition of epinephrine. These drugs are useful for less involved procedures or outpatient surgical procedures. For more extensive surgical procedures requiring hospital admission, longer-acting agents such as bupivacaine or ropivacaine are appropriate. Plain bupivacaine and ropivacaine produce surgical anesthesia lasting 4 to 6 hours; the addition of epinephrine may prolong this period to 8 to 12 hours. The local anesthetic timeline must be considered when prescribing a drug for outpatient infraclavicular block because blocks lasting as long as 18 to 24 hours can result from higher concentrations of bupivacaine with added epinephrine.

Traditional Block Technique

PLACEMENT

Anatomy. At the level of the proximal axilla, where infraclavicular block is performed, the axilla is a pyramid-shaped space with an apex, a base, and four sides (Fig. 6-1A). The base is the concave armpit, and the anterior wall is composed of the pectoralis major and minor muscles and their accompanying fasciae. The posterior wall of the axilla is formed by the scapula and the scapular musculature, the subscapularis and the teres major. The latissimus dorsi muscle abuts the teres major muscle to form the inferior aspect of the posterior wall of the axilla (Fig. 6-1B). The medial wall of the axilla is composed of the serratus anterior muscle and its fascia, and the lateral wall is formed by the converging muscle and tendons of the anterior and posterior walls as they insert into the humerus (see Fig. 6-1B). The apex of the axilla is triangular and is formed by the convergence of the clavicle, the scapula, and the first rib. The neurovascular structures of the limb pass into the pyramid-shaped axilla through its apex (Fig. 6-2A).

The contents of the axilla are blood vessels and nerves—the axillary artery and vein and the brachial plexus, respectively—and lymph nodes and loose areolar tissue. The neurovascular elements are enclosed within the anatomically variable, multipartitioned axillary sheath, a fascial extension of the prevertebral layer of cervical fascia covering the scalene muscles. The axillary sheath adheres to the clavipectoral fascia behind the pectoralis minor muscle and continues along the neurovascular structures until it enters the medial intramuscular septum of the arm (Fig. 6-2B).

The brachial plexus divisions become cords as they enter the axilla. The posterior divisions of all three trunks unite to form the posterior cord; the anterior divisions of the superior and middle trunks form the lateral cord; and the nonunited anterior division of the inferior trunk forms the medial cord. These cords are named according to their relationship to the second part of the axillary artery (Fig. 6-3). From these cords, nerves to the subscapularis, pectoralis major and minor, and latissimus dorsi muscles leave the brachial plexus. The medial brachial cutaneous, medial antebrachial cutaneous, and axillary nerves also leave the brachial plexus from the level of the cords.

At the lateral border of the pectoralis minor muscle (which inserts onto the coracoid process), the three cords

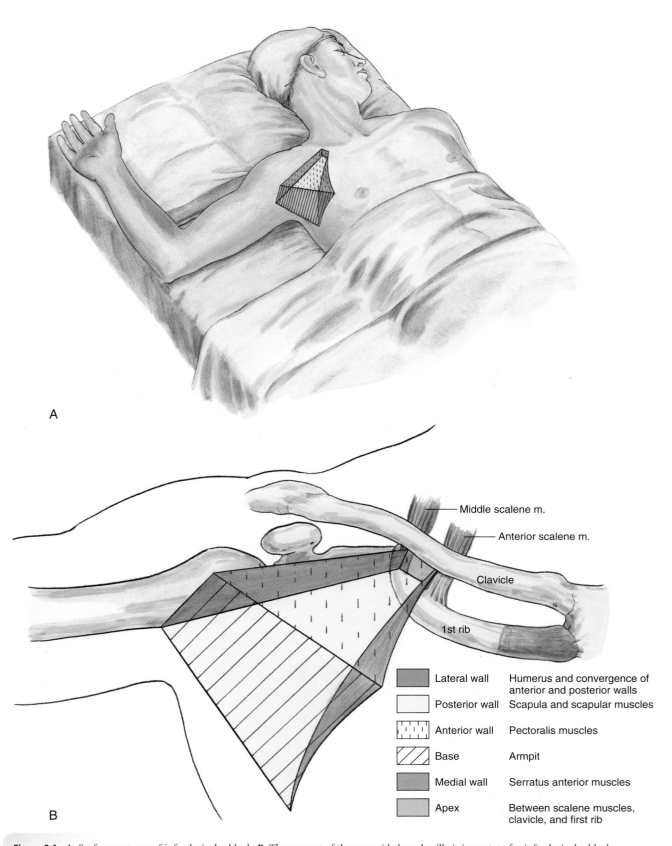

Figure 6-1. **A,** Surface anatomy of infraclavicular block. **B,** The concept of the pyramid-shaped axilla is important for infraclavicular block.

	Lateral wall	Humerus and convergence of anterior and posterior walls
	Posterior wall	Scapula and scapular muscles
	Anterior wall	Pectoralis muscles
	Base	Armpit
	Medial wall	Serratus anterior muscles
	Apex	Between scalene muscles, clavicle, and first rib

Labels in B: Middle scalene m., Anterior scalene m., Clavicle, 1st rib

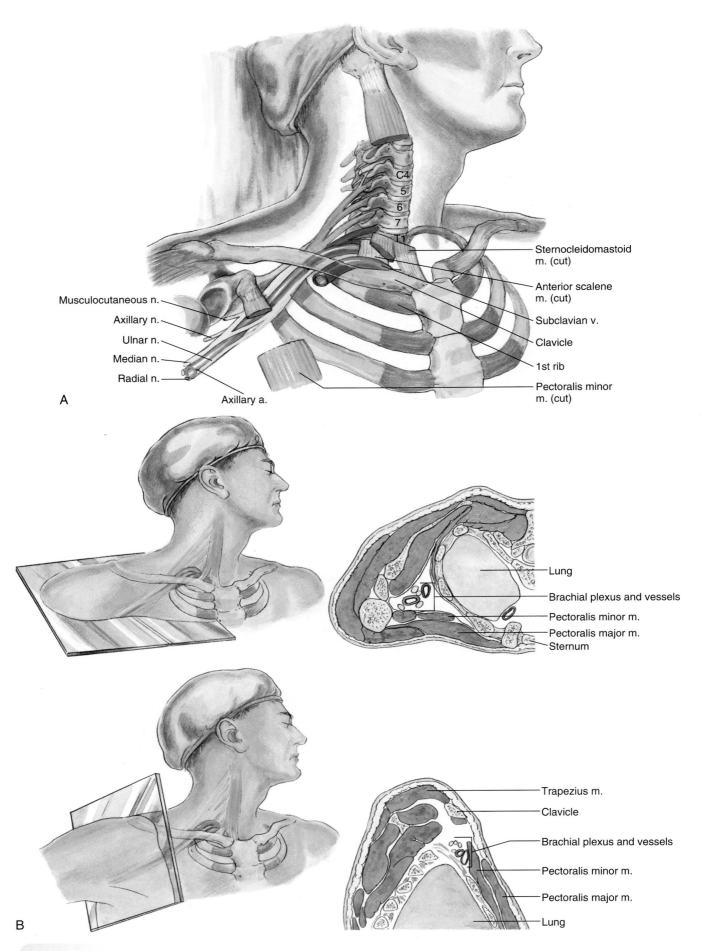

Musculocutaneous n.

Axillary n.

Ulnar n.

Median n.

Radial n.

Axillary a.

C4
5
6
7
T1

Sternocleidomastoid
m. (cut)

Anterior scalene
m. (cut)

Subclavian v.

Clavicle

1st rib

Pectoralis minor
m. (cut)

A

Lung

Brachial plexus and vessels

Pectoralis minor m.

Pectoralis major m.

Sternum

Trapezius m.

Clavicle

Brachial plexus and vessels

Pectoralis minor m.

Pectoralis major m.

Lung

B

Figure 6-2. Anatomy important for infraclavicular block. **A,** Muscles, bones, and neurovascular structures. **B,** Cross-sectional *(top)* and parasagittal *(bottom)* anatomy.

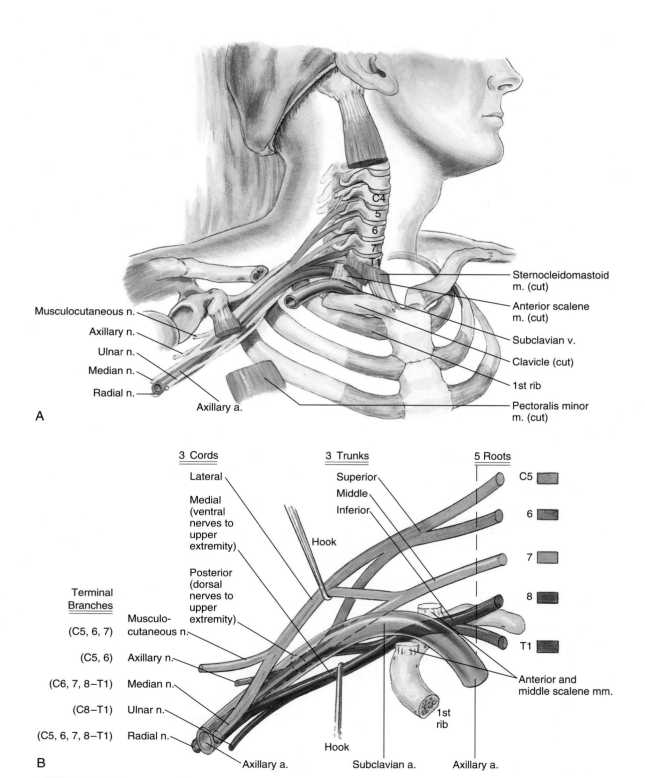

A

Musculocutaneous n.
Axillary n.
Ulnar n.
Median n.
Radial n.
Axillary a.

Sternocleidomastoid m. (cut)
Anterior scalene m. (cut)
Subclavian v.
Clavicle (cut)
1st rib
Pectoralis minor m. (cut)

C4
5
6
7
T1

B

3 Cords
Lateral
Medial (ventral nerves to upper extremity)
Posterior (dorsal nerves to upper extremity)

3 Trunks
Superior
Middle
Inferior
Hook

5 Roots
C5
6
7
8
T1

Terminal Branches

(C5, 6, 7)   Musculo-cutaneous n.
(C5, 6)   Axillary n.
(C6, 7, 8–T1) Median n.
(C8–T1)   Ulnar n.
(C5, 6, 7, 8–T1) Radial n.

Axillary a.
Hook
Subclavian a.
Axillary a.
Anterior and middle scalene mm.
1st rib

Figure 6-3. Brachial plexus anatomy important for infraclavicular block. **A,** Regional anatomy. **B,** Detailed infraclavicular anatomy.

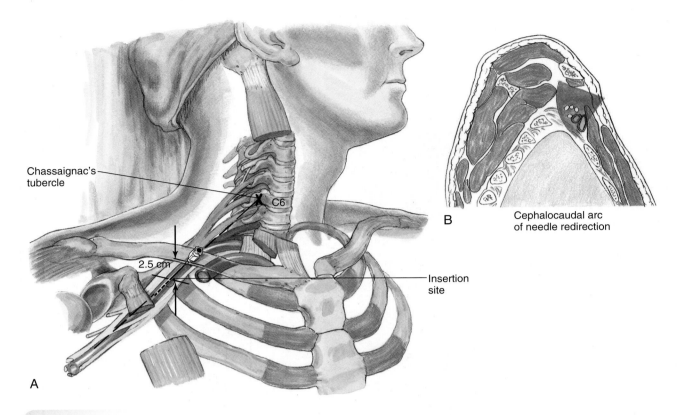

Chassaignac's tubercle

C6

2.5 cm

Insertion site

B

Cephalocaudal arc of needle redirection

A

Figure 6-4. Technique of infraclavicular block. **A,** Surface markings for block. **B,** Parasagittal view showing arc of needle redirection.

reorganize to give rise to the peripheral nerves of the upper extremity. In a simplified scheme, the branches of the lateral and medial cords are all "ventral" nerves to the upper extremity. The posterior cord, in contrast, provides all "dorsal" innervation to the upper extremity. Thus, the radial nerve supplies all the dorsal muscles in the upper extremity below the shoulder. The musculocutaneous nerve supplies muscular innervation in the arm and provides cutaneous innervation to the forearm. In contrast, the median and ulnar nerves are nerves of passage in the arm, but in the forearm and hand they provide the ventral musculature with motor innervation. These nerves can be further categorized: the median nerve innervates more heavily in the forearm, whereas the ulnar nerve innervates more heavily in the hand.

Position. The patient is placed supine, with the arm to be blocked abducted at the shoulder to a 90-degree angle if possible. If pain prevents this, the arm can be left at the patient's side and adjustments can be made with skin markings. The anesthesiologist can stand on the ipsilateral or the contralateral side of the patient, depending on his or her preference and the patient's body habitus. I prefer to stand on the ipsilateral side of the patient.

Needle Puncture. With the arm abducted at the shoulder, the coracoid process is identified by palpation and a skin mark placed at its most prominent portion. The skin entry mark is then made at a point 2 cm medial and 2 cm caudad to the previously marked coracoid process (Fig. 6-4A). Deeper infiltration is then performed with a 25-gauge, 5-cm needle while the needle is directed from the insertion site in a vertical parasagittal plane. Then a 6- to 9.5-cm,

20- to 22-gauge needle is inserted in a direction similar to that taken by the infiltration needle. If a paresthesia technique is used, a distal upper extremity paresthesia is sought; if a nerve stimulator technique is used, a distal upper extremity motor response is sought. If needle redirection is needed to achieve either a paresthesia or a motor response, the needle should be redirected in a cephalocaudad arc (Fig. 6-4B). The depth of contact with the brachial plexus depends on body habitus and needle angulation; it ranges from 2.5 to 3 cm in slender patients and from 8 to 10 cm in larger individuals.

Once adequate needle position has been achieved, either the single-injection dose of local anesthetic is administered incrementally or 20 mL of preservative-free normal saline solution is injected before threading the continuous brachial plexus catheter. For a single-injection technique the block can be administered in a manner similar to that used in either a supraclavicular or an axillary block. For a continuous technique, I currently use a stimulating catheter device to optimize catheter placement.

POTENTIAL PROBLEMS

An infraclavicular block should not cause neuraxial or pulmonary complications. Although vascular compromise (puncture of the axillary artery or vein) is theoretically possible, in my experience this occurs infrequently. If a continuous catheter technique is chosen, there is the possibility that despite adequate initial needle position, the catheter may be threaded too far away from the plexus to result in an effective block. However, the use of stimulating catheters has decreased this concern.

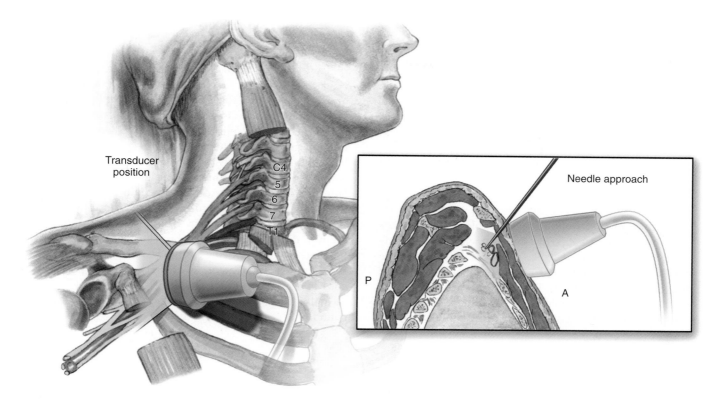

Figure 6-5. Parasagittal section of infraclavicular block with anatomic correlates. A, anterior; P, posterior.

Ultrasonography-Guided Technique

The brachial plexus is farthest from the patient's skin at the typical site of infraclavicular block (5 to 10 cm). The ultrasonographic implications are twofold: (1) the ultrasonography depth settings will have to be adjusted accordingly, and (2) transducer frequency may need to be reduced to improve ultrasound penetration. I use this approach for single-injection blocks for surgery distal to the elbow when a supraclavicular approach is not feasible or warranted. More important, I use this approach for catheter placement for prolonged analgesia in upper extremity surgeries such as elbow replacements or serial débridement; this may also be applicable to patients with chronic pain requiring catheter-assisted analgesia techniques during physical therapy.

To start, the operator should place the transducer inferior to the clavicle, such that a sagittal image slice of the patient is created on the image screen (Fig. 6-5). The subclavian artery and vein should appear in short axis and as circular hypoechoic structures posterior to the pectoralis major and minor muscles. If there is difficulty locating the vessels, the operator should slide the transducer laterally and increase the depth settings. Next, the medial edge of the transducer should be rotated caudad to optimize the short-axis view of the vessels. The three cords of the brachial plexus should be identified around the subclavian artery as hyperechoic circles or ovals with hypoechoic fascicles (Fig. 6-6). The operator should be aware of the

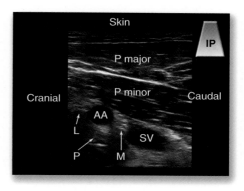

Figure 6-6. Sonogram highlighting the three cords of the brachial plexus (L, lateral; M, medial; P, posterior) viewed during infraclavicular block. P major/minor, pectoralis major/minor; AA, axillary artery; SV, subclavian vein.

amount of pressure being applied to the transducer because it is possible to compress the subclavian vein unintentionally despite the transducer's distance from the vessel.

For the approach, I use the in-plane technique and prefer to insert the needle from the cephalad side of the transducer. However, the needle can be inserted from the caudad side. Regardless of the needle insertion site, the goal is to place the needle near the brachial plexus, posterior to the subclavian artery (i.e., the 6 o'clock position). For single-injection techniques, I seek to generate a circumferential spread of local anesthetic around the subclavian artery. Such a spread of local anesthetic should also incorporate the three cords of the brachial plexus. If this is not observed with the single-injection technique, the needle can be repositioned near the artery as necessary.

For a continuous catheter placement technique, 10 mL can be injected posterior to the subclavian artery as for the single-injection technique. This initial injection helps to confirm needle tip location and facilitates catheter threading. The catheter is than advanced 2 to 3 cm into a portion of the brachial plexus sheath. The catheter is then injected with additional local anesthetic as necessary for the surgical procedure and postoperative analgesia.

PEARLS

To produce an effective infraclavicular block, the operator must be able to visualize the three-dimensional anatomy of the pyramid-shaped axilla and be able to move the needle tip effectively through a cephalocaudad arc to locate the plexus (see Fig. 6-4B). In addition, when placing the needle the operator should strive to obtain a distal upper extremity motor response through nerve stimulation—or obtain a definite distal paresthesia, if that approach is taken—to produce optimal needle position. Once the infraclavicular catheter is placed and secured, it is much more effective than any other brachial plexus continuous catheter technique. This reason alone makes the infraclavicular block my preferred site for continuous catheter brachial plexus analgesia. Because this technique crosses two pectoral muscle fascial planes, it is often more painful than other brachial plexus techniques. I therefore prefer to use a nerve stimulator or ultrasonography for plexus localization combined with heavier sedation than that used with other brachial techniques. The location of the stimulating needle or catheter can be ascertained by observing the motor response of the fifth digit to stimulation with this technique while the arm is in anatomic position. If the fifth digit moves laterally (pronation of the forearm), the lateral cord is being stimulated. If the fifth digit moves posteriorly (extension of the wrist), the posterior cord is being stimulated. Finally, if the fifth digit moves medially (flexion of the wrist), the medial cord is being stimulated.

Axillary Block

David L. Brown

with contributions from

Brian D. Sites and Brian C. Spence

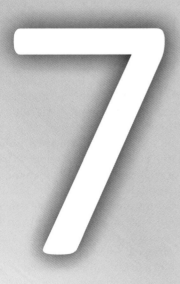

PERSPECTIVE

Axillary brachial plexus block is most effective for surgical procedures distal to the elbow. Some patients can undergo procedures on the elbow or lower humerus with an axillary technique, but strong consideration should be given to a supraclavicular block for those requiring more proximal procedures. It is discouraging to carry out a "successful" axillary block only to find that the surgical procedure extends outside the area of block. This block is appropriate for hand and forearm surgery; thus, it is often the most appropriate technique for outpatients in a busy hand surgery practice. Some anesthesiologists find axillary block suitable for elbow surgical procedures, and continuous axillary catheter techniques may be indicated for postoperative analgesia in these patients. Because this block is carried out distant from both the neuraxial structures and the lung, complications associated with those areas are avoided.

Patient Selection. To undergo an axillary block, patients must be able to abduct the arm at the shoulder. As the experience of the operator increases, the need for abduction decreases, but this block cannot be carried out with the arm at the side. Because the block is most appropriate for forearm and hand surgery, it is a rare patient with a surgical condition at those sites who cannot abduct the arm as needed.

Pharmacologic Choice. Because hand and wrist procedures often require less motor blockade than procedures on the shoulder, the concentration of local anesthetic needed for axillary block can usually be slightly less than that needed for supraclavicular or interscalene block. Appropriate drugs are lidocaine (1% to 1.5%), mepivacaine (1% to 1.5%), bupivacaine (0.5%), and ropivacaine (0.5% to 0.75%). Lidocaine and mepivacaine produce 2 to 3 hours of surgical anesthesia without epinephrine and 3 to 5 hours with the addition of epinephrine. These drugs can be useful for less involved procedures or outpatient surgical procedures. For more extensive surgical procedures requiring hospital admission, a longer-acting agent such as bupivacaine can be chosen. Plain bupivacaine and ropivacaine produce surgical anesthesia that lasts from 4 to 6 hours; the addition of epinephrine may prolong this period to 8 to 12 hours. The local anesthetic timeline must be considered when prescribing a drug for outpatient axillary block because blocks lasting as long as 18 to 24 hours can result from higher concentrations of bupivacaine with added epinephrine. With continuous catheter techniques used for postoperative analgesia or chronic pain syn-

dromes, 0.25% bupivacaine or 0.2% ropivacaine may be used, and even lower concentrations of these drugs may be used after a trial.

Traditional Block Technique

PLACEMENT

Anatomy. At the level of the distal axilla, where the axillary block is undertaken (Fig. 7-1), the axillary artery can be visualized as the center of a four-quadrant neurovascular bundle. I conceptualize these nerves in quadrants like a clock face because multiple injections during axillary block result in more acceptable clinical anesthesia than does injection at a single site. The musculocutaneous nerve is found in the 9- to 12-o'clock quadrant in the substance of the coracobrachialis muscle. The median nerve is most often found in the 12- to 3-o'clock quadrant; the ulnar nerve is "inferior" to the median nerve in the 3- to 6-o'clock quadrant; and the radial nerve is located in the 6- to 9-o'clock quadrant. The block does not need to be performed in the axilla; in fact, needle insertion in the middle to lower portion of the axillary hair patch or even more distal to this is effective. It is clear from radiographic and anatomic study of the brachial plexus and the axilla that separate and distinct sheaths are associated with the plexus at this point. Keeping this concept in mind will help to decrease the number of unacceptable blocks performed. Also, this more distal approach to axillary block is similar to the mid-humeral brachial plexus block.

Position. The patient is placed supine, with the arm forming a 90-degree angle with the trunk, and the forearm forming a 90-degree angle with the upper arm (Fig. 7-2). This position allows the anesthesiologist to stand at the level of the patient's upper arm and palpate the axillary artery, as illustrated in Figure 7-2. A line should be drawn tracing the course of the artery from the mid-axilla to the lower axilla; overlying this line, the index and third fingers of the anesthesiologist's left hand are used to identify the artery and minimize the amount of subcutaneous tissue overlying the neurovascular bundle. In this manner, the anesthesiologist can develop a sense of the longitudinal course of the artery, which is essential for performing an axillary block.

Needle Puncture. While the axillary artery is identified with two fingers, the needle and syringe are inserted as shown in Figure 7-3. Some local anesthetic should be

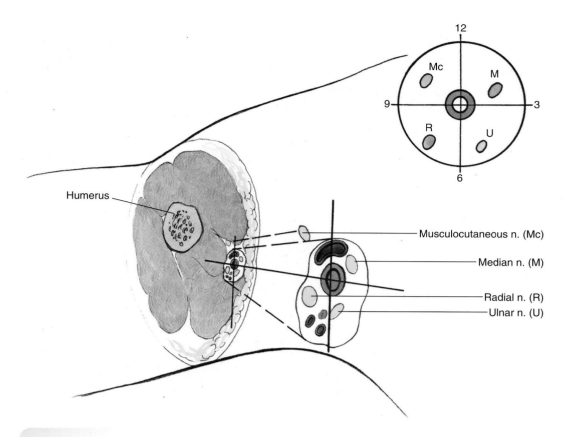

Figure 7-1. Axillary block: functional quadrant anatomy of distal axilla.

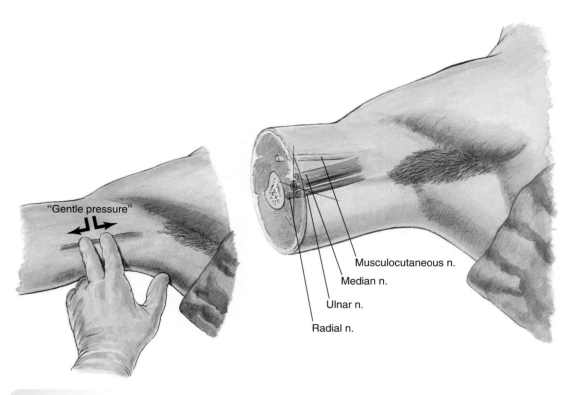

Figure 7-2. Axillary block: position of patient arm and clinician's fingers for palpation of axillary artery.

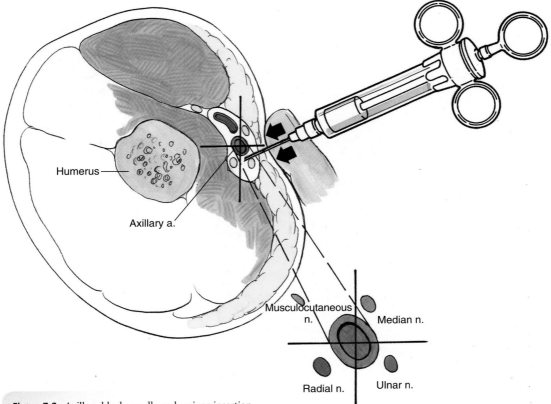

Figure 7-3. Axillary block: needle and syringe insertion.

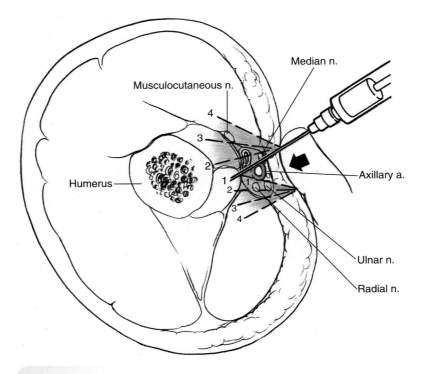

Figure 7-4. Axillary block: fanlike injection pattern using axillary artery as guide.

deposited in each of the quadrants surrounding the axillary artery. If paresthesia is obtained it is beneficial, although undue time should not be expended or patient discomfort incurred from an attempt to elicit a paresthesia. As illustrated in Figure 7-4, effective axillary block is produced by using the axillary artery as an anatomic landmark and infiltrating in a fanlike manner around the artery. Anesthesia of the musculocutaneous nerve is best achieved by infiltrating into the mass of the coracobrachialis muscle. This maneuver can be carried out by identifying the coracobrachialis and injecting anesthetic into its substance, or by inserting a longer needle until it contacts the humerus and injecting in a fanlike manner near the humerus (see Fig. 7-4).

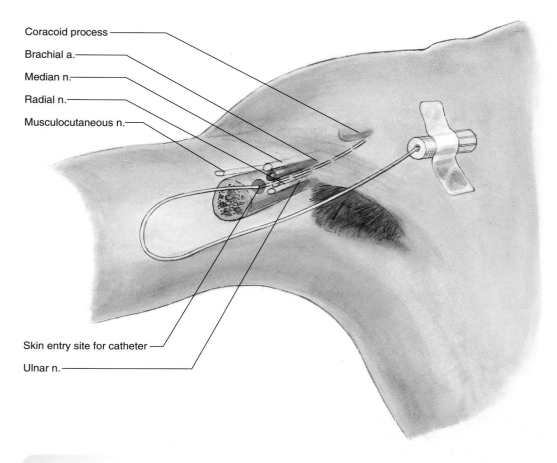

Coracoid process
Brachial a.
Median n.
Radial n.
Musculocutaneous n.

Skin entry site for catheter
Ulnar n.

Figure 7-5. Axillary block: continuous catheter technique after threading 10 cm of catheter proximally.

When using a continuous catheter technique for an axillary block, stimulating or nonstimulating catheter kits may be used; I prefer the stimulating catheter (Fig. 7-5). With the nonstimulating catheter, the epidural needle is positioned either with the assistance of a nerve stimulator or with elicitation of paresthesia as an end point. After the needle is positioned, 20 mL of preservative-free normal saline solution is injected through the needle, and then the appropriate-size catheter is inserted approximately 10 cm past the needle tip. Once the catheter has been secured with a plastic occlusive dressing, the initial bolus of drug is injected and the infusion is started.

POTENTIAL PROBLEMS

Problems with axillary block are infrequent because of the distance of this block from neuraxial structures and the lung. One occasional complication, which can be minimized by using multiple injections rather than a fixed needle, is systemic toxicity. Use of a single immobile needle to inject large volumes of a local anesthetic increases the potential for systemic toxicity relative to the use of smaller volumes of local anesthetic injected at multiple sites. Another potential problem with axillary block is the development of postoperative neuropathy, but one should not assume that axillary block is the cause of all neuropathy after upper extremity surgery. One must follow a logical

and systematic approach when seeking the cause of a neuropathy if we are to understand the true incidence and causes of neuropathy after brachial plexus block and upper extremity surgery.

Ultrasonography-Guided Technique

Ultrasonography-guided axillary block has fallen out of favor at my institution because of our success with ultrasonography-guided supraclavicular nerve block. I believe that the supraclavicular approach is more efficient and predictable in producing surgical anesthesia; however, the following is provided as a guide to those who may wish to carry out an axillary nerve block with ultrasonographic guidance.

The operator should place the ultrasound transducer in the axilla perpendicular to the long axis of the neurovascular bundle (Fig. 7-6). The goal is to obtain an image with the axillary artery in the center as a pulsatile hypoechoic circle. Before needle insertion, the operator should attempt to identify the four major nerves of the brachial plexus at this level (Fig. 7-7). The musculocutaneous nerve may not be visualized in the same image with the other three nerves because it is often several centimeters anterior and lateral used to confirm the impression of a nerve. I typically inject 5 to 8 mL of local anesthetic for each nerve blocked (see *Video 7: Axillary Nerve Block* on the Expert Consult Website).

To visually locate the musculocutaneous nerve, the operator should slide the transducer anterolaterally and locate the coracobrachialis muscle. The musculocutaneous nerve appears as a hyperechoic oval or circle lying between the coracobrachialis and biceps muscles (see Fig. 7-7). A separate needle insertion site is needed to block this nerve. The needle is advanced through the biceps muscle using the in-plane technique. We also use 5 to 8 mL of local anesthetic to block the musculocutaneous nerve identified by ultrasonography.

PEARLS

To perform axillary block effectively, the operator must understand the organization of the peripheral nerves at the level of the lower axilla. The axillary sheath at this level is discontinuous, and multiple injections may be required to allow the axillary block to reach full effectiveness. This does not mean that a single injection cannot produce acceptable surgical anesthesia; however, the most consistently effective axillary blocks result from depositing smaller amounts of local anesthetic in multiple sites.

Another reminder when using a paresthesia-seeking axillary technique is that a radial paresthesia is obtained infrequently. Thus, the anesthesiologist should not persist in attempting to produce one but instead should inject the anesthetic in its expected position and let the local anesthetic volume produce the block. Further, because the four-quadrant axillary approach uses a "field block" to anesthetize the musculocutaneous nerve, it also does not require elicitation of a paresthesia to be effective. Because the median and ulnar nerves are more superficial when the arm is in an axillary block position, they are the nerves that paresthesia is most likely to affect. Nevertheless, unnecessarily seeking a paresthesia for an extended time, even for median or ulnar sites, may result in anesthetic delays and patient discomfort and will discourage anesthesiologists from carrying out this block. If one keeps in mind the quadrant approach to axillary block, this technique should be accomplished in an efficient manner.

A mnemonic that is useful for remembering the position of the nerves at the level of the axillary block is "M&Ms are tops" (i.e., median and musculocutaneous nerves lie more cephalad in the abducted arm). Everyone can relate the "top-notch" candy M&Ms to the cephalad position of the two "m" nerves.

When using a continuous catheter technique for postoperative analgesia or treatment of chronic pain, carefully securing the catheter will help prevent its unintentional removal. Also, the ability to place an infraclavicular catheter minimizes the number of axillary catheters needed in the anesthesiologist's practice and is likely to improve her or his confidence in performing continuous brachial techniques.

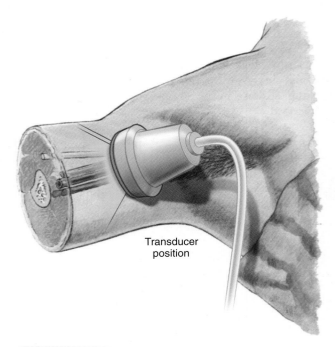

Figure 7-6. Axillary block: orientation of transducer in axilla for ultrasonography-guided block.

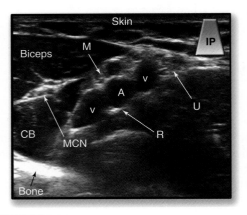

Figure 7-7. Axillary block: sonogram showing axillary block structures identified from typical transducer location. A, artery; CB, coracobrachialis muscle; M, median nerve; MCN, musculocutaneous nerve; R, radial nerve; U, ulnar nerve; v, vein.

to the axillary artery; there is a high degree of variability in the axillary neurovascular structures.

Once the four nerves have been identified, color-flow Doppler mode should be used over the projected individual needle paths to rule out unsuspected vascularity. If vascularity is present, the operator should slide the transducer either more distally or more proximally to provide a clearer path for needle insertion. The needle approach is an in-plane technique, from either edge of the transducer. My experience suggests that manipulating the needle to ensure local anesthetic spread around all target nerves increases the success of the blocks. If the appearance of a neural structure is equivocal, nerve stimulation can be

Distal Upper Extremity Block

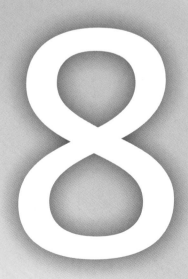

Ulnar, Median, and Radial Block at the Elbow

PERSPECTIVE

In general, distal upper extremity blocks—those at the elbow or wrist—are not frequently required if facility with more proximal blocks is gained. These more distal peripheral blocks are perceived to be associated with a slightly higher likelihood of nerve injury, perhaps because many of the peripheral branches are anatomically located in sites where the nerve is contained within bony and ligamentous surroundings. Although it is not difficult to localize the nerves at these peripheral sites, especially with ultrasonographic guidance, the "entrapment" of these nerves makes more proximal blocks, such as the axillary block, my preferred approach. Further, because a significant portion of hand and forearm surgery is carried out using an upper arm tourniquet, use of more distal blocks mandates significantly heavier sedation so that the patient can tolerate tourniquet inflation pressures.

Patient Selection. Few patients should require distal upper extremity block; an exception might be those needing supplementation after brachial plexus block. In any event, comprehensive anesthesia care should be possible without frequent use of these blocks.

Pharmacologic Choice. These peripheral blocks are usually considered for superficial surgery; thus, lower concentrations of local anesthetic are appropriate because motor blockade should not be an issue. Therefore, 0.75% to 1% mepivacaine or lidocaine, or 0.25% bupivacaine, or 0.2% ropivacaine should be sufficient.

PLACEMENT

At the Elbow

Anatomy. Of the three major nerves at the elbow—radial, median, and ulnar—the ulnar is most predictable in location. As illustrated in Figure 8-1, the ulnar nerve is located in the ulnar groove, which is a bony fascial canal between the medial epicondyle of the humerus and the olecranon

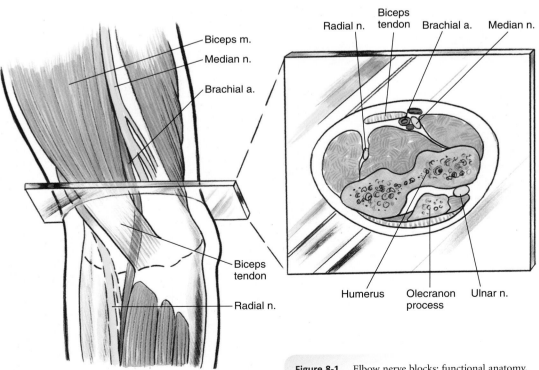

Figure 8-1. Elbow nerve blocks: functional anatomy.

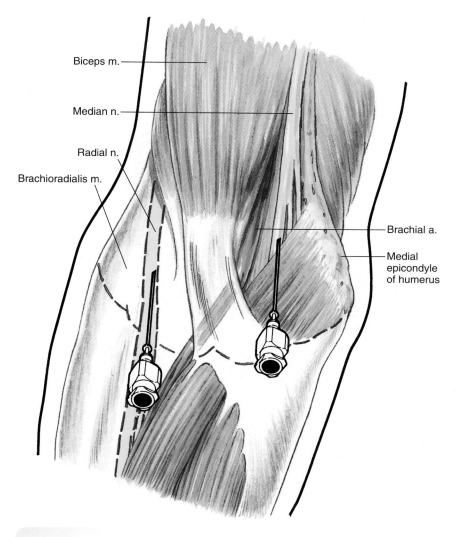

Figure 8-2. Elbow nerve blocks: median and radial nerves.

process. This area is extremely well protected by fibrous tissue and, although it may seem at first like an easy site to carry out block, the nerve is well protected (and potentially vulnerable) in the ulnar groove. The median nerve at the elbow lies medial to the brachial artery, which lies just medial to the biceps muscle. Conversely, the radial nerve has a somewhat variable course; it pierces the lateral intramuscular septum on its way to the forearm, and lies between the brachialis muscle and the brachioradialis muscle in the distal aspect of the upper arm. It is more effectively blocked in the axilla than at the elbow.

Position. All three of these nerves are blocked with the patient in the supine position and the arm supinated and abducted at the shoulder at a 90-degree angle. In addition, when the ulnar nerve block is performed, the forearm is flexed on the upper arm to more easily identify the ulnar groove (as illustrated in Fig. 8-3).

Needle Puncture: Median Nerve Block. A line should be drawn between the medial and lateral epicondyles of the humerus (at the level of the "pane of glass" shown in Fig. 8-1). Immediately medial to the brachial artery, the needle is inserted in the plane of the pane of glass, and a paresthesia is sought or a nerve stimulator or ultrasonographic

guidance is used to direct the needle (Fig. 8-2). After the needle is positioned, 3 to 5 mL of solution is injected medial to the brachial artery.

Needle Puncture: Radial Nerve Block. The radial nerve is likewise blocked at the level of the pane of glass in Figure 8-1. The biceps tendon at that level should be identified, and then a mark is made 1 to 2 cm lateral to the tendon. Again, a small-gauge, 3-cm needle is inserted through the mark in the plane of the pane of glass, and a paresthesia is sought or a nerve stimulator or ultrasonographic guidance is used to direct the needle, and 3 to 5 mL of solution is injected at that site (see Fig. 8-2).

Needle Puncture: Ulnar Nerve Block. As illustrated in Figure 8-3, the forearm is flexed on the upper arm and the ulnar groove is palpated. At a point approximately 1 cm proximal to a line drawn between the olecranon process and the medial epicondyle, a small-gauge, 2-cm needle is inserted. A paresthesia should be easily obtainable, and once it is, the needle is withdrawn 1 mm, and 3 to 5 mL of local anesthetic is injected through the needle. A larger volume of solution should not be injected directly into the ulnar groove because high pressure in this tightly contained fascial space may increase the risk of nerve injury.

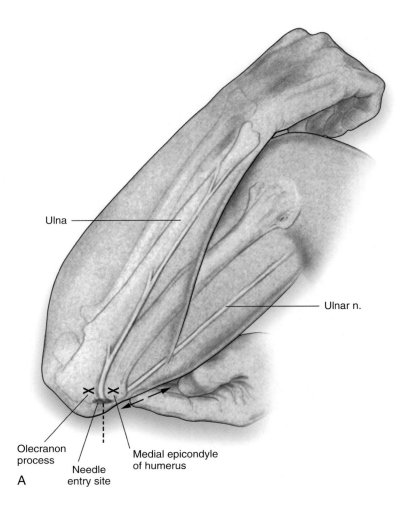

Ulna

Ulnar n.

Olecranon
process

Needle
entry site

Medial epicondyle
of humerus

A

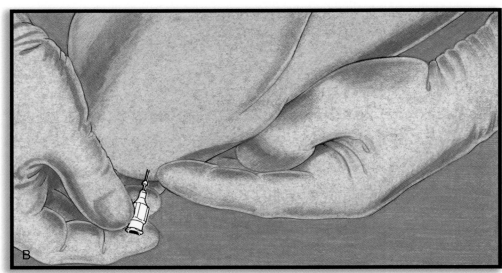

B

Figure 8-3. Ulnar nerve block: positioning. **A,** Palpation of the ulnar groove. **B,** Needle insertion.

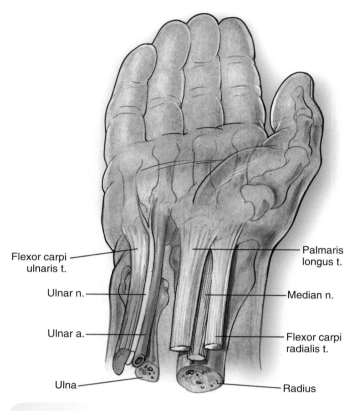

Figure 8-4. Wrist nerve blocks: functional anatomy.

Labels on figure:
Flexor carpi ulnaris t.
Ulnar n.
Ulnar a.
Ulna
Palmaris longus t.
Median n.
Flexor carpi radialis t.
Radius

At the Wrist

Anatomy. The ulnar nerve lies immediately lateral to the tendon of the flexor carpi ulnaris muscle and immediately medial to the ulnar artery (Fig. 8-4). The median nerve lies between the tendon of the palmaris longus muscle and the tendon of the flexor carpi radialis muscle. That places the median nerve in the long axis of the radius. The radial nerve at the wrist has already divided into a number of its peripheral branches, and effective radial block requires a field block along the radial aspect of the wrist.

Position. For a peripheral block at the wrist, the patient rests supine while the arm is extended at the shoulder and supported on an arm board (Fig. 8-5). The wrist is flexed over a small support, and the most effective position for the anesthesiologist is to stand in the long axis of the arm board. Thus, while performing the block, the anesthesiologist may observe the patient's face.

Needle Puncture: Ulnar Nerve Block. It should be easy to palpate the tendon of the flexor carpi ulnaris and the ulnar artery immediately proximal to the ulnar styloid process. A small-gauge, short-bevel needle can be inserted perpendicular to the wrist at this site, and a paresthesia should be easy to elicit. Three to 5 mL of solution can be injected at this site; if no paresthesia is obtained, a similar amount can be injected in a fanlike manner between those two structures with near certainty of block.

Needle Puncture: Median Nerve Block. On a line between the styloid process of the ulna and the prominence of the distal radius, the palmaris longus tendon and the tendon of the flexor carpi radialis are identified. These tendons can be accentuated by having the patient flex the wrist while making a fist. The median nerve lies deep and between those structures, so a blunt-beveled, small-gauge, short needle is inserted between the tendons. If a paresthesia is obtained, 3 to 5 mL of solution is injected; if none is obtained, a similar amount is injected in a fanlike manner between the two tendons.

Needle Puncture: Radial Nerve Block. Blocking the radial nerve at the wrist requires infiltration of its multiple peripheral branches, which descend along the dorsal and radial aspect of the wrist. A field block is performed at the subcutaneous level in and around the anatomic snuffbox. The injection should be carried out superficial to the extensor pollicis longus tendon, which is easily identified by having the patient extend the thumb. This block may require from 5 to 6 mL of local anesthetic and is used infrequently.

POTENTIAL PROBLEMS

As outlined, problems with peripheral blocks primarily involve the potential for compression nerve injury and possibly a slightly increased incidence of neuropathy. Theoretically, this occurs because of the tight fascial compartments in which these nerves run through the distal arm, forearm, and wrist. Likewise, blocking these distal nerves does not allow for tourniquet use, which is often the clinically limiting factor.

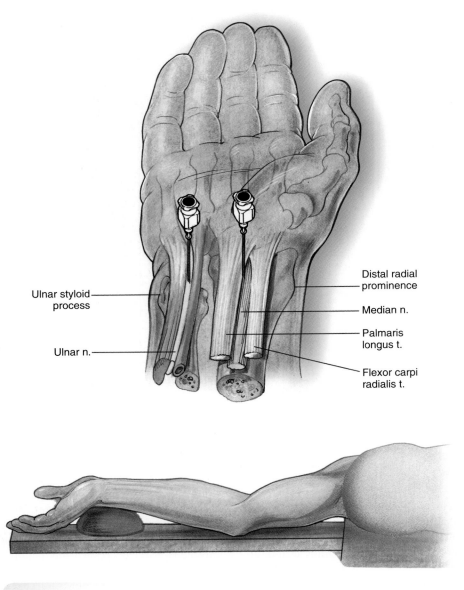

Ulnar styloid process

Ulnar n.

Distal radial prominence

Median n.

Palmaris longus t.

Flexor carpi radialis t.

Figure 8-5. Wrist nerve blocks: needle insertion and arm positioning.

Suggestions for the successful use of these blocks involve avoiding them, when possible. Understanding the concepts outlined for the axillary nerve block (see Chapter 7, Axillary Block) should make the necessity for these blocks infrequent.

Digital Nerve Block

PERSPECTIVE

Digital nerve block is commonly used in emergency departments but is not frequently used by anesthesiologists. It can be used for any surgery that requires a digital operation. However, its widest use is in repair of lacerations.

Patient Selection. The most common use for this block is in emergency departments, although its use may be appropriate in an occasional elective surgical patient with a single-digit surgical problem.

Pharmacologic Choice. As with any of the more peripheral upper extremity blocks, lower concentrations of any of the amide local anesthetics are appropriate for digital block, with the strong recommendation to avoid epinephrine-containing solutions.

PLACEMENT

Anatomy. As illustrated in Figure 8-6, the digital nerves can be conceptualized as running at the "corners" of the proximal phalanx. The nerves run near arteries and veins and are the distal continuations of both the median and ulnar nerves.

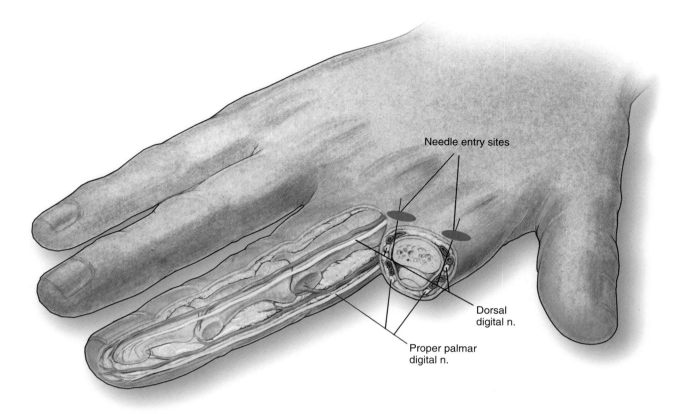

Needle entry sites

Dorsal
digital n.

Proper palmar
digital n.

Figure 8-6. Digital nerve block: anatomy and needle insertion.

Position. Digital nerve block is most effectively carried out with the hand pronated. The skin over the dorsum of the finger is less tightly fixed to the underlying structures than it is on the ventral surface.

Needle Puncture. Skin wheals are raised at the dorsolateral borders of the proximal phalanx, and a blunt-beveled, small-gauge, short needle is inserted at the dorsal surface of the lateral border of the phalanx. Infiltration of both the dorsal and the ventral branches of the digital nerve is carried out bilaterally, and a total of 1 to 2 mL at each site should be sufficient for block.

POTENTIAL PROBLEMS

Epinephrine-containing solutions should not be used for digital nerve block.

PEARLS

These blocks should be used principally for emergency department procedures, and comprehensive anesthesia care requires at least familiarity with the technique.

Intravenous Regional Block

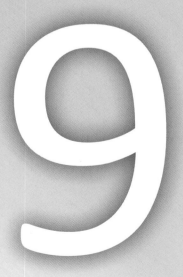

PERSPECTIVE

Intravenous (IV) regional anesthesia was introduced by Bier in 1908. As illustrated in Figure 9-1, in the initial description a surgical procedure was required to cannulate a vein, and both proximal and distal tourniquets were used to contain the local anesthetic in the venous system. After its introduction, the technique fell into disuse until the less toxic amino amides became available in the mid-20th century. This technique can be used for a variety of upper extremity operations, including both soft tissue and orthopedic procedures, primarily in the hand and forearm. The technique has also been used for foot procedures with a calf tourniquet.

Patient Selection. The technique is best suited for patients in whom there is no disruption of the venous system of the involved upper extremity because the technique relies on an intact venous system. It can be used for distal orthopedic fractures and soft tissue operations. IV regional block may not be appropriate for patients in whom movement of the upper extremity causes significant pain because movement of the upper extremity is required to exsanguinate blood from the venous system adequately.

Pharmacologic Choice. The most commonly used agent for IV regional anesthesia is a dilute concentration of lidocaine; however, prilocaine has also been successfully used.

Lidocaine is used in a 0.5% concentration; approximately 50 mL is used for an upper extremity IV regional block.

PLACEMENT

Anatomy. The only anatomic detail necessary for clinical use of the IV regional block is identification of a peripheral vein; one must be cannulated in the involved extremity.

Position. The patient should be resting supine on the operating table with an IV tube already established in the nonsurgical arm. The involved arm should be extended on an arm board near available supplies (Fig. 9-2).

Needle Puncture. Before placement of the IV catheter in the operative extremity, a tourniquet, either double or single, should be placed around the upper arm of the patient. An IV cannula is then inserted in the operative extremity, as distally as possible, most commonly in the dorsum of the hand (Fig. 9-3). There are two methods for exsanguinating the venous blood from the operative extremity. The traditional technique requires the wrapping of an Esmarch bandage from distal to proximal (Fig. 9-4). When the Esmarch bandage is not available or the patient is in too much pain to allow its placement, another method is to raise the arm for 3 to 4 minutes to allow gravity to exsanguinate the operative upper extremity (Fig. 9-5).

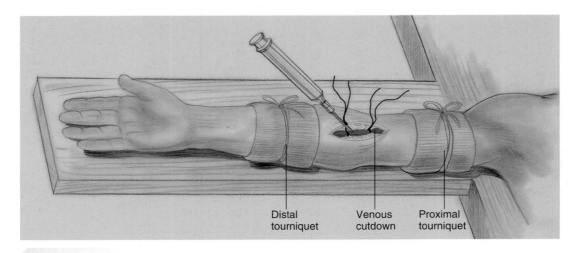

Distal tourniquet   Venous cutdown   Proximal tourniquet

Figure 9-1. Early Bier block: surgical technique.

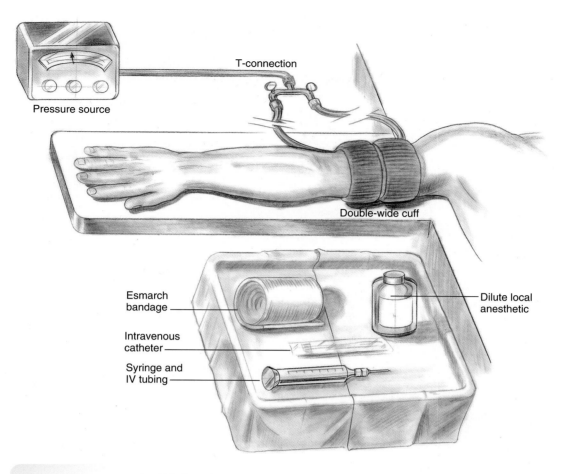

Figure 9-2. Intravenous regional block: equipment.

Pressure source

T-connection

Double-wide cuff

Esmarch bandage

Dilute local anesthetic

Intravenous catheter

Syringe and IV tubing

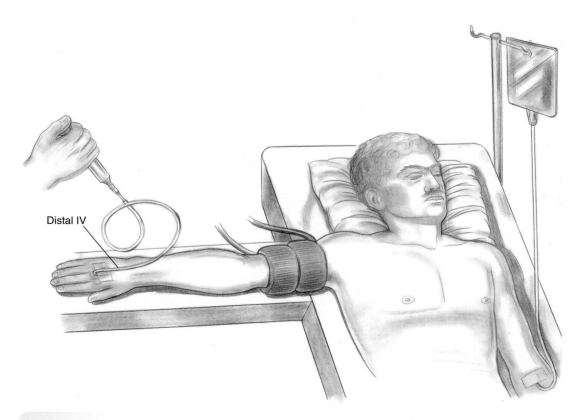

Figure 9-3. Intravenous regional block: distal IV site.

Distal IV

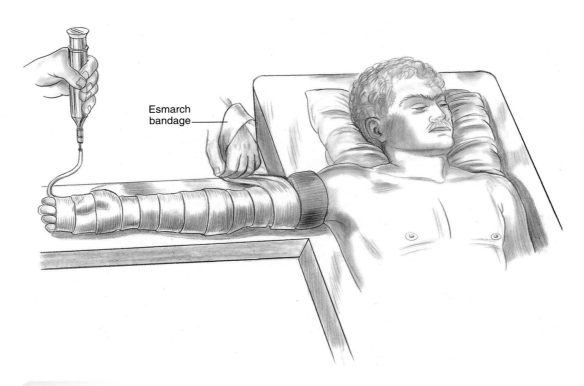

Esmarch
bandage

Figure 9-4. Intravenous regional block: venous exsanguination with Esmarch bandage.

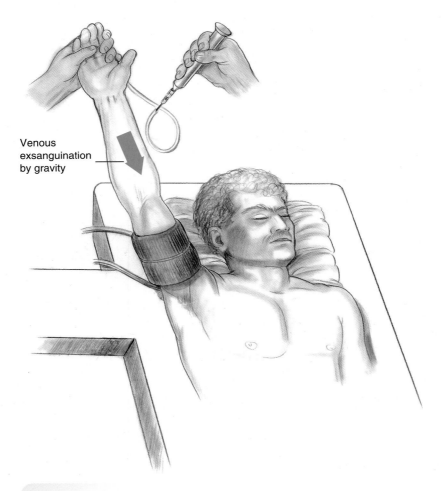

Venous
exsanguination
by gravity

Figure 9-5. Intravenous regional block: venous exsanguination by gravity.

After the blood has been exsanguinated from the upper extremity, the tourniquet is inflated. If a double tourniquet is used, only the upper tourniquet is inflated. Recommendations for tourniquet inflation pressures range from 50 mm Hg above systolic blood pressure with a wide cuff, to a cuff pressure double the systolic blood pressure, to 300 mm Hg regardless of blood pressure. Until more information is available, I caution against using pressures greater than 300 mm Hg during upper extremity block.

If an Esmarch bandage has been used, the elastic bandage is then unwrapped, and in the average adult 50 mL of 0.5% lidocaine without a vasoconstrictor is injected. Onset of the block usually occurs within 5 minutes, and the block is effective for procedures lasting as long as 90 to 120 minutes. This time limit is due to tourniquet time constraints rather than to diminution of the local anesthetic effect. The IV cannula is removed before preparation for operation. The block persists as long as the cuff is inflated and disappears shortly after deflation.

POTENTIAL PROBLEMS

The principal disadvantage of IV regional anesthesia is that physicians unfamiliar with treating local anesthetic toxicity may use the technique when appropriate resuscitation measures are not available. Although some workers report successful use of IV regional anesthesia for lower extremity surgery, especially if a calf tourniquet is used for foot surgery, its use is not widespread. During upper extremity use, a considerable number of patients complain about tourniquet pressure even when a double tourniquet is used, and this is often the clinically limiting feature of this technique. Appropriate use of IV sedatives is important for patient comfort.

PEARLS

Figure 9-6 illustrates the two complementary theories of how IV regional anesthesia produces block. The figure

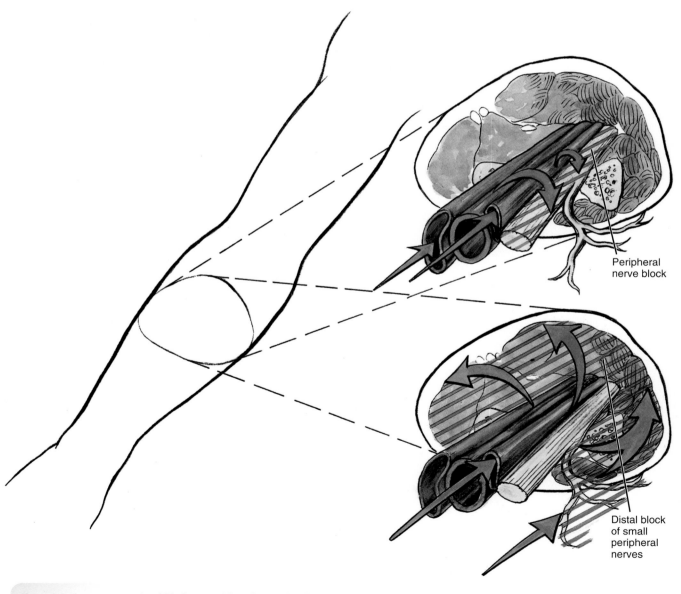

Peripheral nerve block

Distal block of small peripheral nerves

Figure 9-6. Intravenous regional block: potential mechanism(s) of action.

conceptualizes local anesthetic entering the venous system and producing block by blocking the peripheral nerves running with the venous structures. It also outlines a theory that may be complementary—that is, the local anesthetic leaves the veins and blocks small distal branches of peripheral nerves. It is likely that both of these theories are operative. If IV regional anesthesia is to be used successfully, all members of the operating team should understand the importance of tourniquet integrity because the most significant problems with the technique involve unintentional deflation of the tourniquet.

SECTION III:
Lower Extremity Blocks

Lower Extremity Block Anatomy

10

Anesthesiologists are more comfortable carrying out lower extremity regional block than upper extremity regional block because of the ease and simplicity of blocking the lower extremities with neuraxial techniques. Also, in no anatomic site outside the neuraxis are the lower extremity plexuses as compactly packaged as are the nerves to the upper extremity in the brachial plexus. If one compares the path of lower extremity nerves over the pelvic brim to the path of the brachial plexus over the first rib, it is clear that the four major nerves to the lower extremity exit from four widely differing sites (Figs 10-1 and 10-2). Thus, regional block of the lower extremity focuses on block of individual peripheral nerves, and my approach to anatomy will follow that concept.

Two major nerve plexuses innervate the lower extremity: the lumbar plexus and the lumbosacral plexus. The lumbar plexus primarily innervates the ventral aspect, whereas the lumbosacral plexus primarily innervates the dorsal aspect of the lower extremity (see Fig. 10-2).

The lumbar plexus is formed from the ventral rami of the first three lumbar nerves and part of the fourth lumbar nerve. In approximately half of patients, a small branch from the twelfth thoracic nerve joins the first lumbar nerve. The lumbar plexus forms from the ventral rami of these nerves anterior to the transverse processes of the lumbar vertebrae deeply within the psoas muscle (Fig. 10-3). The cephalad portion of the lumbar plexus (i.e., the first lumbar nerve, and often a portion of the twelfth thoracic nerve)

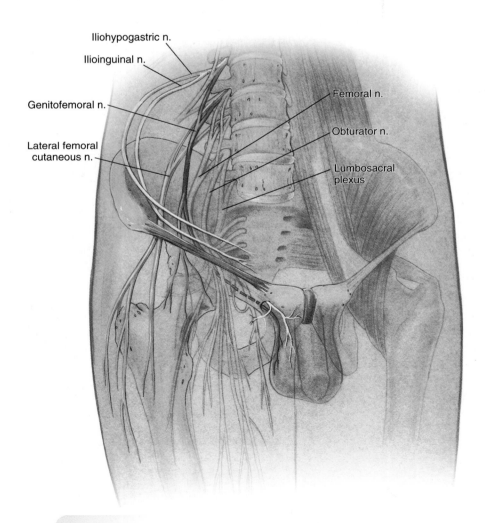

Figure 10-1. Lower extremity anatomy: major nerves, anterior oblique view.

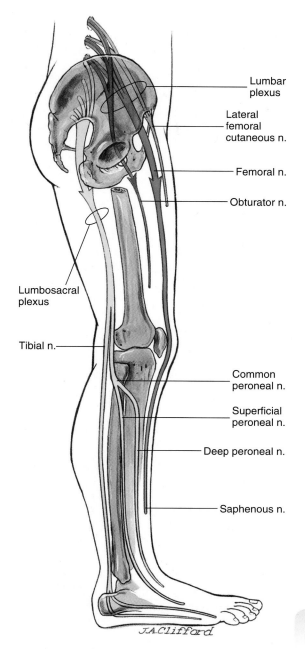

Lumbar
plexus

Lateral
femoral
cutaneous n.

Femoral n.

Obturator n.

Lumbosacral
plexus

Tibial n.

Common
peroneal n.

Superficial
peroneal n.

Deep peroneal n.

Saphenous n.

J.A.Clifford

Figure 10-2. Lower extremity anatomy: major nerves, lateral view.

Figure 10-3. Lumbar plexus anatomy: cross-sectional view. Ao, aorta; VC, vena cava.

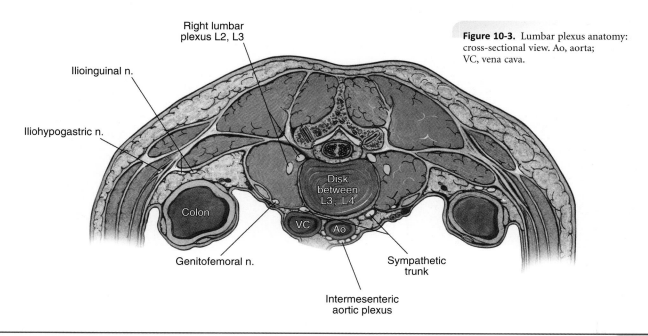

Right lumbar
plexus L2, L3

Ilioinguinal n.

Iliohypogastric n.

Disk
between
L3, L4

Colon

VC

Ao

Genitofemoral n.

Sympathetic
trunk

Intermesenteric
aortic plexus

splits into superior and inferior branches. The superior branch redivides into the iliohypogastric and ilioinguinal nerves, and the smaller inferior branch unites with a small superior branch of the second lumbar nerve to form the genitofemoral nerve (see Fig. 10-1).

The iliohypogastric nerve penetrates the transversus abdominis muscle near the crest of the ilium and supplies motor fibers to the abdominal musculature. It ends in an anterior cutaneous branch to the skin of the suprapubic region and a lateral cutaneous branch in the hip region (Fig. 10-4).

The ilioinguinal nerve courses slightly inferior to the iliohypogastric nerve. It then traverses the inguinal canal and ends cutaneously in branches to the upper and medial parts of the thigh and near the anterior scrotal nerves, which supply the skin at the root of the penis and the anterior part of the scrotum in males (see Fig. 10-4). In females, the comparable anterior labial nerves supply the skin of the mons pubis and labia majora.

The genitofemoral nerve divides at a variable level into genital and femoral branches. The genital branch is small; it enters the inguinal canal at the deep inguinal ring and supplies the cremaster muscle, small branches to the skin and fascia of the scrotum, and adjacent parts of the thigh.

The femoral branch is the more medial of the two branches and continues under the inguinal ligament on the anterior surface of the external iliac artery. Below the inguinal ligament, it pierces the femoral sheath and passes through the saphenous opening to supply the skin over the femoral triangle lateral to that supplied by the ilioinguinal nerve (see Fig. 10-4). These three nerves are clinically important during regional block for inguinal herniorrhaphy or other groin procedures carried out under regional block.

Caudal to these three nerves are three major nerves of the lumbar plexus that exit from the pelvis anteriorly and innervate the lower extremity. These are the lateral femoral cutaneous, femoral, and obturator nerves (see Figs. 10-1 and 10-2).

The lateral femoral cutaneous nerve passes under the lateral end of the inguinal ligament. It may be superficial or deep to the sartorius muscle and it descends at first deep to the fascia lata. It provides cutaneous innervation to the lateral portion of the buttock distal to the greater trochanter and to the proximal two thirds of the lateral aspect of the thigh.

The obturator nerve descends along the medial posterior aspect of the psoas muscle and through the pelvis to the obturator canal into the thigh. This nerve supplies the

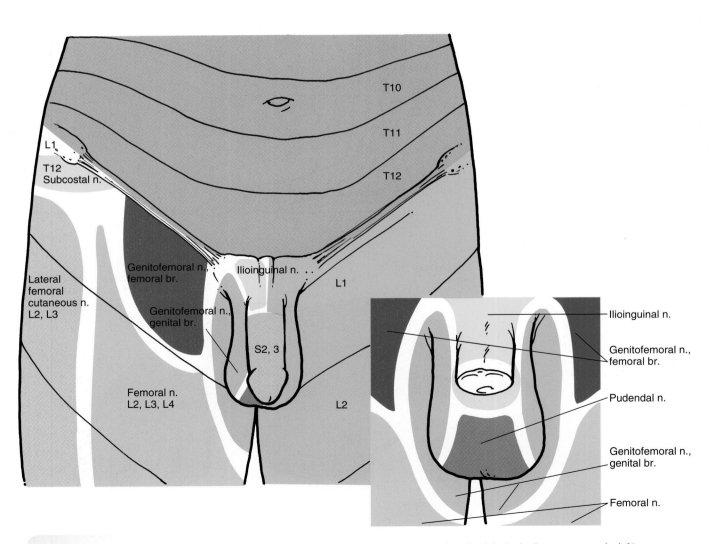

Figure 10-4. Lower extremity anatomy: proximal innervation (peripheral nerves labeled on right side of the body, dermatomes on the left).

adductor group of muscles, the hip and knee joints, and often the skin on the medial aspect of the thigh proximal to the knee.

The femoral nerve is the largest branch of the lumbar plexus. It emerges through the fibers of the psoas muscle at the muscle's lower lateral border and descends in the groove between the psoas and the iliacus muscles. It passes under the inguinal ligament within this groove. Slightly before, or on, entering the femoral triangle of the upper thigh, the femoral nerve breaks into numerous branches supplying the muscles and skin of the anterior thigh, knee, and hip joints.

The lumbosacral plexus is formed by the ventral rami of the lumbar fourth and fifth and the sacral first, second, and third nerves. Occasionally, a portion of the fourth sacral nerve contributes to the sacral plexus. The nerve from the plexus that is of primary interest to anesthesiologists during lower extremity block is the sciatic nerve. The posterior femoral cutaneous nerve is sometimes listed as an additional branch important to anesthesiologists. In reality, the sciatic nerve is the combination of two major nerve trunks:

the first is the tibial nerve, derived from the anterior branches of the ventral rami of the fourth and fifth lumbar and the first, second, and third sacral nerves, whereas the second is the common peroneal nerve, derived from the dorsal branches of the ventral rami of the same five nerves. These two major nerve trunks pass as the sciatic nerve through the upper leg to the popliteal fossa, where they divide into their terminal branches, the tibial and common peroneal nerves.

Figures 10-5 and 10-6 illustrate the cutaneous innervation of the peripheral nerves of the lower extremity. This subject is illustrated with the patient's lower extremity in both the anatomic and the lithotomy positions for greatest clinical utility. Figure 10-7 illustrates the dermatomal innervation of the lower extremities in a similar manner. Figure 10-8 illustrates the osteotome pattern of lower extremity innervation and will be most useful to anesthesiologists who are providing anesthesia for orthopedic procedures. Figure 10-9 helps clarify the cross-sectional anatomy pertinent to regional block of the lower extremity.

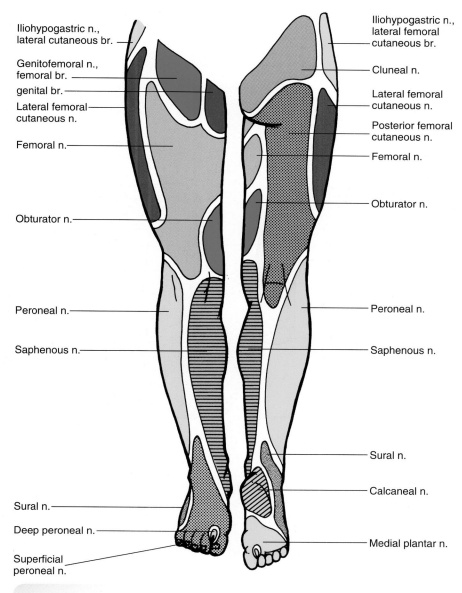

Figure 10-5. Lower extremity anatomy: proximal and distal innervation.

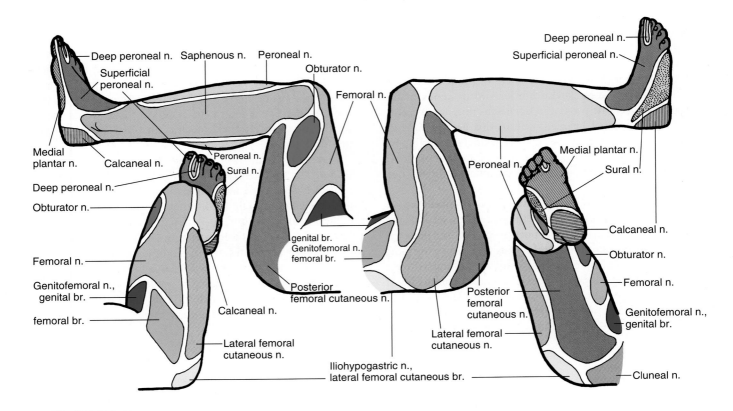

Figure 10-6. Lower extremity anatomy in lithotomy position: proximal and distal peripheral nerves.

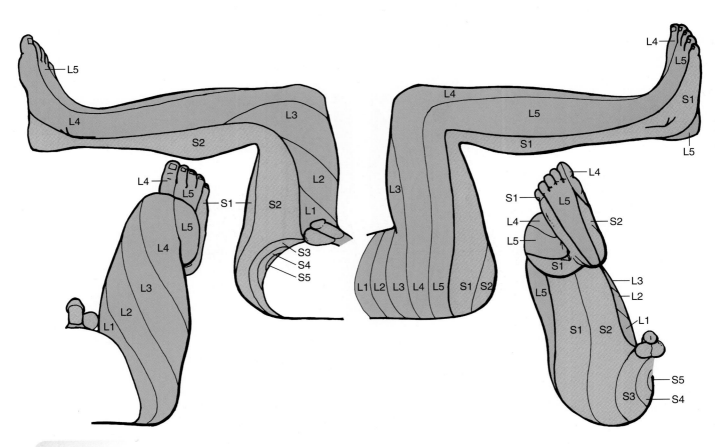

Figure 10-7. Lower extremity anatomy in lithotomy position: dermatomes.

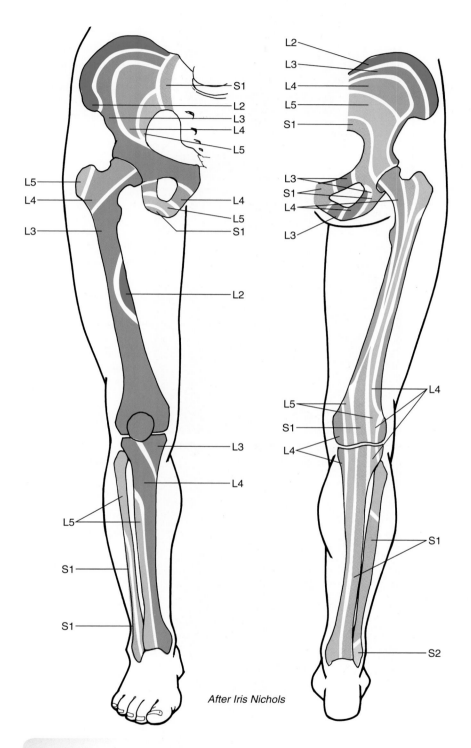

Figure 10-8. Lower extremity anatomy: osteotomes.

After Iris Nichols

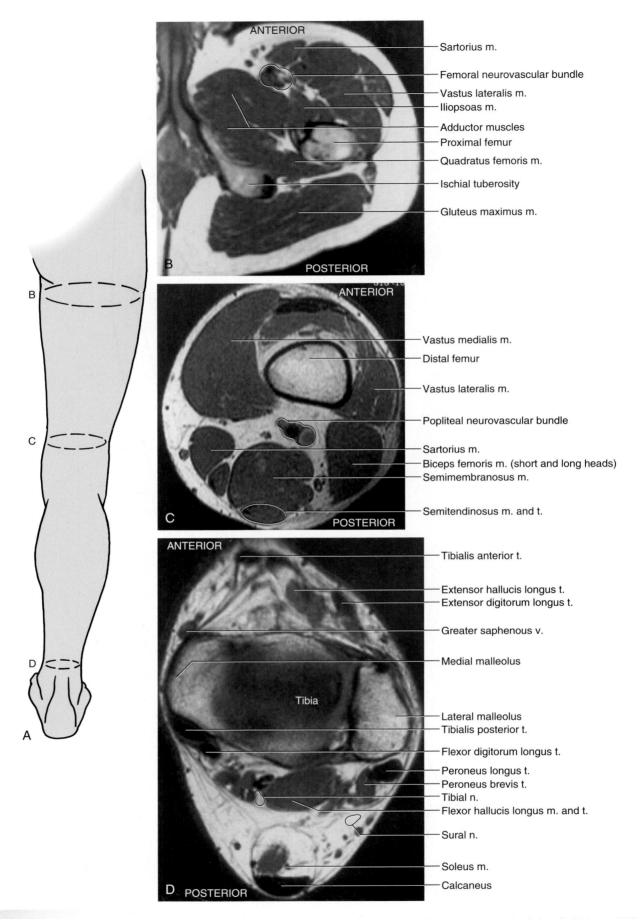

Figure 10-9. Lower extremity anatomy: cross-sectional magnetic resonance images. **A,** Location of sections. **B,** Upper leg (below the hip). **C,** Middle leg (above the knee). **D,** Lower leg (above the ankle).

Lumbar Plexus Block

11

Inguinal Perivascular Block (Three-in-One Block)

PERSPECTIVE

The inguinal perivascular block is based on the concept of injecting local anesthetic near the femoral nerve in an amount sufficient to track proximally along fascial planes to anesthetize the lumbar plexus. The three principal nerves of the lumbar plexus pass from the pelvis anteriorly: the lateral femoral cutaneous, the femoral, and the obturator nerves. As illustrated in Figure 11-1, the theory behind this block presumes that the local anesthetic will track in the fascial plane between the iliacus and the psoas muscles to reach the region of the lumbar plexus roots.

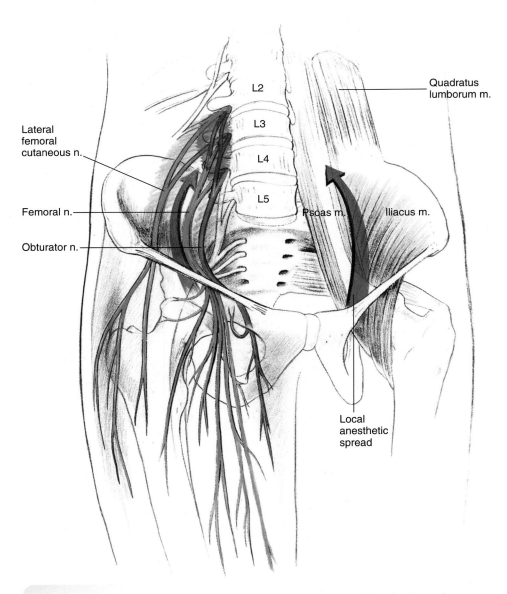

Figure 11-1. Lumbar plexus anatomy: proposed mechanism of proximal local anesthetic spread.

Patient Selection. As outlined, lower extremity block is often most effectively and efficiently performed with neuraxial blocks. Nevertheless, in some patients avoidance of bilateral block or sympathectomy may make an alternative approach necessary.

Pharmacologic Choice. Local anesthetics should be selected by deciding whether a primarily sensory or a sensory and motor block is needed. Any of the amino amides can be used. It has been suggested that the volume of local anesthetic needed for adequate lumbar plexus block from this approach can be estimated by dividing the patient's height, in inches, by three. That number is the volume of local anesthetic in milliliters that theoretically will provide lumbar plexus block.

PLACEMENT

Anatomy. The concept behind this block is that the only anatomy one needs to visualize is the extension of sheath-like fascial planes that surround the femoral nerve.

Position. The patient should be placed supine on the operating table with the anesthesiologist standing at the patient's side in position to palpate the ipsilateral femoral artery.

Needle Puncture. A short-beveled, 22-gauge, 5-cm needle is inserted immediately lateral to the femoral artery, caudal to the inguinal ligament in the lower extremity to be blocked. It is advanced with cephalad angulation until a femoral paresthesia occurs; alternatively, nerve stimulation or ultrasonographic guidance is used to identify correct perineural location of the needle tip. At this point, the needle is firmly fixed, and while the distal femoral sheath is digitally compressed, the entire volume of local anesthetic is injected.

POTENTIAL PROBLEMS

My clinical experience suggests that the principal problem with this technique is a lack of predictability. In addition, whenever a large volume of local anesthetic is injected through a fixed "immobile" needle, the risk of systemic toxicity is increased. If the technique is used, incremental injection of local anesthetic, accompanied by frequent aspiration for blood, should be carried out.

PEARLS

This block should be used when the goal is lower extremity analgesia, not anesthesia during an operation. I do not believe one needs to master this technique to provide comprehensive regional anesthesia care.

Psoas Compartment Block

PERSPECTIVE

In concept, the psoas compartment block produces block of all lumbar and some sacral nerves, thus providing anesthesia of the anterior thigh. This block is described in Chapter 37, Paravertebral Block. It is best termed a lumbar paravertebral block.

Sciatic Block

12

PERSPECTIVE

The sciatic nerve is one of the largest nerve trunks in the body, yet few surgical procedures can be performed with sciatic block alone. It is most often combined with femoral, lateral femoral cutaneous, or obturator nerve blocks. The block is also effective for analgesia of the lower leg and may provide pain relief from ankle fractures or tibial fractures before operative intervention.

Patient Selection. This block may be indicated for patients needing analgesia before transport for definitive orthopedic surgical repair of lower leg or ankle fractures. For patients in whom it may be desirable to avoid the sympathectomy accompanying neuraxial block, sciatic block combined with femoral nerve block often allows ankle and foot procedures to be carried out. One group of patients in whom this block is often useful are those undergoing distal amputations of the lower extremity who have vascular compromise based on diabetes or peripheral vascular disease.

Pharmacologic Choice. Sciatic nerve block requires from 20 to 25 mL of local anesthetic solution. When this volume is added to that required for other lower extremity peripheral blocks, the total may reach the upper end of an acceptable local anesthetic dose range. Conversely, uptake of local anesthetic from these lower extremity sites is not as rapid as with epidural or intercostal block; thus, a larger mass of local anesthetic may be appropriate in this region. If motor blockade is desired with this block, 1.5% mepivacaine or lidocaine may be necessary, whereas 0.5% bupivacaine or 0.5% to 0.75% ropivacaine will be effective.

Traditional Block Technique

PLACEMENT

Anatomy. The sciatic nerve is formed from L4 through S3 roots. These roots of the sacral plexus form on the anterior surface of the lateral sacrum and are assembled into the sciatic nerve on the anterior surface of the piriformis muscle. The sciatic nerve results from the fusion of two major nerve trunks. The "medial" sciatic nerve is functionally the tibial nerve, which forms from the ventral branches of the ventral rami of L4-L5 and S1-S3; the posterior branches of the ventral rami of these same nerves form the "lateral" sciatic nerve, which is functionally the peroneal nerve. As the sciatic nerve exits the pelvis, it is anterior

to the piriformis muscle and is joined by another nerve, the posterior cutaneous nerve of the thigh. At the inferior border of the piriformis, the sciatic and posterior cutaneous nerves of the thigh lie posterior to the obturator internus, the gemelli, and the quadratus femoris. At this point, these nerves are anterior to the gluteus maximus. Here, the nerve is approximately equidistant from the ischial tuberosity and the greater trochanter (Figs. 12-1 to 12-3). The nerve continues downward through the thigh to lie along the posteromedial aspect of the femur. At the cephalad portion of the popliteal fossa, the sciatic nerve usually divides to form the tibial and common peroneal nerves. Occasionally, this division occurs much higher, and sometimes the tibial and peroneal nerves are separate through their entire course. In the popliteal fossa, the tibial nerve continues downward into the lower leg, whereas the common peroneal nerve travels laterally along the medial aspect of the short head of the biceps femoris muscle.

Classic Approach

Position. The patient is positioned laterally, with the side to be blocked nondependent. The nondependent leg is flexed and its heel placed against the knee of the dependent leg (Fig. 12-4). The anesthesiologist is positioned to allow insertion of the needle, as shown in Figure 12-4.

Needle Puncture. A line is drawn from the posterior superior iliac spine to the midpoint of the greater trochanter. Perpendicular to the midpoint of this line, another line is extended caudomedially for 5 cm. The needle is inserted through this point (Fig. 12-5). As a cross-check for proper placement, an additional line may be drawn from the sacral hiatus to the previously marked point on the greater trochanter. The intersection of this line with the 5-cm perpendicular line should coincide with the needle insertion site.

At this site, a 22-gauge, 10- to 12-cm needle is inserted, as illustrated in Figure 12-4. The needle should be directed through the entry site toward an imaginary point where the femoral vessels course under the inguinal ligament. The needle is inserted until a paresthesia is elicited or until bone is contacted. If bone is encountered before a paresthesia is elicited, the needle is redirected along the line joining the sacral hiatus and the greater trochanter until a paresthesia or motor response is elicited. During this needle redirection, the needle should not be inserted more than 2 cm past the depth at which bone was originally contacted, or the needle tip will be placed anterior to the site of the sciatic nerve. Once a paresthesia or motor response is elicited, 20 to 25 mL of local anesthetic is injected.

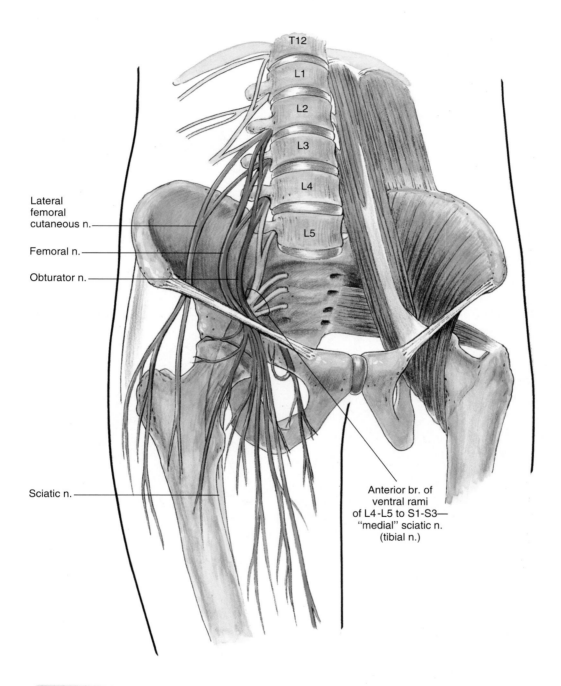

Figure 12-1. Sciatic nerve anatomy: anterior oblique view.

Labels:
- T12
- L1
- L2
- L3
- L4
- L5
- Lateral femoral cutaneous n.
- Femoral n.
- Obturator n.
- Sciatic n.
- Anterior br. of ventral rami of L4-L5 to S1-S3— "medial" sciatic n. (tibial n.)

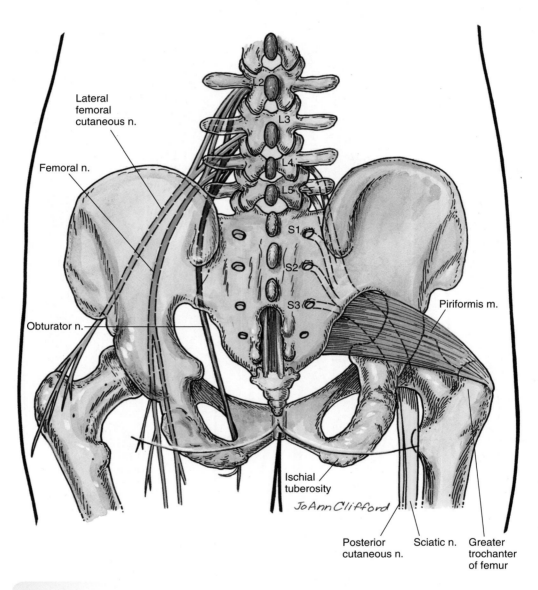

Figure 12-2. Sciatic nerve anatomy: posterior view.

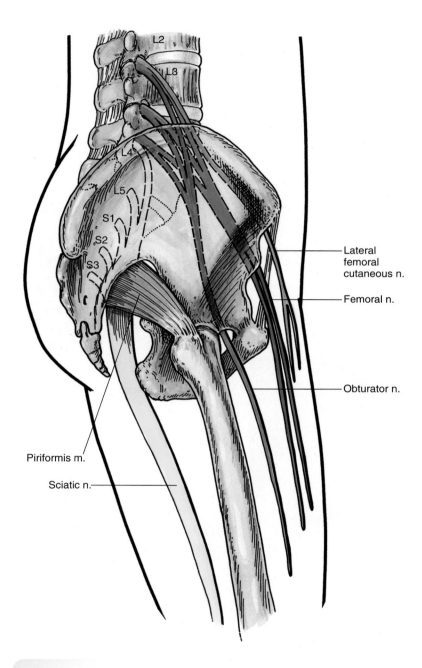

Lateral femoral cutaneous n.

Femoral n.

Obturator n.

Piriformis m.

Sciatic n.

L2

L3

L4

L5

S1

S2

S3

Figure 12-3. Sciatic nerve anatomy: lateral view.

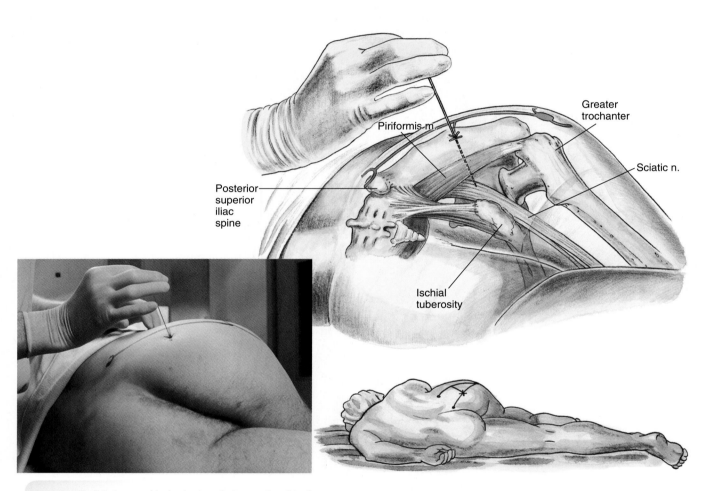

Labels in figure:

Piriformis m.

Posterior superior iliac spine

Greater trochanter

Sciatic n.

Ischial tuberosity

Figure 12-4. Sciatic nerve block: classic technique and positioning.

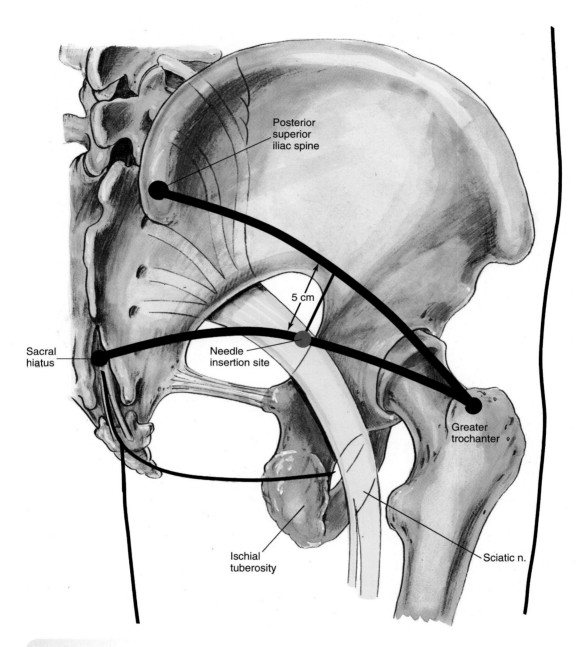

Figure 12-5. Sciatic nerve block: surface markings technique.

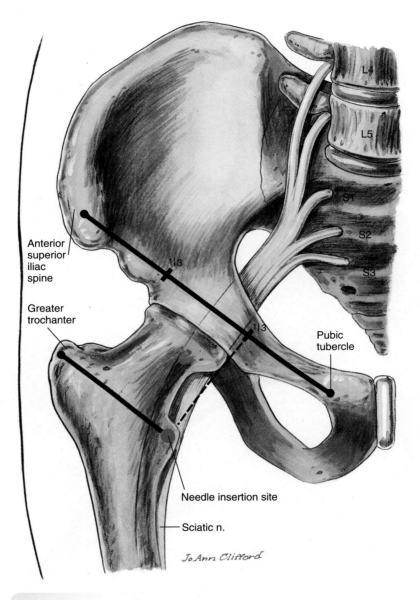

Anterior
superior
iliac
spine

Greater
trochanter

1|3

1|3

L4

L5

S1

S2

S3

Pubic
tubercle

Needle insertion site

Sciatic n.

JoAnn Clifford

Figure 12-6. Sciatic nerve block: anterior technique.

Anterior Approach

Position. The anterior block of the sciatic nerve can be carried out in the supine patient whose leg is in the neutral position. The anesthesiologist should be at the patient's side, similar to positioning during femoral nerve block.

Needle Puncture. In the supine patient, a line should be drawn from the anterior superior iliac spine to the pubic tubercle. Another line should be drawn parallel to this line from the midpoint of the greater trochanter inferomedially, as illustrated in Figure 12-6. The first line is trisected,

and a perpendicular line is drawn caudolaterally from the juncture of the medial and middle thirds, as shown in Figure 12-6. At the point where the perpendicular line crosses the more caudal line, a 22-gauge, 12-cm needle is inserted so that it contacts the femur at its medial border. Once the needle has contacted the femur, it is redirected slightly medially to slide off the medial surface of the femur. At approximately 5 cm past the depth required to contact the femur, a paresthesia or motor response should be sought to ensure successful block (Fig. 12-7). Once a paresthesia or motor response is obtained, 20 to 25 mL of local anesthetic is injected.

ANTERIOR

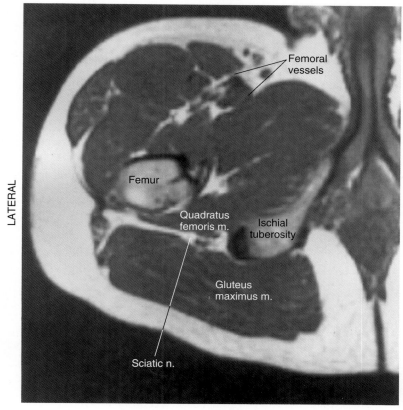

Femoral
vessels

Femur

Quadratus
femoris m.

Ischial
tuberosity

LATERAL

Gluteus
maximus m.

Sciatic n.

POSTERIOR

Figure 12-7. Magnetic resonance image (cross-sectional) at level of anterior sciatic nerve.

POTENTIAL PROBLEMS

In patients in whom the block is being used for an injury to the lower extremity, the classic position is sometimes difficult to use. This block can also be of long duration, and patients should be warned of this before surgery. Although it is unsubstantiated, some consider that dysesthesias may be more common after this block than after other peripheral blocks. The same problems pertaining to the classic approach should be considered with the anterior approach.

PEARLS

Classic Approach

The keys to making this block work are adequate positioning of the patient and a systematic redirection of the needle until a paresthesia is obtained.

Anterior Approach

Although the anterior approach is conceptually simple, I am able to produce anesthesia using it slightly less often than when using the classic approach. Perhaps with additional experience this difference would not be as apparent. One observation that may help to improve one's success rate with this block is to make sure that the lower extremity

to be blocked is maintained in the neutral position and is not allowed to assume either a medially or a laterally rotated position. This block may be useful in supine patients who are in significant discomfort and cannot be positioned for the classic approach.

Ultrasonography-Guided Technique

The transgluteal approach to the sciatic nerve using ultrasonographic guidance can be very challenging because of its depth, resulting in significant ultrasound attenuation, lack of tissue penetration, and poor image quality. Therefore, most ultrasonographic approaches to block the proximal sciatic nerve occur in the subgluteal region, at the crease formed by the gluteus muscles.

Subgluteal Approach

With the patient in the lateral or prone position, the operator should palpate the infragluteal crease to feel for the ropelike complex of the biceps femoris tendon. The transducer should be placed over this region (Fig. 12-8). The first objective is to identify one or both bony landmarks. At this level, the sciatic nerve is flanked by the greater

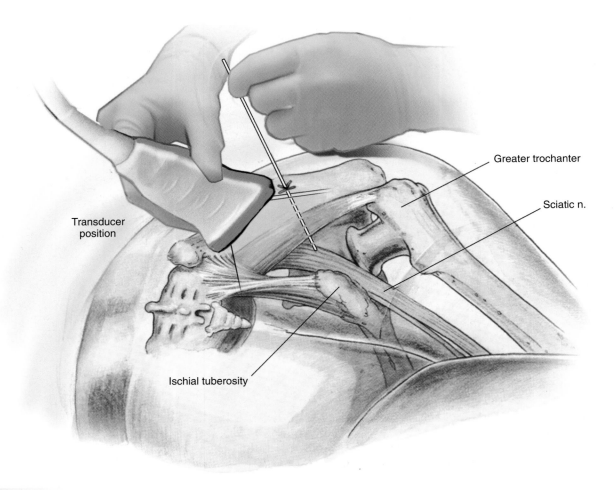

Greater trochanter

Sciatic n.

Transducer
position

Ischial tuberosity

Figure 12-8. Subgluteal ultrasound transducer positioning for sciatic nerve block.

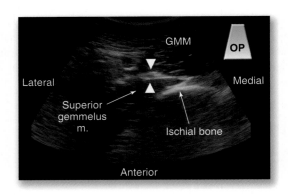

Figure 12-9. Sciatic nerve appearing as oval hyperechoic structure *(arrowheads)* with subgluteal ultrasound transducer positioning. GMM, gluteus maximus muscle.

trochanter laterally and the ischial tuberosity medially, both of which appear as highly reflective hyperechoic structures. The sciatic nerve should appear as a hyperechoic oval 1 to 2 cm in diameter and slightly lateral to the tendon of the biceps femoris muscle, which may also appear as an oval hyperechoic structure (Fig. 12-9). Using either the in-plane or out-of-plane technique, the needle is advanced toward the sciatic nerve. Local anesthetic is deposited by injection in a circumferential pattern around the nerve.

PEARLS

The supine popliteal approach to the sciatic nerve is ergonomically more challenging than the prone position. The operator should take time to position the patient and himself or herself. Many operators find it helpful to sit, with the bed at chest level and the ultrasonography machine on the contralateral side at eye level.

A curved transducer with a frequency of 8 MHz or less tends to be favored for the subgluteal block. The curved transducer allows a larger field of view to include reference structures such as the greater trochanter and the ischial tuberosity. The lower frequency facilitates better penetration given the often deeper nature of the nerve at this location compared with the popliteal approach.

To generate surgical anesthetic conditions, multiple injections are often necessary to ensure circumferential coverage of local anesthetic around the sciatic nerve.

Femoral Block

David L. Brown

with contributions from

Brian D. Sites and Brian C. Spence

13

PERSPECTIVE

This block is useful for surgical procedures carried out on the anterior thigh, both superficial and deep. It is most frequently combined with other lower extremity peripheral blocks to provide anesthesia for operations on the lower leg and foot. As an analgesic technique, it is used for femoral fracture analgesia or for prolonged continuous catheter analgesia after surgery on the knee or femur.

Patient Selection. Because the patient is supine when this block is carried out, virtually any patient undergoing a surgical procedure of the lower extremity is a candidate. Because elicitation of paresthesia is not necessary to carry out femoral block, even anesthetized patients are candidates.

Pharmacologic Choice. As with all lower extremity blocks, a decision must be made about the extent of sensory and motor blockade desired. If motor blockade is necessary, higher concentrations of local anesthetic are needed. As with concerns about local anesthetic use in the sciatic block, the desire for motor blockade must be balanced against the volume of local anesthetic necessary if femoral, sciatic, lateral femoral cutaneous, and obturator blocks are combined. Approximately 20 mL of local anesthetic should be adequate to produce femoral block. With continuous catheter techniques used for postoperative analgesia, 0.25% bupivacaine or 0.2% ropivacaine may be used, and even lower concentrations of these drugs may be useful after a trial. With this technique, a rate of 8 to 10 mL per hour usually suffices.

Traditional Block Technique

PLACEMENT

Anatomy. The femoral nerve travels through the pelvis in the groove between the psoas and the iliacus muscles, as illustrated in Figure 13-1. It emerges beneath the inguinal ligament, posterolateral to the femoral vessels, as illustrated in Figure 13-2. It frequently divides into its branches at or above the level of the inguinal ligament.

Position. The patient is in a supine position, and the anesthesiologist should stand at the patient's side to allow easy palpation of the femoral artery.

Needle Puncture. A line is drawn connecting the anterior superior iliac spine and the pubic tubercle, as illustrated in Figure 13-3. The femoral artery is palpated on this line, and a 22-gauge, 4-cm needle is inserted, as illustrated in Figure 13-4. The initial insertion should abut the femoral artery in a perpendicular fashion, as shown in Figure 13-5 (position 1); a "wall" of local anesthetic is developed by redirecting the needle in a fanlike manner in progressive steps to position 2. (Ultrasonography highlights that the nerve is deep to the fascia iliaca, something difficult to appreciate without imaging guidance.) Approximately 20 mL of local anesthetic is injected incrementally in this fashion. It may also be useful to displace the needle entry site laterally 1 cm, direct the needle tip to lie immediately posterior to the femoral artery, and then inject an additional 2 to 5 mL of drug. This allows block of those fibers that may be in a more posterior relationship to the femoral artery. Elicitation of paresthesia is variable with this block; however, if one does occur, the mediolateral injection should still be carried out because the nerve often divides into branches cephalad to the inguinal ligament.

When using a continuous catheter technique, either stimulating catheter block kits or traditional epidural needles and matched catheters may be used in adults (Fig. 13-6). In the latter situation, the epidural needle is positioned either with the assistance of a nerve stimulator or with paresthesia elicitation as an end point. After the needle is positioned, 20 mL of preservative-free normal saline solution is injected through the needle, and then the appropriate-size catheter is inserted approximately 10 cm past the needle tip. Once the catheter has been secured with a plastic occlusive dressing, the initial bolus injection of drug is carried out and the infusion is started.

POTENTIAL PROBLEMS

Patients with peripheral vascular disease often require unilateral lower extremity block; thus, a number of patients with prosthetic femoral arteries may be suitable candidates for this block. If lower extremity peripheral regional block has been chosen in a patient who has recently undergone placement of a prosthetic femoral artery, efforts should be made to avoid the prosthesis.

PEARLS

Because a traditional block is actually a field block, enough "soak time" must be allowed to produce satisfactory

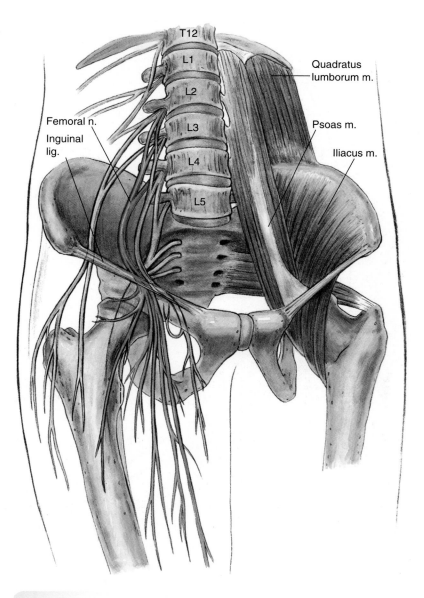

Figure 13-1. Femoral nerve anatomy: anterior oblique view.

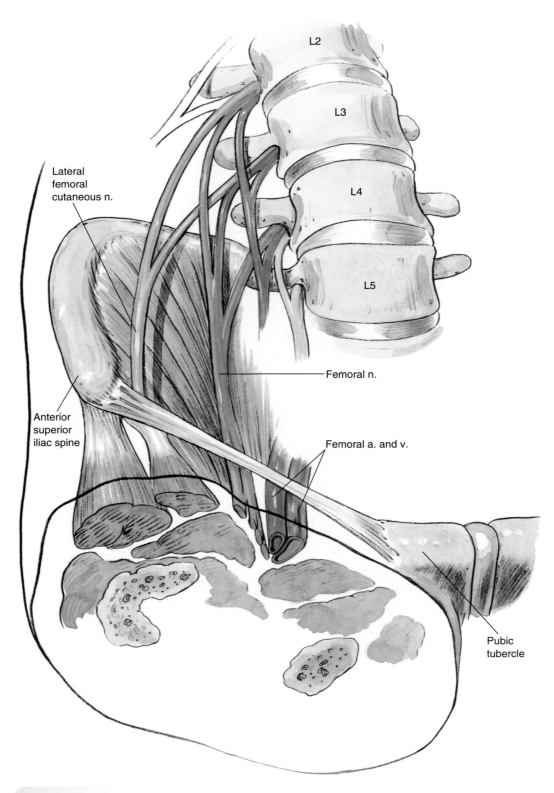

Lateral
femoral
cutaneous n.

Anterior
superior
iliac spine

L2

L3

L4

L5

Femoral n.

Femoral a. and v.

Pubic
tubercle

Figure 13-2. Femoral nerve anatomy: at inguinal ligament.

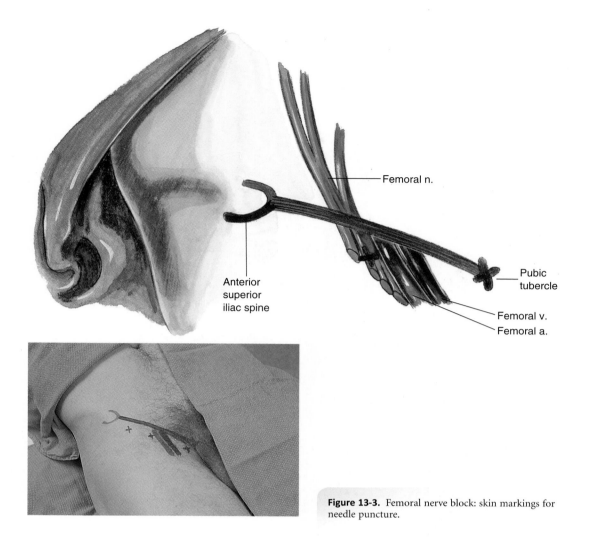

Femoral n.

Anterior
superior
iliac spine

Pubic
tubercle

Femoral v.

Femoral a.

Figure 13-3. Femoral nerve block: skin markings for needle puncture.

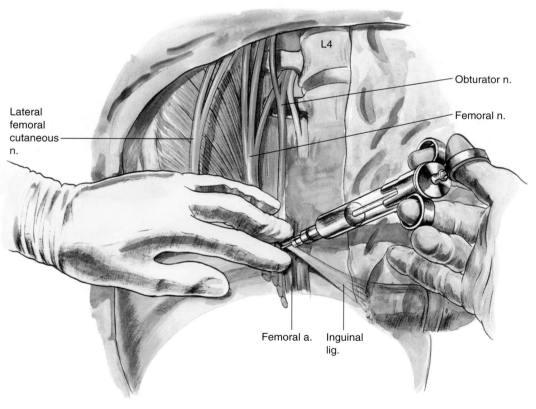

L4

Obturator n.

Femoral n.

Lateral
femoral
cutaneous
n.

Femoral a.   Inguinal
lig.

Figure 13-4. Femoral nerve block: needle puncture.

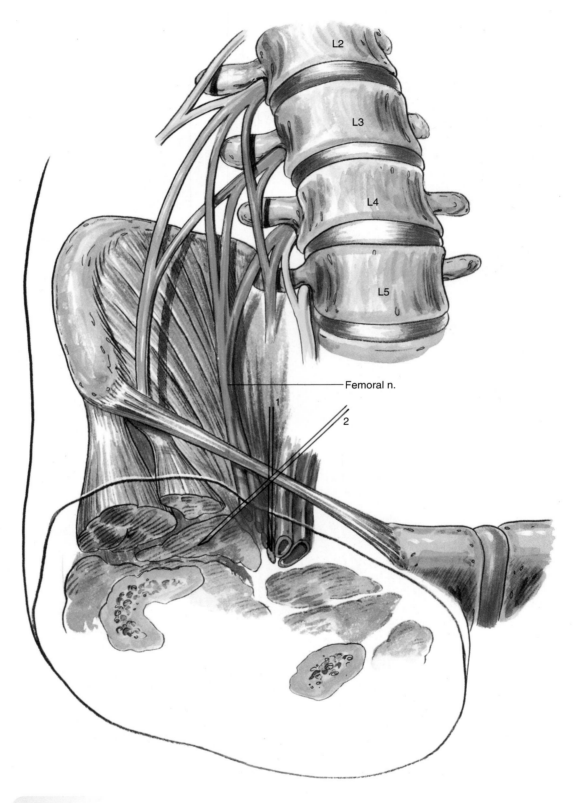

Femoral n.

1

2

L2

L3

L4

L5

Figure 13-5. Femoral nerve block: local anesthetic injection.

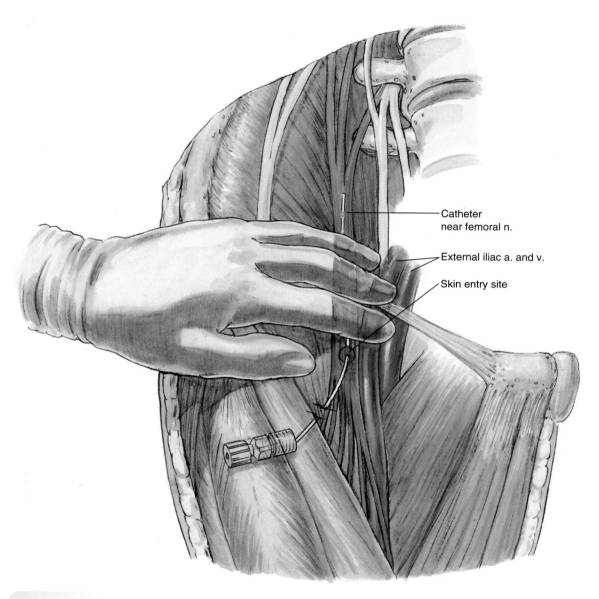

Figure 13-6. Femoral nerve block: use of continuous catheter.

Catheter
near femoral n.

External iliac a. and v.

Skin entry site

anesthesia. When sciatic and femoral blocks are combined, it is often helpful to place the femoral block before the sciatic block, thus allowing extra soak time. Increasingly, patients undergoing surgery on the knee are effectively being offered femoral block as part of the postoperative analgesia regimen. Most often this is provided as a single-shot technique; however, some practitioners provide the analgesia using a continuous catheter method.

Ultrasonography-Guided Technique

The transducer should be placed in the infrainguinal region (Fig. 13-7) with the goal of imaging the femoral artery in its true short axis (i.e., it appears as a complete circle). If the patient is obese or there is difficulty locating the femoral artery, engaging the Doppler function may help in locating the femoral artery as a pulsatile structure.

Once the artery has been located, the nerve can be identified as an oval hyperechoic structure lying just lateral to the artery (Fig. 13-8). A key structure to identify is the fascia iliaca, which appears as a hyperechoic line extending off the iliopsoas muscle. The local anesthetic must be injected below the fascia iliaca to generate an effective block.

The needle is inserted at a roughly 45-degree angle using the in-plane technique, as depicted in Figure 13-7. The primary objective for this block is to visualize the needle or needle-related motion puncturing below the fascia iliaca and adjacent to the femoral nerve (see Fig. 13-7). There is a characteristic spread of local anesthetic (Fig. 13-9; see Fig. 13-8), which confirms correct needle tip location (see *Video 10: Femoral Nerve Block: Correct Spread of Local Anesthetic Under the Fascia Iliaca* on the Expert Consult Website).

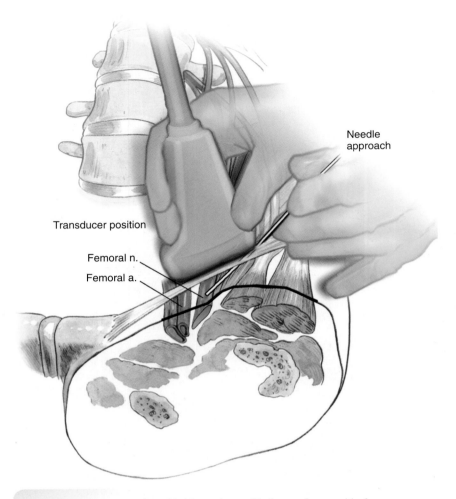

Figure 13-7. Ultrasonography-guided femoral nerve block: transducer positioning.

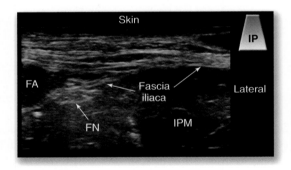

Figure 13-8. Ultrasonography-guided femoral nerve block: femoral nerve (FN) as hypoechoic structure. FA, femoral artery; IPM, iliopsoas muscle.

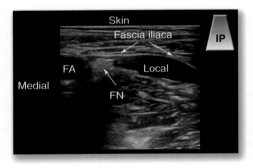

Figure 13-9. Ultrasonography-guided femoral nerve block: spread of local anesthetic. FA, femoral artery; FN, femoral nerve.

The femoral nerve is consistently located lateral to the femoral artery at a level defined by a straight line drawn through the 3- to 9-o'clock positions on the artery. The femoral artery and femoral nerve are *not* in the same anatomic compartment. Therefore, if local anesthetic solution is seen spreading in a perivascular location, the needle should be repositioned to produce local anesthetic spread below the fascia iliaca.

There is no reason the needle must contact the femoral nerve with this block. When the local anesthetic is deposited under the fascia iliaca, a solid block should result. As shown in Figure 13-7, I often inject 1 to 3 cm lateral to the femoral nerve (see *Video 11: Femoral Nerve Block: In-Plane Technique* on the Expert Consult Website).

Lateral Femoral Cutaneous Block

14

PERSPECTIVE

When this block is combined with other lower extremity blocks, it allows lower leg procedures to be carried out with fewer complaints of tourniquet pain. It also allows superficial procedures on the lateral thigh, including skin graft harvesting. In a pain practice, it allows the diagnosis of myalgia paresthetica, which is a neuralgia involving the lateral femoral cutaneous nerve.

Patient Selection. Like femoral nerve block, this block is carried out with the patient in the supine position. Thus, almost any patient is a candidate for a lateral femoral cutaneous block.

Pharmacologic Choice. The same concerns about local anesthetic choice that were outlined for sciatic and femoral blocks (Chapters 12 and 13, respectively) apply to the lateral femoral cutaneous block. If multiple lower extremity blocks are being used, the operator must consider the total dosage being administered. Because the lateral femoral cutaneous nerve does not have motor components, a lower concentration of 10 to 15 mL of local anesthetic is effective.

PLACEMENT

Anatomy. As shown in Figure 14-1, the lateral femoral cutaneous nerve emerges along the lateral border of the

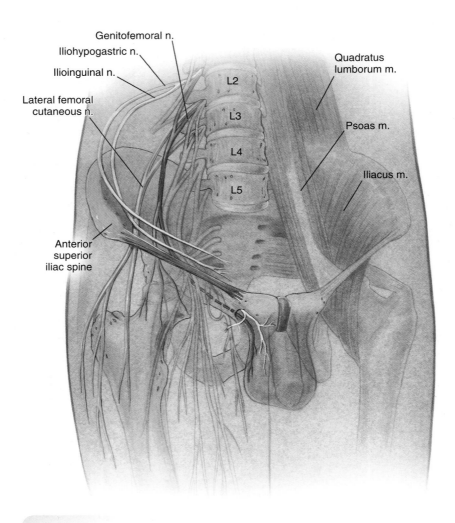

Figure 14-1. Lateral femoral cutaneous nerve: anatomy.

psoas muscle immediately caudad to the ilioinguinal nerve. It courses deep to the iliac fascia and anterior to the iliacus muscle to emerge from the fascia immediately inferior and medial to the anterior superior iliac spine, as shown in Figure 14-2. After passing beneath the inguinal ligament, it crosses or passes through the origin of the sartorius muscle and travels beneath the fascia lata, dividing into anterior and posterior branches at variable distances below the inguinal ligament. The anterior branch supplies the skin over the anterolateral thigh, whereas the posterior branch supplies the skin over the lateral thigh from the greater trochanter to the midthigh.

Position. The patient is in a supine position with the anesthesiologist at the patient's side, similar to the position taken for the femoral nerve block.

Needle Puncture. The anterior superior iliac spine is marked in the supine patient, and a 22-gauge, 4-cm needle is inserted at a site 2 cm medial and 2 cm caudal to the

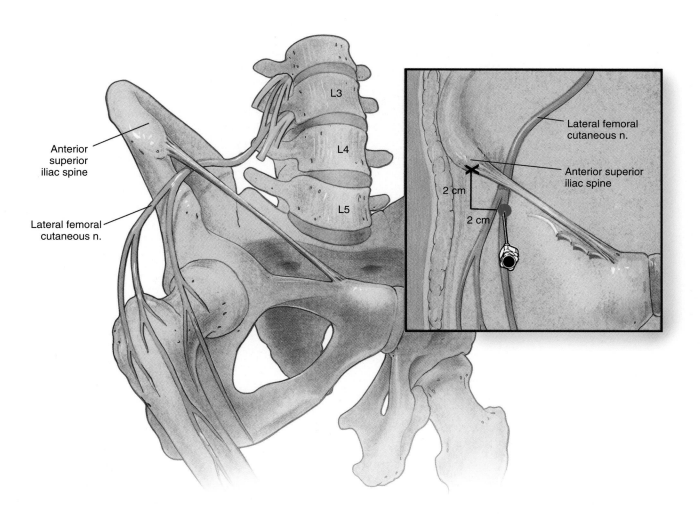

Figure 14-2. Lateral femoral cutaneous nerve block: technique.

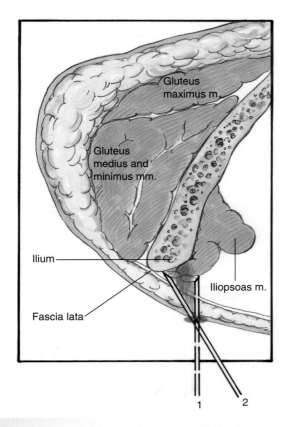

Figure 14-3. Lateral femoral cutaneous nerve block: cross-sectional technique for local anesthetic injection.

mark (see Fig. 14-2). As shown in Figure 14-3, the needle is advanced until a "pop" is felt as the needle passes through the fascia lata. Local anesthetic is then injected in a fanlike manner above and below the fascia lata, from medial (*position 1*) to lateral (*position 2*), as illustrated in Figure 14-3.

POTENTIAL PROBLEMS

The superficial nature of this block allows one to avoid most problems associated with regional blocks.

PEARLS

An adequate volume of local anesthetic should be used for this block (i.e., 10 to 15 mL). Because this is a sensory nerve, low concentrations of local anesthetics are useful, such as 0.5% to 0.75% mepivacaine or lidocaine, 0.25% bupivacaine, or 0.2% ropivacaine. By keeping the concentration lower for this portion of a three- or four-nerve lower extremity block, adequate volumes and concentrations of local anesthetic can be maintained for the sciatic and femoral nerves. If this block is used to provide anesthesia for a skin graft harvest site on the lateral thigh, it is useful to perform the block, wait until sensory changes develop, and then outline the peripheral innervation of the lateral femoral cutaneous nerve in that specific patient before any skin is harvested.

Obturator Block

15

PERSPECTIVE

This block is most often combined with the sciatic, femoral, and lateral femoral cutaneous nerve blocks to allow surgical procedures on the lower extremities. If an operation on the knee using these peripheral blocks is planned, the obturator block is often essential. Another use for this block is in patients who have hip pain. It can be used diagnostically to help identify the cause of pain because obturator nerve

block may provide considerable pain relief if the nerve's articular branch to the hip is involved in pain transmission. The block also may be useful in the evaluation of lower extremity spasticity or chronic pain syndromes.

Patient Selection. As with femoral and lateral femoral cutaneous nerve blocks, elicitation of paresthesias is not essential for obturator block. Any patient able to lie supine is a candidate.

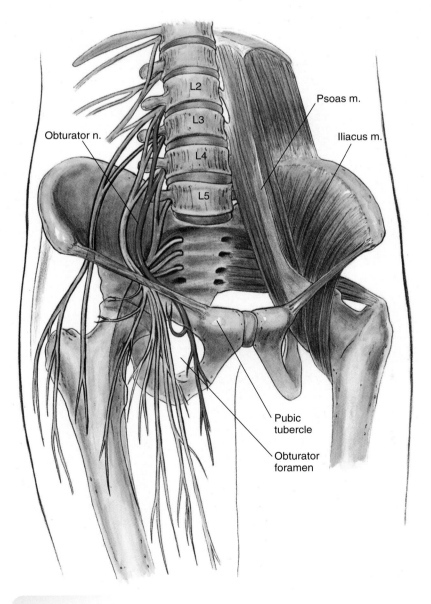

Figure 15-1. Obturator nerve: functional anatomy.

Pharmacologic Choice. Motor blockade is most often not necessary for surgical patients receiving obturator nerve block; thus, lower concentrations of local anesthetics are appropriate for obturator block: 0.75% to 1.0% lidocaine or mepivacaine, 0.25% bupivacaine, or 0.2% ropivacaine.

PLACEMENT

Anatomy. The obturator nerve emerges from the medial border of the psoas muscle at the pelvic brim and travels along the lateral aspect of the pelvis anterior to the obturator internus muscle and posterior to the iliac vessels and ureter. It enters the obturator canal cephalad and anterior to the obturator vessels, which are branches from the internal iliac vessels. In the obturator canal, the obturator nerve divides into anterior and posterior branches (Fig. 15-1). The anterior branch supplies the anterior adductor muscles and sends an articular branch to the hip joint and a cutaneous area on the medial aspect of the thigh. The

posterior branch innervates the deep adductor muscles and sends an articular branch to the knee joint. In 10% of patients an accessory obturator nerve may be found.

Position. The patient should be supine with the legs positioned in a slightly abducted position. The genitalia should be protected from antiseptic solutions.

Needle Puncture. The pubic tubercle should be located and an "X" marked 1.5 cm caudad and 1.5 cm lateral to the tubercle (Fig. 15-2). The needle is inserted at this point, and at a depth of approximately 1.5 to 4 cm it contacts the horizontal ramus of the pubis. The needle is then withdrawn, redirected laterally in a horizontal plane, and inserted 2 to 3 cm deeper than the depth of the initial contact with bone. The needle tip now lies within the obturator canal (see Fig. 15-2) With the needle in this position, 10 to 15 mL of local anesthetic solution is injected while the needle is advanced and withdrawn slightly to ensure development of a "wall" of local anesthetic in the canal.

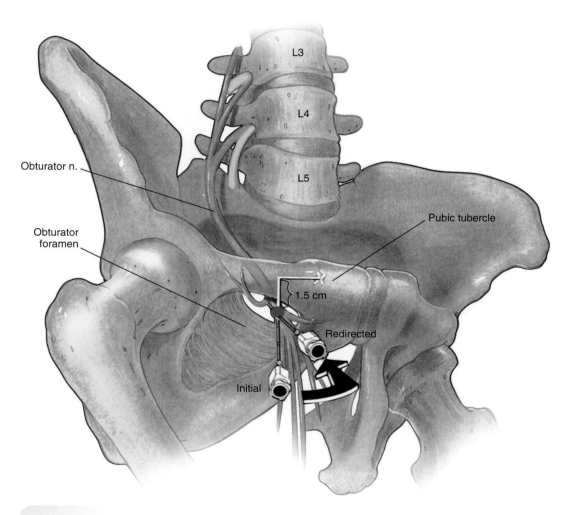

Figure 15-2. Obturator nerve block: technique.

POTENTIAL PROBLEMS

The obturator canal is a vascular location; thus, the potential exists for intravascular injection or hematoma formation, although these are more theoretical than clinical concerns.

PEARLS

This block, even in trained hands, has a variable success rate. My experience suggests that one must rely on volume of anesthetic delivered rather than on absolute accuracy of needle position. Fortunately, use of an obturator block with the other lower extremity peripheral nerve blocks is not an absolute requirement for most surgical procedures. If this block is used diagnostically for patients with chronic pain, it is helpful to use a nerve stimulator to guide needle placement. This will minimize diagnostic confusion when pain relief is produced with a small volume of local anesthetic. Large-volume injections (approximately 15 mL) are performed with this block for many surgical procedures.

Popliteal and Saphenous Block

16

PERSPECTIVE

The nerves blocked in the popliteal fossa—the tibial and peroneal nerves—are extensions of the sciatic nerve. The principal use of this block is for foot and ankle surgery. The addition of a saphenous nerve block improves comfort for many patients undergoing the popliteal block because medial lower leg and ankle sensory blockade makes tourniquets and medial ankle surgery more comfortable.

Patient Selection. To use the classic form of this block, the patient must be able to assume the prone position. Elicitation of a paresthesia or motor response is desirable but not essential; however, block effectiveness decreases without these end points.

Pharmacologic Choice. The principal use of these blocks is to provide sensory analgesia; thus, lower concentrations of

a local anesthetic are practical, in contrast to situations in which motor blockade is essential. Concentrations of 1% lidocaine, 1% mepivacaine, 0.25% to 0.5% bupivacaine, and 0.2% to 0.5% ropivacaine are effective.

Traditional Block Technique

PLACEMENT

Anatomy. As illustrated in Figure 16-1, the cephalad popliteal fossa is defined by the semimembranosus and semitendinosus muscles medially and the biceps femoris muscle laterally. Its caudad extent is defined by the gastrocnemius muscles both medially and laterally. If this quadrilateral area is bisected, as shown in Figure 16-1, the area of interest to the anesthesiologist is the cephalolateral quadrant

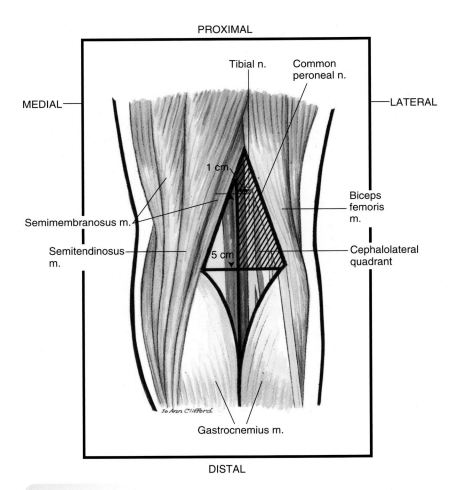

Figure 16-1. Popliteal fossa: surface anatomy and technique for popliteal block.

(*hatched area*). Here, both tibial and common peroneal nerve block is possible. The tibial nerve is the larger of these two nerves; it separates from the common peroneal nerve at the upper limit of the popliteal fossa and sometimes higher. The tibial nerve continues the straight course of the sciatic nerve and runs lengthwise through the popliteal fossa immediately under the popliteal fascia. Inferiorly, it passes between the heads of the gastrocnemius muscles. The common peroneal nerve follows the tendon of the biceps femoris muscle along the cephalolateral margin of the popliteal fossa, as illustrated in Figure 16-2. After the common peroneal nerve leaves the popliteal fossa, it travels around the head of the fibula and divides into the superficial peroneal and deep peroneal nerves.

Position. The patient is placed in a prone position and the anesthesiologist stands at the patient's side to allow palpation of the borders of the popliteal fossa.

Needle Puncture. With the patient in the prone position, he or she is asked to flex the leg at the knee, which allows more accurate identification of the popliteal fossa. Once the popliteal fossa has been defined, it is divided into equal medial and lateral triangles, as shown in Figure 16-1. An "X" is placed 5 to 7 cm superior to the skin crease of the popliteal fossa and 1 cm lateral to the midline of the triangles, as shown in Figure 16-1. Through this site, a 22-gauge, 4- to 6-cm needle is advanced at an angle of 45 to 60 degrees to the skin while being directed anterosuperiorly (Fig. 16-3). A paresthesia or motor response is sought; when obtained, 30 to 40 mL of local anesthetic is injected.

When a saphenous block is added for foot and ankle surgery, the patient's knee is bent at approximately a 45-degree angle, and the medial aspect of the leg is exposed. Two primary techniques are used for saphenous block. A superficial ring of local anesthetic may be injected just distal to the medial surface of the tibial condyle. Often 5 to 10 mL of local anesthetic is needed. Conversely, a more proximal technique (at the cross-sectional level of the superior border of the patella) is possible (Fig. 16-4). In this case, a 22- to 25-gauge, 3- to 4-cm needle is inserted immediately deep to the sartorius muscle in the plane between the vastus medialis and the sartorius muscles, and 10 mL of local anesthetic is injected.

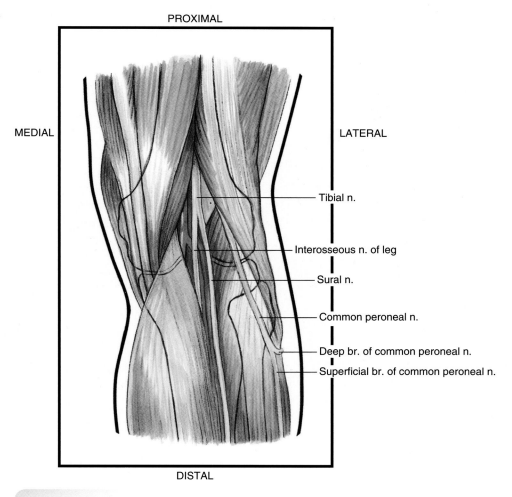

PROXIMAL

MEDIAL

LATERAL

Tibial n.

Interosseous n. of leg

Sural n.

Common peroneal n.

Deep br. of common peroneal n.

Superficial br. of common peroneal n.

DISTAL

Figure 16-2. Popliteal fossa: neural anatomy.

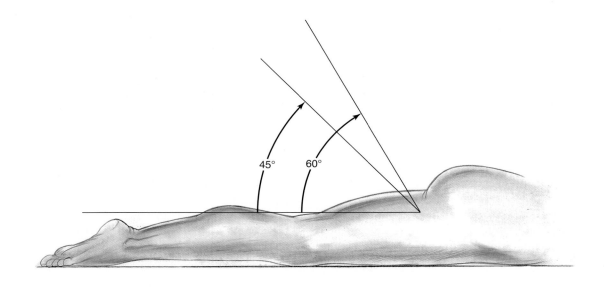

Figure 16-3. Popliteal fossa: needle angle technique for popliteal block.

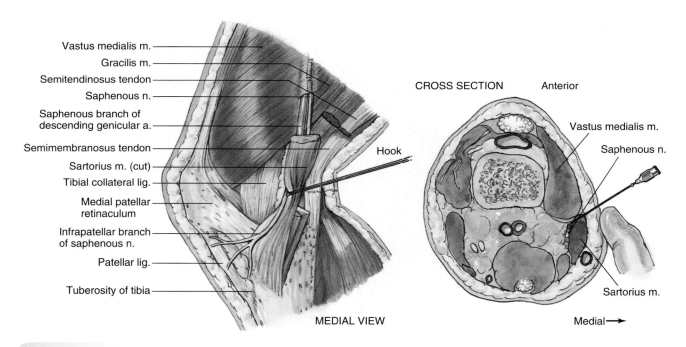

Vastus medialis m.
Gracilis m.
Semitendinosus tendon
Saphenous n.
Saphenous branch of descending genicular a.
Semimembranosus tendon
Sartorius m. (cut)
Tibial collateral lig.
Medial patellar retinaculum
Infrapatellar branch of saphenous n.
Patellar lig.
Tuberosity of tibia

Hook

MEDIAL VIEW

CROSS SECTION   Anterior

Vastus medialis m.
Saphenous n.
Sartorius m.

Medial →

Figure 16-4. Saphenous nerve block: anatomy and proximal technique.

POTENTIAL PROBLEMS

Although vascular structures also occupy the popliteal fossa, intravascular injection should be infrequent if the usual precautions are taken. Hematoma formation is possible.

Ultrasonography-Guided Technique

POPLITEAL BLOCK

The patient can be placed in either the supine or prone position (Fig. 16-5). The first objective is to define the popliteal artery or the popliteal vein; the former is a pulsatile hypoechoic circle and the latter is a compressible hypoechoic circle. The vein typically lies more posterior than the artery. Immediately posterior to the vessels is the tibial nerve, appearing as a distinct hyperechoic circle with internal hypoechoic fascicles. Moving the transducer in a proximal direction, the operator will soon see a smaller hyperechoic circle joining the tibial component from the lateral aspect of the screen (Fig. 16-6; see *Video 8: Popliteal Anatomy* on the Expert Consult Website). This second structure is the common peroneal nerve. This is the location where most practitioners perform the block.

With the patient in the prone position, the needle is inserted using the in-plane needle insertion technique. Typically, the needle is inserted at a roughly 45-degree angle with respect to the skin (see Fig. 16-5). The needle is advanced and contact is made with the outermost hyperechoic layer of the sciatic nerve. There is often a tactile and visual "popping" sensation as the needle penetrates a tissue layer just external to the epineurium. The end result of the injection is the circumferential spread of local anesthetic around the sciatic nerve (see *Video 9: Popliteal Nerve Block: In-Plane Technique* on the Expert Consult Website).

When the patient is in the supine position, the needle is also inserted using the in-plane technique. However, the needle is placed completely parallel with the faceplate of the transducer. With this approach, the needle acts as a strong specular reflector, thus generating the clearest and brightest image of the needle possible (Fig. 16-7).

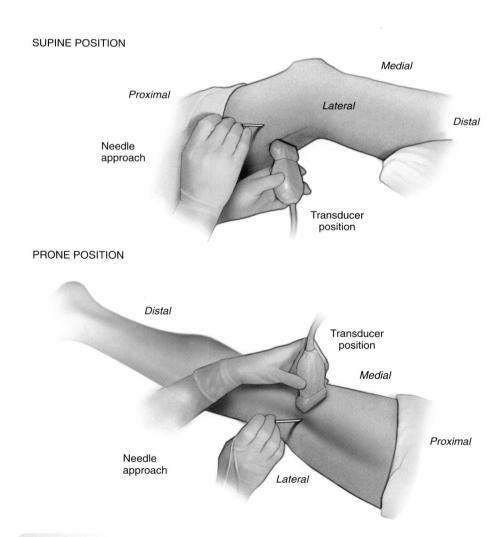

Figure 16-5. Ultrasonography-guided popliteal block: patient and transducer positioning.

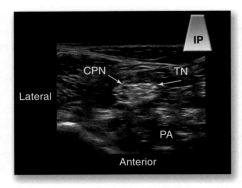

Figure 16-6. Ultrasonography-guided popliteal block: tibial and peroneal nerve hyperechoic structures. CPN, common peroneal nerve; PA, popliteal artery; TN, tibial nerve.

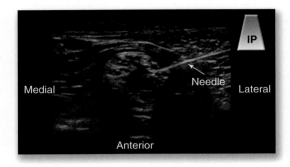

Figure 16-7. With the patient in the supine position, the needle acts as a strong specular reflector.

PEARLS

An increasing number of centers report using popliteal nerve block, especially with ultrasonographic guidance. Excellent results are reported by the centers that have effectively incorporated this technique into a busy foot and ankle surgical practice. As with many other lower extremity peripheral nerve blocks, local anesthetic volume seems to be the key to making this block useful.

It also is apparent from watching many resident physicians perform this block that if the needle is initially misdirected, it is directed too far medially. Usually all that is needed is to redirect the needle to a more lateral position. Finally, some groups are promoting a lateral approach to the popliteal block, and time will tell whether maintaining the patient in a supine position for this lateral technique will increase the interest of anesthesiologists in popliteal blocks.

The saphenous nerve block appears to require a higher volume of local anesthetic than many physicians use, so one should be generous in the volume used with this block, keeping in mind that the popliteal block requires 30 to 40 mL of local anesthetic to produce a block reliably.

Ankle Block

17

PERSPECTIVE

This block is often used for surgical procedures carried out on the foot, especially for those not requiring high lower-leg tourniquet pressure.

Patient Selection. The ankle block is principally an infiltration block and does not require elicitation of paresthesia. Thus, patient cooperation is not mandatory. Although the block is most efficient for the anesthesiologist if the patient can assume the prone as well as the supine position, this is not essential.

Pharmacologic Choice. Because motor blockade is not often needed for procedures carried out during ankle block, lower concentrations of local anesthetics may be used. Practical choices are 1% lidocaine, 1% mepivacaine, 0.25% to 0.5% bupivacaine, and 0.2% to 0.5% ropivacaine. Many physicians suggest that epinephrine should not be used during ankle block, especially if injection is circumferential.

PLACEMENT

Anatomy. The peripheral nerves requiring block during ankle block are derived from the sciatic nerve, with the exception of a terminal branch of the femoral nerve, the saphenous nerve. The saphenous nerve is the only branch of the femoral nerve below the knee; it courses superficially anterior to the medial malleolus, providing cutaneous innervation to an area of the medial ankle and foot. The remaining nerves requiring block at the ankle are terminal branches of the sciatic nerve—the common peroneal and tibial nerves. The tibial nerve divides into the posterior

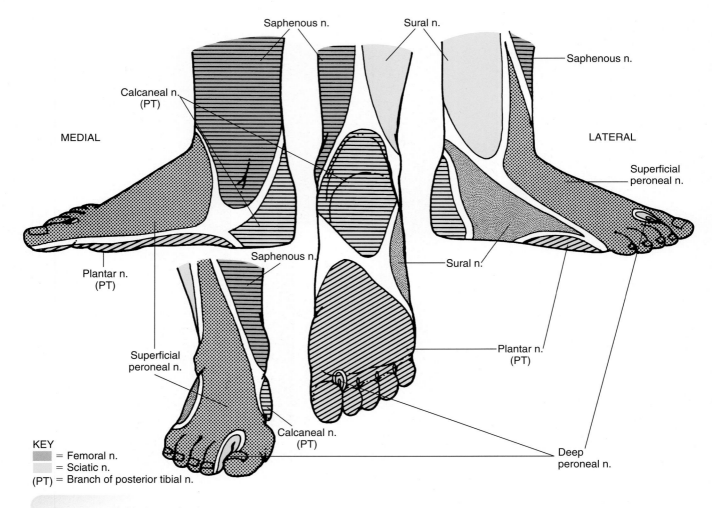

Figure 17-1. Ankle block: peripheral innervation.

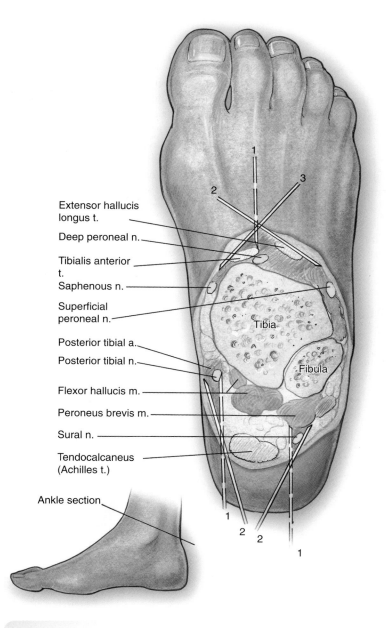

Extensor hallucis
longus t.

Deep peroneal n.

Tibialis anterior
t.

Saphenous n.

Superficial
peroneal n.

Posterior tibial a.

Posterior tibial n.

Flexor hallucis m.

Peroneus brevis m.

Sural n.

Tendocalcaneus
(Achilles t.)

Ankle section

Tibia

Fibula

Figure 17-2. Ankle block: cross-sectional anatomy and technique.

tibial and sural nerves, which provide cutaneous innervation as outlined in Figure 17-1. The common peroneal nerve divides into its terminal branches, the superficial and deep peroneal nerves, in the proximal portion of the lower leg. Their cutaneous innervation is also illustrated in Figure 17-1. Figure 17-2 identifies the locations of these nerves in a cross-sectional view at the level of ankle block.

Needle Puncture: General. It is often helpful (although not necessary) to have the patient in the prone position initially to facilitate block of the posterior tibial and sural nerves. Once these two nerves have been blocked, the patient assumes the supine position so that block of the saphenous and peroneal nerves can be carried out. The block can be performed with the patient in the supine position if the lower leg is placed on a padded support, and this position facilitates appropriate intravenous sedation.

Needle Puncture: Posterior Tibial Nerve. With the patient in the prone position, the ankle to be blocked is supported on a pillow. A 22-gauge, 4-cm needle is directed anteriorly at the cephalad border of the medial malleolus, just medial to the Achilles tendon, as shown in Figure 17-2. The needle is inserted near the posterior tibial artery, and if a paresthesia is obtained, 3 to 5 mL of local anesthetic is injected. If no paresthesia is obtained, the needle is allowed to contact the medial malleolus, and 5 to 7 mL of local anesthetic is deposited near the posterior tibial artery.

Needle Puncture: Sural Nerve. The sural nerve is blocked with the patient positioned as for the posterior tibial nerve block. As illustrated in Figure 17-2, the sural nerve is blocked by inserting a 22-gauge, 4-cm needle anterolaterally immediately lateral to the Achilles tendon at the cephalad border of the lateral malleolus. If no paresthesia is obtained, the needle is allowed to contact the lateral malleolus, and 5 to 7 mL of local anesthetic is injected as the needle is withdrawn.

Needle Puncture: Deep Peroneal, Superficial Peroneal, and Saphenous Nerves. After the patient assumes the supine position, the anterior tibial artery pulsation is located at the superior level of the malleoli. A 22-gauge, 4-cm needle is advanced posteriorly and immediately lateral to this point (see Fig. 17-2). An alternative is to insert the needle between the tendons of the anterior tibial and the extensor hallucis longus muscles. Approximately 5 mL of local anesthetic is injected into this area. From this midline skin wheal, a 22-gauge, 8-cm needle is advanced subcutaneously laterally and medially to the malleoli, injecting 3 to 5 mL of local anesthetic in each direction. These lateral and medial approaches block the superficial peroneal and saphenous nerves, respectively.

POTENTIAL PROBLEMS

While the ankle block can be painful if the patient is not adequately sedated, this should not be an issue because an alert patient is not essential for the block.

PEARLS

As mentioned, patients should be adequately sedated during this block because it is primarily a "volume" block. Although the medial and lateral malleoli approaches to an ankle block appear similar, there are differences. The sural nerve (lateral ankle) is found in a more superficial position relative to the malleolus than is the tibial nerve (medial ankle). The anesthesiologist should make sure to perform the sural portion of the block with this distinction in mind. The block should not be chosen if high tourniquet pressures are required to carry out the surgical procedure. Epinephrine-containing solutions should be avoided in circumferential injections of the ankle. Outpatient foot surgery patients often can walk with assistance after ankle block, which facilitates earlier discharge of these patients from the outpatient surgery center, while still experiencing effective postoperative analgesia.

SECTION IV:
Head and Neck Blocks

Head and Neck Block Anatomy

18

Use of regional anesthesia for head and neck surgery declined rapidly after general anesthesia and tracheal intubation became available and accepted. One reason for the decline is that small doses of local anesthetic can easily produce systemic toxicity. Nevertheless, in few other areas in the body can such small doses of local anesthetic provide such effective regional block. There are still circumstances in which head and neck block is useful. Many of these involve the diagnosis or treatment of pain syndromes. Also, many plastic surgical procedures on superficial structures can be managed easily with effective block of the nerves of the head and neck. One crucial aspect of head and neck block for anesthesiologists is expertise in airway anatomy and innervation. In some circumstances in an anesthetic practice, proper airway management, including airway blocks, can be lifesaving.

Sensory innervation of the face is provided by the trigeminal nerve. Three branches of the trigeminal—the ophthalmic, maxillary, and mandibular—provide innervation, as illustrated in Figure 18-1. The cutaneous innervation of the posterior head and neck is from the cervical nerves. The dorsal ramus of the second cervical nerve ends in the greater occipital nerve, which provides cutaneous innervation to the larger portion of the posterior scalp (see Fig. 18-1). The greater occipital nerve is a continuation of the medial branch of the dorsal ramus of the second cervical

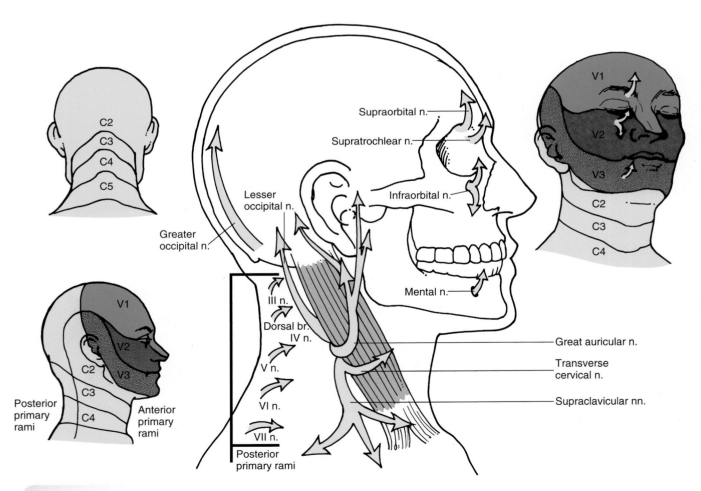

Figure 18-1. Head and neck anatomy: innervation.

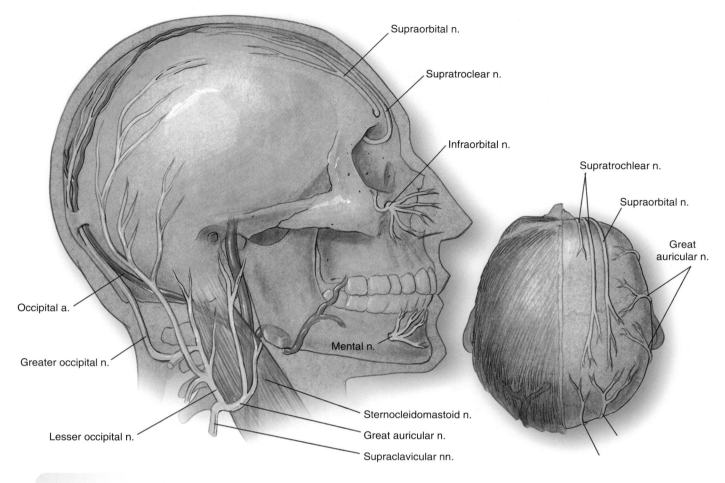

Figure 18-2. Head and neck anatomy: peripheral nerves.

nerve and ascends from the cervical vertebrae to the muscles of the neck in company with the occipital artery. The greater occipital nerve becomes subcutaneous in its course with the occipital artery immediately lateral to the inion, slightly inferior to the superior nuchal line (Fig. 18-2). The ventral rami of cervical nerves II, III, and IV provide the majority of cutaneous innervation to the anterior and lateral portions of the neck, with cervical nerve II providing innervation to the scalp through both the lesser occipital and the posterior auricular nerves (see Fig. 18-1). The superficial cervical plexus is formed as cervical nerves II, III, and IV leave the vertebral transverse processes and follow a course in which they become subcuta-

neous at the midpoint of the posterior border of the sternocleidomastoid muscle (see Fig. 18-2). At this point, the superficial cervical plexus can be easily blocked by infiltration.

The trigeminal nerve is a mixed motor and sensory nerve, although the majority of it involves sensory innervation. The only motor fibers are the branches that supply the muscles of mastication through the mandibular nerve. The trigeminal nerve is organized in the cranium within the trigeminal ganglion (gasserian or semilunar ganglion). From this ganglion, the ophthalmic nerve exits from the cranium through the superior orbital fissure, the maxillary nerve through the foramen rotundum, and the mandibular

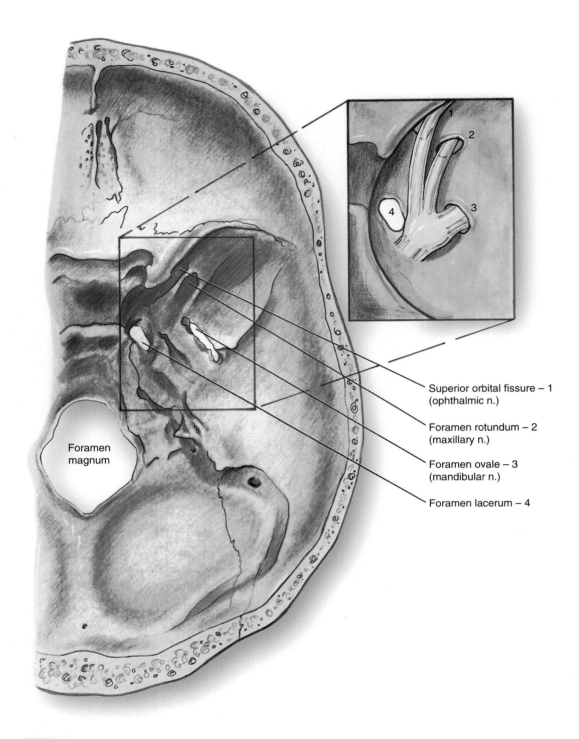

Superior orbital fissure – 1
(ophthalmic n.)

Foramen rotundum – 2
(maxillary n.)

Foramen ovale – 3
(mandibular n.)

Foramen lacerum – 4

Foramen
magnum

Figure 18-3. Intracranial anatomy: trigeminal nerve and branches.

nerve through the foramen ovale (Fig. 18-3). After leaving these foramina, the maxillary and mandibular nerves follow courses that place them in the immediate proximity of the lateral pterygoid plate. The pterygoid plate is an important landmark for effective maxillary or mandibular block (Fig. 18-4). The terminal branches of the trigeminal nerve end in the supraorbital, infraorbital, and mental nerves. These exit through bony foramina that occur on a line perpendicular through the pupil, as illustrated in Figure 18-5.

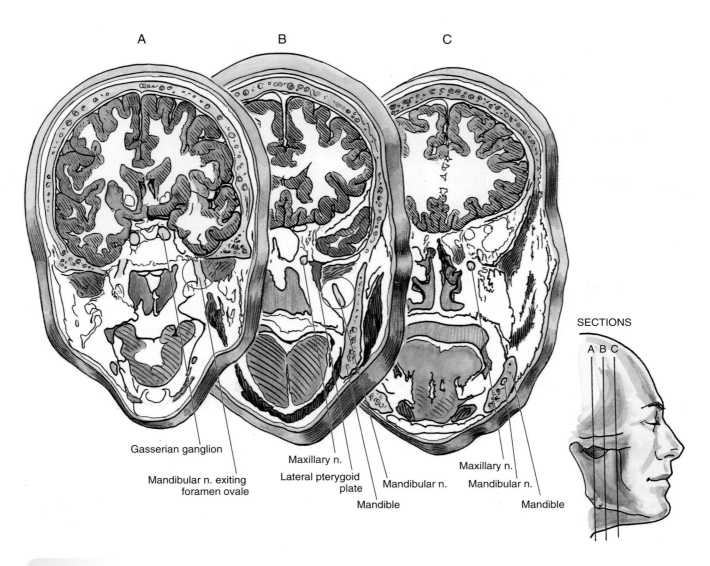

A   B   C

Gasserian ganglion

Mandibular n. exiting
foramen ovale

Maxillary n.

Lateral pterygoid
plate

Mandibular n.

Mandible

Maxillary n.

Mandibular n.

Mandible

SECTIONS

A B C

Figure 18-4. Coronal anatomy: peripterygoid relationships of maxillary and mandibular nerves.

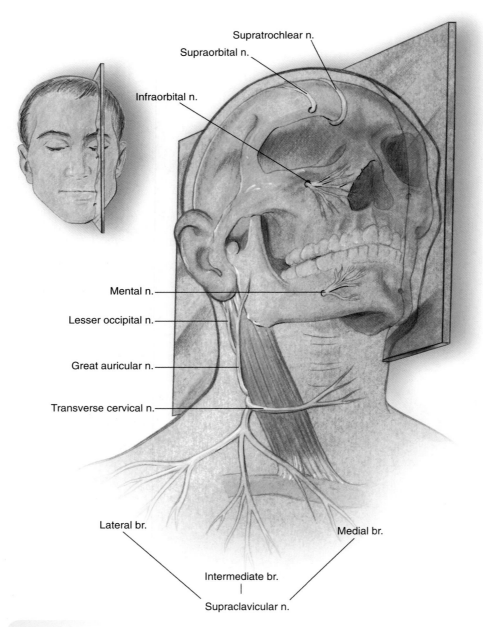

Figure 18-5. Head and neck anatomy: superficial neural relationships.

Occipital Block

19

PERSPECTIVE

Occipital nerve block is most frequently used in the diagnosis and treatment of occipital neuralgia. It is also useful when combined with other head and neck blocks to provide scalp anesthesia when infiltration alone will not suffice.

Patient Selection. Most candidates for occipital nerve block will be experiencing symptoms consistent with occipital neuralgia. These patients are often at the end of a long and frustrating medical evaluation and thus may need a detailed explanation of what to expect during the block.

Pharmacologic Choice. This block requires only 3 to 5 mL of local anesthetic, so virtually any local anesthetic can be used.

PLACEMENT

Anatomy. The greater occipital nerve arises from the dorsal rami of the second cervical nerve and travels deep to the cervical musculature until it becomes subcutaneous slightly inferior to the superior nuchal line. It emerges on this line in association with the occipital artery, which is the most useful landmark for locating the greater occipital nerve (Fig. 19-1).

Position. The most effective patient position for the greater occipital block is the sitting position, with the chin flexed on the chest. A short, 25-gauge needle is inserted through the skin at the level of the superior nuchal line to develop a "wall" of local anesthetic surrounding the posterior occipital artery. The artery is commonly found approximately one third of the distance between the external

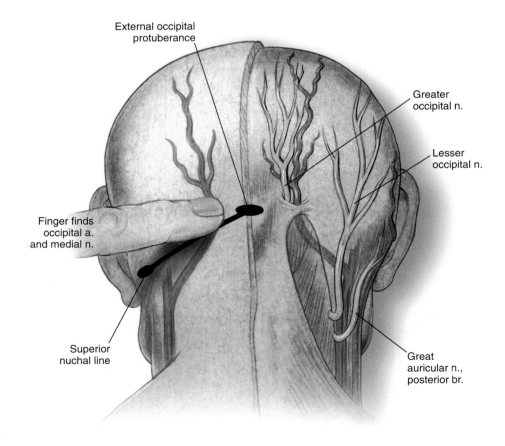

Figure 19-1. Occipital nerve block: anatomy and technique.

occipital protuberance and the mastoid process on the superior nuchal line. Injection of 3 to 5 mL of local anesthetic in this area will produce satisfactory anesthesia.

POTENTIAL PROBLEMS

The superficial nature of this block should make complications infrequent. However, it is important to ask the patient whether he or she has undergone any posterior cranial surgery because total spinal anesthesia has occurred after occipital nerve block in patients who have had such surgery.

PEARLS

To make this block effective for pain diagnosis and therapy, the anesthesiologist must make the expectations for the block clear to the patient before performing the block. Often patients reach the anesthesiologist only after a long and arduous trial of alternative pain therapies; thus, it is as important for the anesthesiologist to handle the psychosocial implications of the procedure as it is to discuss the technical features.

When a diagnostic block is planned, it is important to keep the dose of local anesthetic small to minimize confusion with relief of myofascial pain. Similarly, relief of ipsilateral retro-orbital or temporal pain after an occipital block does not rule out the possibility of occipital neuralgia as the cause of the pain syndrome because pain relief is produced outside the typical sensory distribution of the occipital nerve. In some of these cases, owing to brain stem and spinal cord interneuronal connections between the trigeminal nucleus and the second cervical spinal nerve, retro-orbital pain is frequently relieved with a greater occipital nerve block.

Trigeminal (Gasserian) Ganglion Block

20

PERSPECTIVE

Although the trigeminal ganglion block can be used for surgical procedures involving the face, its principal use is as a diagnostic block before trigeminal neurolysis in patients with facial neuralgia. Even after the anesthesiologist successfully identifies the trigeminal nerve as the cause of facial pain, neurolysis is most often carried out today using thermocoagulation techniques rather than neurolytic solutions.

Patient Selection. Current practice patterns virtually guarantee that patients undergoing this block will be experiencing facial neuralgia. Patients with severe underlying cardiopulmonary disease who require more than minor facial surgery may be candidates for local anesthetic trigeminal ganglion blocks.

Pharmacologic Choice. Trigeminal ganglion block can be carried out with 1 to 3 mL of local anesthetic; thus, almost any of the local anesthetics is an option.

PLACEMENT

Anatomy. The trigeminal ganglion is located intracranially and measures approximately 1 × 2 cm. In its intracranial location, it lies lateral to the internal carotid artery and cavernous sinus and slightly posterior and superior to the foramen ovale, through which the mandibular nerve leaves the cranium (Fig. 20-1). From the trigeminal ganglion, the fifth cranial nerve divides into its three principal divisions: the ophthalmic, maxillary, and mandibular nerves. These nerves provide sensation to the region of the eye and forehead, upper jaw (midface), and lower jaw, respectively (see Fig. 20-1). The mandibular division carries motor fibers to the muscles of mastication, but otherwise these nerves are wholly sensory. The trigeminal ganglion is partially contained within a reflection of dura mater, Meckel's cave. Figures 20-2 and 20-3 show that the foramen ovale is approximately in the horizontal plane of the zygoma, and in the frontal plane is roughly at the level of the mandibular notch. The foramen ovale is slightly less than 1 cm in diameter and is situated immediately dorsolateral to the pterygoid process.

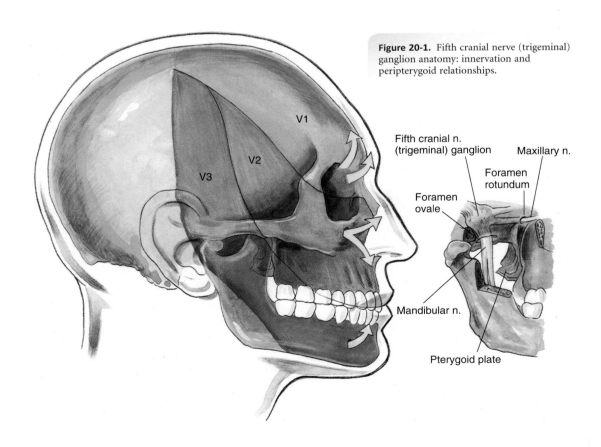

Figure 20-1. Fifth cranial nerve (trigeminal) ganglion anatomy: innervation and peripterygoid relationships.

V1

V2

V3

Fifth cranial n. (trigeminal) ganglion

Maxillary n.

Foramen rotundum

Foramen ovale

Mandibular n.

Pterygoid plate

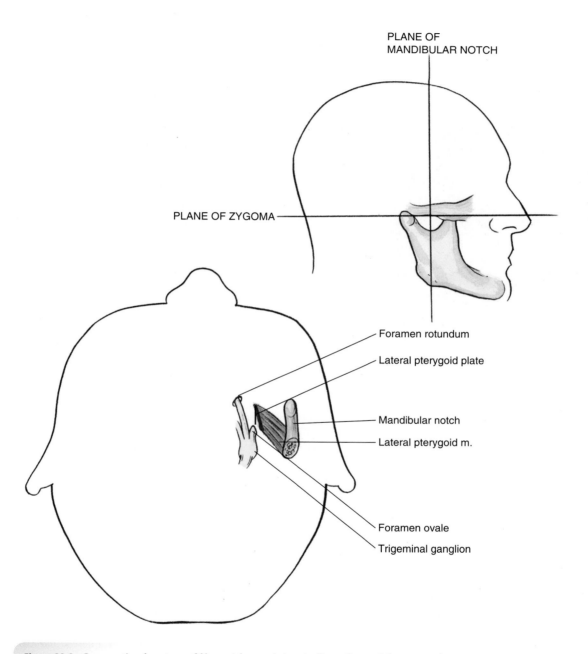

PLANE OF
MANDIBULAR NOTCH

PLANE OF ZYGOMA

Foramen rotundum

Lateral pterygoid plate

Mandibular notch

Lateral pterygoid m.

Foramen ovale

Trigeminal ganglion

Figure 20-2. Cross-sectional anatomy: fifth cranial nerve (trigeminal) ganglion and foramen ovale.

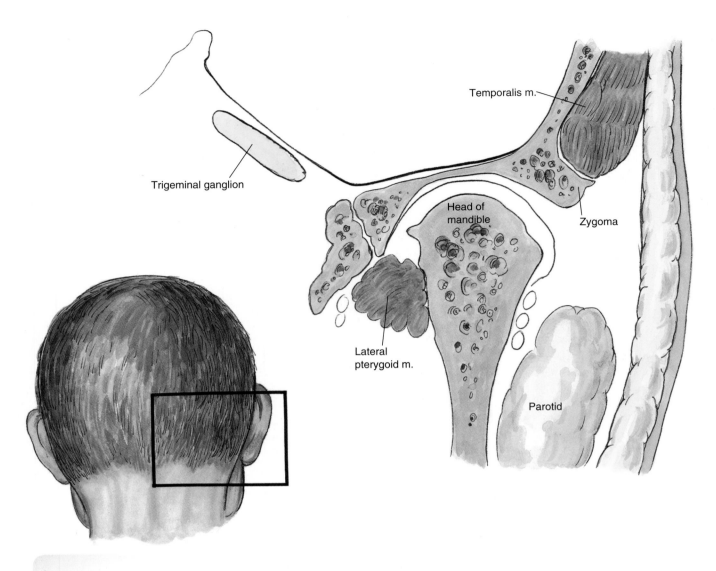

Figure 20-3. Coronal anatomy: section through fifth cranial nerve (trigeminal) ganglion.

Position. Patients are placed in a supine position and asked to fix their gaze straight ahead, as if they were looking off into the distance. The anesthesiologist should be positioned at the patient's side, slightly below the level of the shoulder, so that by looking toward the patient's face, the perspective shown in Figure 20-4 is observed.

Needle Puncture. A skin wheal is raised immediately medial to the masseter muscle, which can be located by asking the patient to clench his or her teeth. (It will most often be located approximately 3 cm lateral to the corner of the mouth.) Through this site, as illustrated in Figure 20-5, a 22-gauge, 10-cm needle is inserted as shown at *position 1*, aided by fluoroscopic guidance. The plane of insertion should be in line with the pupil, as illustrated in Figure 20-4. This will allow the needle tip to contact the infratemporal surface of the greater wing of the sphenoid bone, immediately anterior to the foramen ovale. This

occurs at a depth of 4.5 to 6 cm. Once the needle is firmly positioned against this infratemporal region, it is withdrawn and redirected in a stepwise manner until it enters the foramen ovale at a depth of approximately 6 to 7 cm, or 1 to 1.5 cm past the needle length required to contact the bone initially (*position 2*).

As the foramen is entered, a mandibular paresthesia is often elicited. By advancing the needle slightly, one may also elicit paresthesia in the distribution of the ophthalmic or maxillary nerves. These additional paresthesias should be sought in order to verify a periganglionic position of the needle tip. If the only paresthesia obtained is in the mandibular distribution, the needle tip may not have entered the foramen ovale but may be inferior to it while it abuts the mandibular nerve.

Before injection of local anesthetic, careful aspiration of the needle should be performed to check for cerebrospinal fluid (CSF) because the ganglion's posterior two thirds is

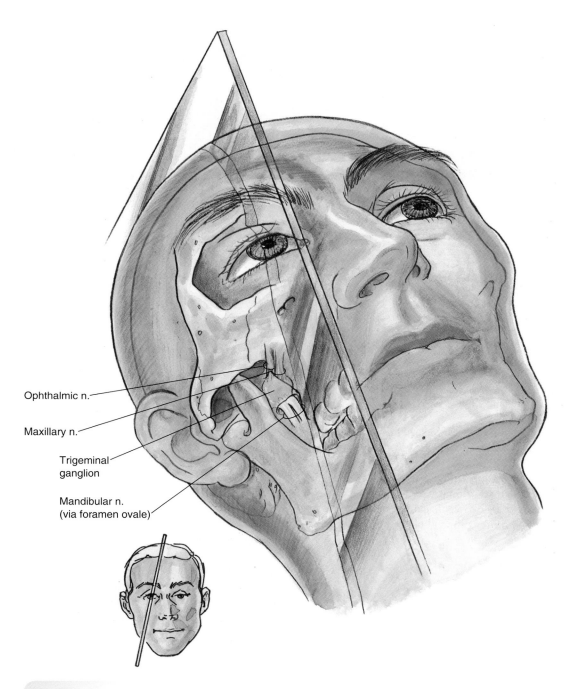

Ophthalmic n.

Maxillary n.

Trigeminal
ganglion

Mandibular n.
(via foramen ovale)

Figure 20-4. Trigeminal ganglion block: anatomy and needle insertion plane.

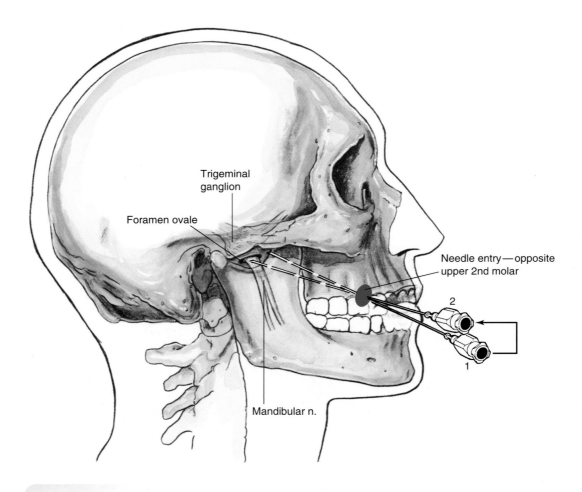

Figure 20-5. Trigeminal ganglion block: anatomy and technique.

enveloped in a reflection of dura, Meckel's cave. If trigeminal block is being undertaken diagnostically before neurolysis, 1 mL of local anesthetic should now be injected. Nerve block should develop within 5 to 10 minutes; if the block is incomplete, an additional 1 to 2 mL of local anesthetic can be injected or the needle can be repositioned in an effort to obtain a more complete block.

POTENTIAL PROBLEMS

Subarachnoid injection of local anesthetic is possible with this block owing to the close anatomic relationship between the trigeminal ganglion and the dural reflection, Meckel's cave. Likewise, the needle will pass through highly vascular regions on its way to the foramen ovale, and hematoma formation is a possibility. The block can also be painful for the patient and may require effective sedation before final needle placement.

PEARLS

As with all regional block techniques, it is important not to develop a sense of "time pressure" when performing this block. This is especially pertinent to trigeminal ganglion block because doses of 1% lidocaine as small as 0.25 mL have produced unconsciousness when unintentionally injected into the CSF during the block. Because this block can be uncomfortable, sufficient time is needed to allow the patient to become comfortable with the approach and appropriate sedation to occur. In addition, skill with fluoroscopic guidance of the technique should be developed.

Maxillary Block

21

PERSPECTIVE

Local anesthetic block of the maxillary nerve in its peripterygoid location is most commonly used to evaluate facial neuralgia. However, it can be used to facilitate surgical procedures in the nerve's cutaneous distribution (Fig. 21-1). Injection of neurolytic solution from the lateral approach to the maxillary nerve in its peripterygoid location should be undertaken with extreme caution owing to its location near the orbit.

Patient Selection. This block is principally used diagnostically in the workup of facial neuralgia. For patients with significant cardiopulmonary disease who require a surgical procedure in the distribution of the maxillary nerve, it can be used for surgical anesthesia.

Pharmacologic Choice. The maxillary nerve can be blocked with a low volume of local anesthetic (<5 mL); thus, virtually any local anesthetic can be chosen.

PLACEMENT

Anatomy. The maxillary nerve is entirely sensory and passes through the foramen rotundum to exit from the cranium. The nerve passes through the pterygopalatine fossa, medial to the lateral pterygoid plate, on its way to the infraorbital fissure. As illustrated in Figure 21-2, it is accessible to the anesthesiologist through a lateral approach as it passes into the pterygopalatine fossa.

Position. The patient is placed in the supine position with the head and neck rotated away from the side to be blocked. While the anesthesiologist palpates the mandibular notch, the patient is asked to open and close his or her mouth gently to make the notch even more obvious.

Needle Puncture. A 22-gauge, 8-cm needle is inserted through the mandibular notch in a slightly cephalomedial direction, as illustrated in Figure 21-3. This allows the needle to impinge on the lateral pterygoid plate at a depth

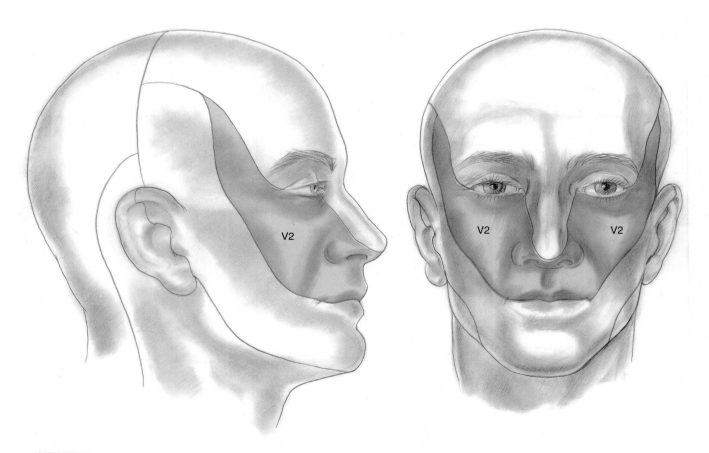

Figure 21-1. Maxillary nerve (V2): cutaneous innervation.

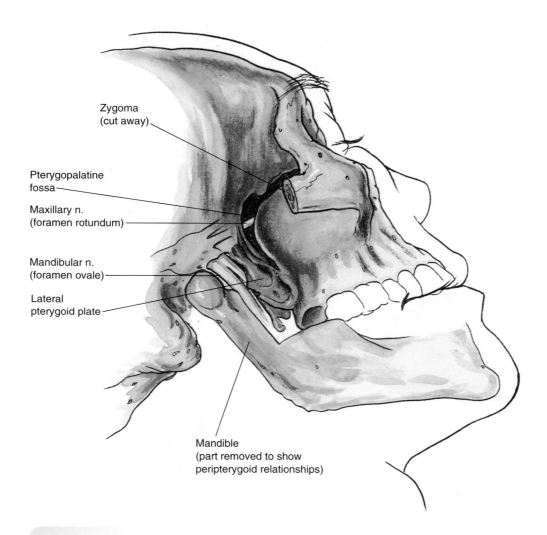

Zygoma
(cut away)

Pterygopalatine
fossa

Maxillary n.
(foramen rotundum)

Mandibular n.
(foramen ovale)

Lateral
pterygoid plate

Mandible
(part removed to show
peripterygoid relationships)

Figure 21-2. Maxillary block anatomy: peripterygoid relationships.

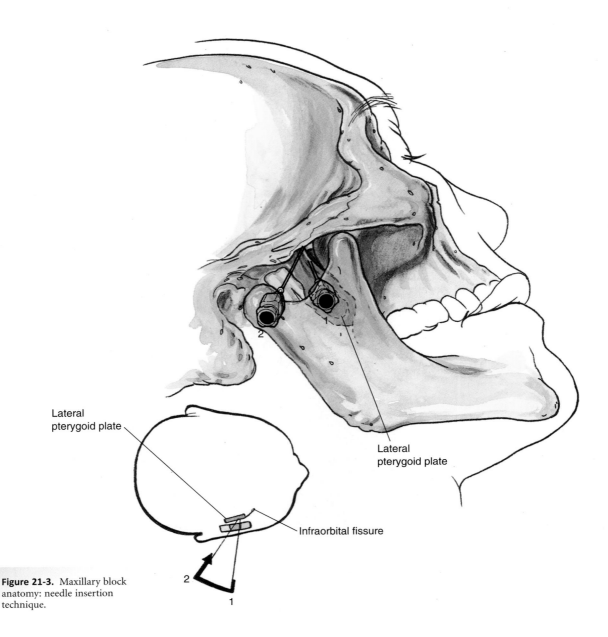

Lateral
pterygoid plate

Lateral
pterygoid plate

Infraorbital fissure

Figure 21-3. Maxillary block anatomy: needle insertion technique.

of approximately 5 cm (*needle position 1*). The needle is then withdrawn and redirected in a stepwise manner toward *position 2* (the pterygopalatine fossa). The needle should not be advanced more than 1 cm past the depth of initial contact with the pterygoid plate. As the needle is "walked off" the pterygoid plate, a sense of walking into the pterygopalatine fossa should be appreciated. Once the needle is adequately positioned, 5 mL of local anesthetic is injected.

POTENTIAL PROBLEMS

Owing to the close proximity of the maxillary nerve to the infraorbital fissure, some spill of local anesthetic into the orbit is possible; thus, patients should be warned that eye movement or vision might be affected. The lateral approach to the maxillary nerve also involves insertion of the needle through a vascular region, and hematoma formation is possible. Again, owing to the close association of the pterygopalatine fossa with the orbit, patients frequently develop a "black eye" after this block.

PEARLS

To become comfortable and clinically successful with this block, the anesthesiologist should find the time to examine the relationship of the foramen rotundum, pterygoid plate, and pterygopalatine fossa. An understanding of the peripterygoid anatomy will promote the anesthesiologist's confidence and the clinical efficacy of this block.

Mandibular Block

22

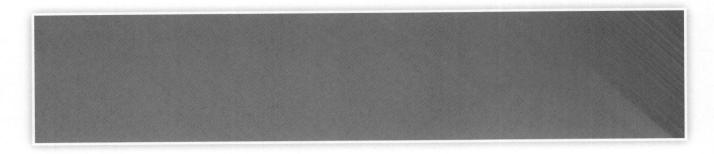

PERSPECTIVE

This block is most often used for diagnosis of facial neuralgias; however, it can be used for surgical procedures on the skin overlying the lower jaw, except at the jaw's angle. Dental procedures on the lower jaw can also be carried out, although dentists more commonly use the intraoral approach to the mandibular nerve to perform this block.

Patient Selection. Patients appropriate for this block are those with facial neuralgias and those with significant cardiopulmonary disease who require a surgical procedure in the region innervated by the mandibular nerve.

Pharmacologic Choice. Because small volumes (5 mL) of local anesthetic will produce regional block of the man-

dibular nerve, virtually any local anesthetic agent is an acceptable choice.

PLACEMENT

Anatomy. The mandibular nerve is a mixed motor-sensory nerve, although it is primarily sensory. It exits from the cranium through the foramen ovale and parallels the posterior margin of the lateral pterygoid plate as it descends inferiorly and laterally toward the mandible (Figs. 22-1 and 22-2). The anterior division of the mandibular nerve is principally motor and supplies the muscles of mastication, whereas the posterior division is principally sensory and supplies the skin and mucous membranes overlying the lower jaw and skin anterior and superior to the ear (Fig. 22-3).

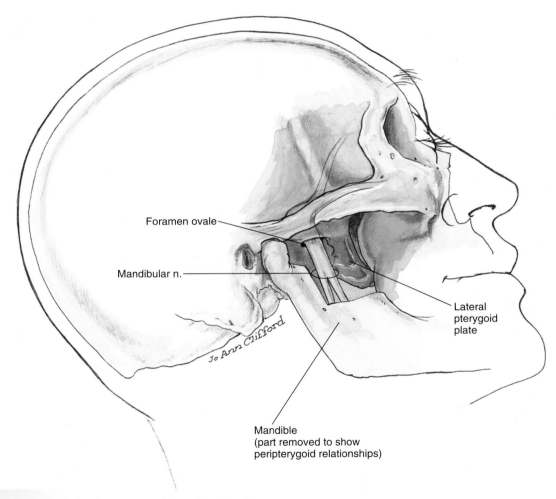

Foramen ovale

Mandibular n.

Lateral pterygoid plate

Mandible (part removed to show peripterygoid relationships)

Figure 22-1. Mandibular block anatomy: peripterygoid relationships.

A   B   C

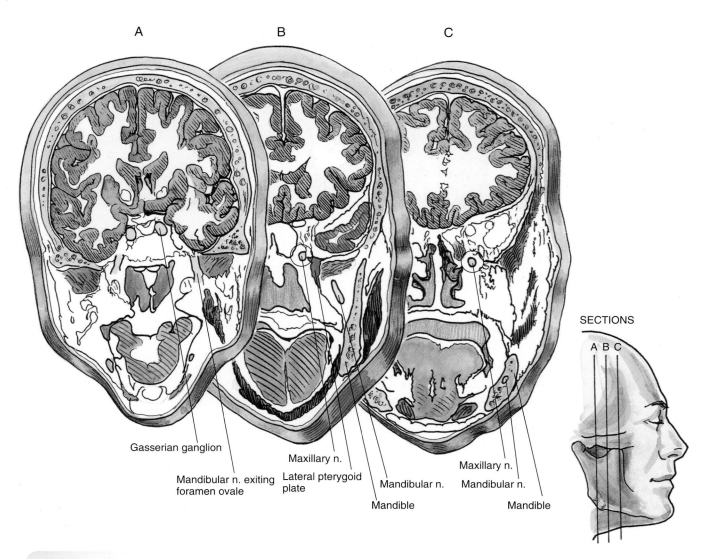

SECTIONS

A B C

Gasserian ganglion

Mandibular n. exiting   Maxillary n.
foramen ovale   Lateral pterygoid   Maxillary n.
                       plate   Mandibular n.   Mandibular n.

                                      Mandible   Mandible

Figure 22-2. Coronal anatomy: peripterygoid relationships.

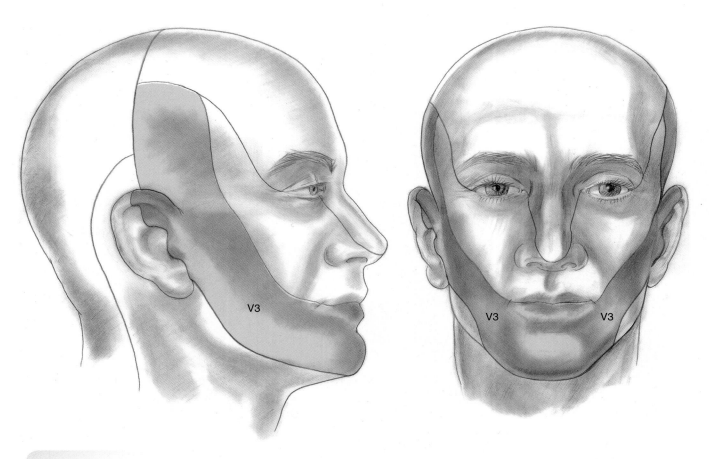

Figure 22-3. Mandibular nerve (V3): cutaneous innervation.

Sensory branches of the mandibular nerve are the buccal, auriculotemporal, lingual, and inferior alveolar nerves. The *buccal nerve* is exclusively sensory and supplies the mucous membranes of the cheek. The *auriculotemporal nerve* passes posterior to the neck of the mandible to supply the skin anterior to the ear and extends into the scalp's temporal region. The *lingual nerve* is joined by the chorda tympani branch of the facial nerve, and together they supply taste and general sensation to the anterior two thirds of the tongue and sensation to the floor of the mouth, including the lingual aspect of the lower gingivae. The *inferior alveolar nerve* supplies the lower teeth and terminates as the mental nerve, which supplies sensation to the lower labial mucous membranes and skin of the chin.

Position. The patient is placed in the supine position, with the head and neck turned away from the side to be blocked. As in the approach used for maxillary block, the patient is asked to open and close his or her mouth gently while the anesthesiologist palpates the mandibular notch to identify it more clearly.

Needle Puncture. The needle is inserted in the midpoint of the mandibular notch and directed to reach the lateral pterygoid plate by taking a slightly cephalomedial angle through the notch, as shown in Figure 22-4. The 22-gauge, 8-cm needle will impinge on the lateral pterygoid plate at a depth of approximately 5 cm (*needle position 1*). The needle is then withdrawn and redirected in small steps to "walk off" the posterior border of the lateral pterygoid plate in a horizontal plane (*needle position 2*), as shown in Figure 22-4. The needle should not be advanced more than 0.5 cm past the depth of the pterygoid plate because the superior constrictor muscle of the pharynx is easily pierced; thus, the needle will enter the pharynx if it is inserted more deeply. Once the needle tip is appropriately positioned, 5 mL of local anesthetic is administered.

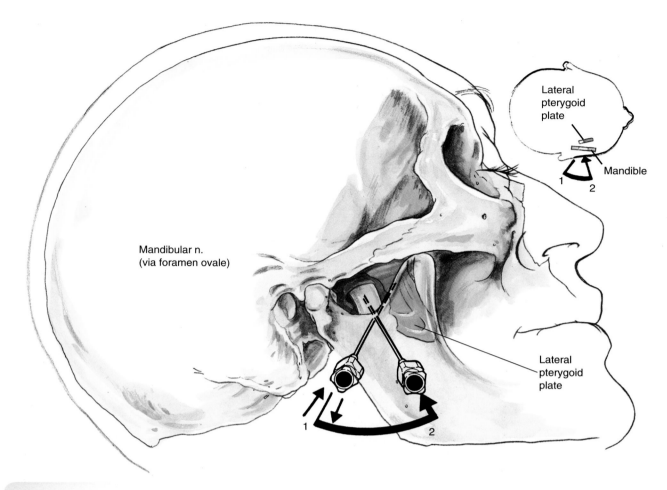

Mandibular n.
(via foramen ovale)

Lateral
pterygoid
plate

Mandible

1
2

Lateral
pterygoid
plate

1
2

Figure 22-4. Mandibular block anatomy: needle insertion technique.

POTENTIAL PROBLEMS

As with maxillary nerve block, the lateral approach to the mandibular nerve requires needle insertion through a vascular region. Thus, hematoma formation is possible. If a hematoma does occur, most often watchful waiting is all that is required. Although it is more difficult to enter the cerebrospinal fluid (CSF) through the foramen ovale from the lateral approach, one must be constantly aware that if a needle is inserted through the foramen ovale into Meckel's cave, small doses of local anesthetic in the CSF can produce unconsciousness.

PEARLS

As with maxillary nerve block, anesthesiologists should develop a thorough understanding of the peripterygoid anatomy before carrying out this block. Needle movements with the mandibular block involve fewer planes than with the maxillary block because the needle is moved primarily in the horizontal plane once it has made contact with the pterygoid plate. Therefore, in some ways, this block is less complex than the maxillary block. Also, because the mandibular nerve is more distant from the orbital structures, there is less risk in using neurolytic solutions with this block.

Distal Trigeminal Block

23

PERSPECTIVE

This block can be used for the diagnosis of facial neuralgia; however, more frequently it is used for superficial surgical procedures that require more than simple infiltration for anesthesia.

Patient Selection. Almost all patients are candidates for distal trigeminal blocks because the bony foramina—supraorbital, infraorbital, and mental—are easily palpable.

Pharmacologic Choice. Owing to the small volumes of local anesthetic necessary for this block, almost any local anesthetic agent may be chosen.

PLACEMENT

Anatomy. The distal branches of the three divisions of the trigeminal nerve—ophthalmic (supraorbital), maxillary (infraorbital), and mandibular (mental)—exit from the skull through their respective foramina on a line that runs almost vertically through the pupil (Fig. 23-1).

Position. The patient is placed in the supine position with the anesthesiologist at the patient's side, approximately at the level of the shoulder.

Needle Puncture. For this block, as illustrated in Figure 23-2, once the respective foramina are identified by palpation, a short, 25-gauge needle is inserted in a cephalomedial direction near each foramen, and approximately 2 to 3 mL of local anesthetic is injected at each site. If a paresthesia is obtained, the local anesthetic can be deposited at that point.

POTENTIAL PROBLEMS

This block is superficial and thus carries with it few complications. One should be cautious about entering the foramina to inject the local anesthetic because intraneural injection is probably more frequent with that approach.

PEARLS

The anesthesiologist should ensure that the patient is properly sedated and should clearly identify the foramina to be blocked, so that accurate needle placement is achieved.

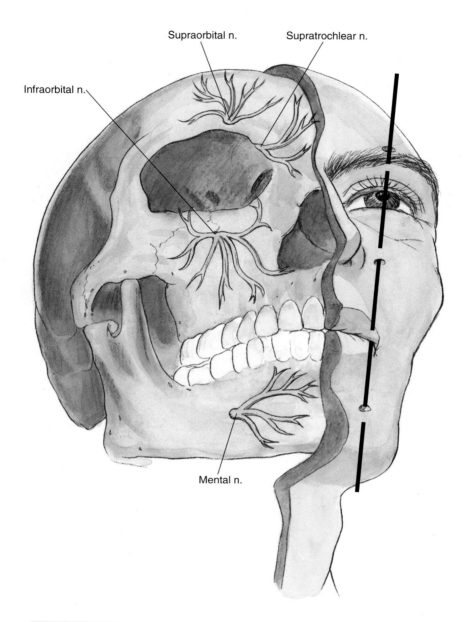

Infraorbital n.

Supraorbital n.

Supratrochlear n.

Mental n.

Figure 23-1. Distal trigeminal nerve: anatomy.

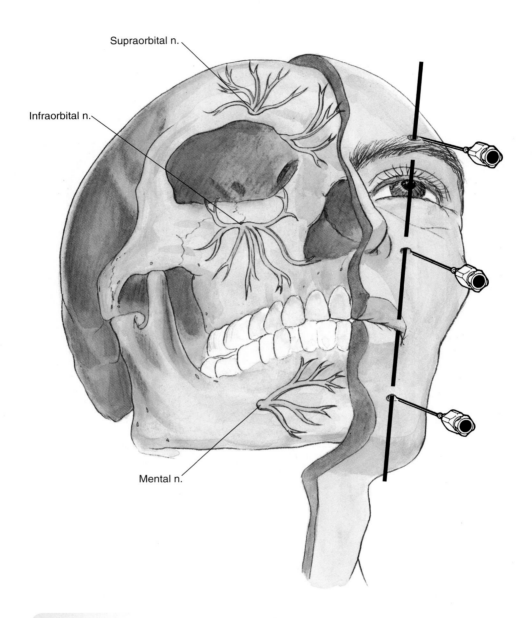

Supraorbital n.

Infraorbital n.

Mental n.

Figure 23-2. Distal trigeminal nerve block: technique.

Retrobulbar (Peribulbar) Block

24

PERSPECTIVE

This block is performed more often by ophthalmologists than by anesthesiologists. The combination of retrobulbar anesthesia and block of the orbicularis oculi muscle allows most intraocular surgery to be performed. This regional block is most useful for corneal, anterior chamber, and lens procedures.

Patient Selection. Patients who require retrobulbar (peribulbar) anesthesia are principally older patients who are undergoing ophthalmic operations.

Pharmacologic Choice. If retrobulbar block is used, 2 to 4 mL of local anesthetic is all that is required to produce adequate retrobulbar anesthesia. Conversely, if the peribulbar approach is chosen (i.e., the needle tip is not purposely inserted through the cone of extraocular muscles), slightly larger volumes, 4 to 6 mL, may be necessary. Almost any of the local anesthetic agents are applicable, with many ophthalmic anesthetists using combinations of bupivacaine and lidocaine.

PLACEMENT

Anatomy. Sensation to the eye is provided by the ophthalmic nerve through the long and short posterior ciliary nerves. Autonomic innervation is provided by the same nerves, and sympathetic fibers traveling with the arteries

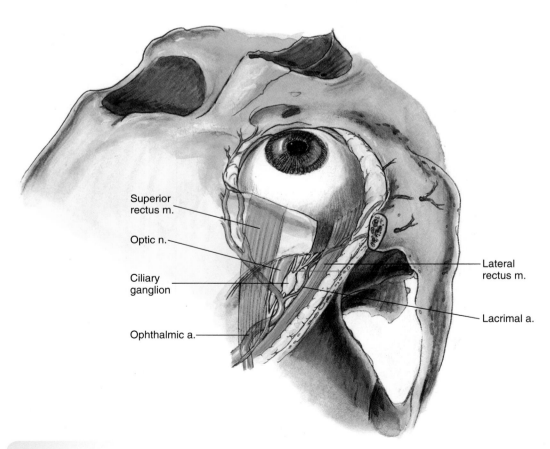

Figure 24-1. Orbital anatomy.

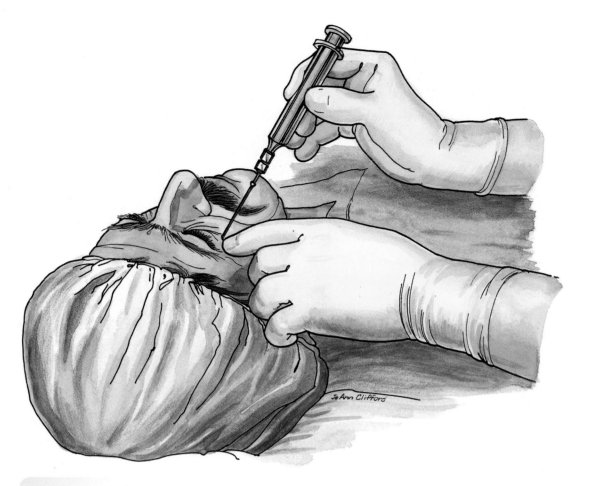

Figure 24-2. Retrobulbar (peribulbar) block: position.

and parasympathetic fibers carried by the inferior branch of the oculomotor nerve provide additional autonomic innervation. Because the innervation of the orbicularis oculi muscle is through the facial nerve, blockade of these fibers is required to ensure a quiet eye during ophthalmic operations. The ciliary ganglion, measuring approximately 2 to 3 mm in length, lies deep in the orbit just lateral to the optic nerve and medial to the lateral rectus muscle. From this ganglion, the long and short ciliary nerves extend forward in the orbit. Immediately posterior to the ciliary ganglion, the ophthalmic artery can be found at the lateral side of the optic nerve as it crosses superior to it and passes forward medially (Fig. 24-1).

Position. Patients are placed in the supine position and are instructed to maintain their primary gaze directly ahead, not "up and in," as in earlier recommendations. With the globe in primary gaze, the optic nerve position minimizes potential intraneural injection. The anesthesiologist is positioned for the injection as illustrated in Figure 24-2.

Needle Puncture. While the patient's gaze is directed cephalad and opposite to the site of injection, a 27-gauge, 31-mm, sharp-beveled needle is inserted at the inferolateral border of the bony orbit and directed toward the

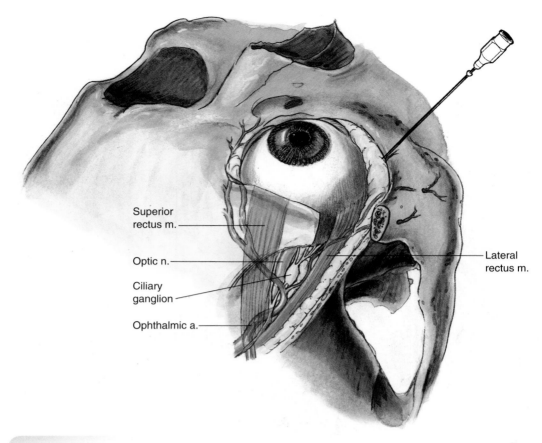

Superior
rectus m.

Optic n.

Ciliary
ganglion

Ophthalmic a.

Lateral
rectus m.

Figure 24-3. Retrobulbar (peribulbar) block: needle puncture.

apex of the orbit, as illustrated in Figure 24-3. The needle should be oriented so that the bevel opening faces toward the globe. A "pop" may be appreciated as the needle tip traverses the bulbar fascia and enters the orbital muscle cone. Before 2 to 4 mL of local anesthetic is injected, careful needle aspiration should be carried out. After retrobulbar block, 5 to 10 minutes should be allowed to pass before the operation is started. This helps to avoid operating on patients who develop retrobulbar hematomas. During these 5 to 10 minutes, the anesthesiologist can apply gentle pressure to the globe, principally to facilitate lowering the intraocular pressure. If a peribulbar technique is chosen, needle insertion begins like that used for retrobulbar (inferotemporal) injection; however, the operator inserts the needle parallel and lateral to the lateral rectus muscle and bulbar fascia rather than making an effort to puncture it. Many practitioners also now suggest making

a second injection of 3 to 5 mL for a peribulbar block either in the superomedial orbit or at the extreme medial side of the palpebral fissure. To complete the local block for ocular surgery, the orbicularis oculi muscle must be blocked to produce an immobile eye. This is carried out by blocking the facial nerve fibers that innervate the muscle.

There are many ways of performing blocks of these facial nerve fibers, and the method illustrated in Figure 24-4 is the example of Van Lint. In this block, a 25-gauge, 4-cm needle is inserted at *needle position 1* until the lower inferolateral orbital rim is reached. While the needle tip contacts bony surface, 1 mL of local anesthetic is injected. Through this skin wheal, the needle is repositioned along the lateral and inferior margins of the orbit (*needle positions 2 and 3*), and 2 to 3 mL of local anesthetic is injected along each needle path.

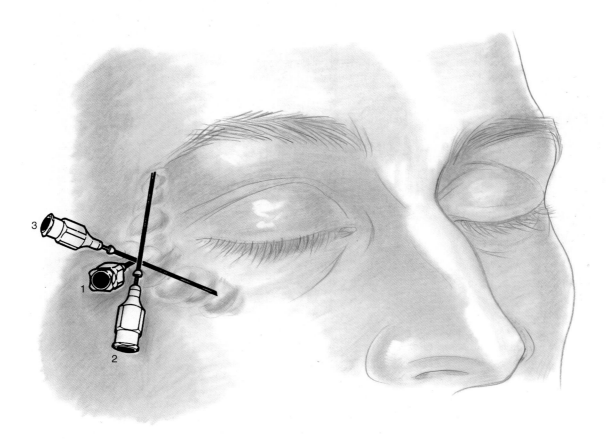

Figure 24-4. Regional block of orbicularis oculi muscle: Van Lint method.

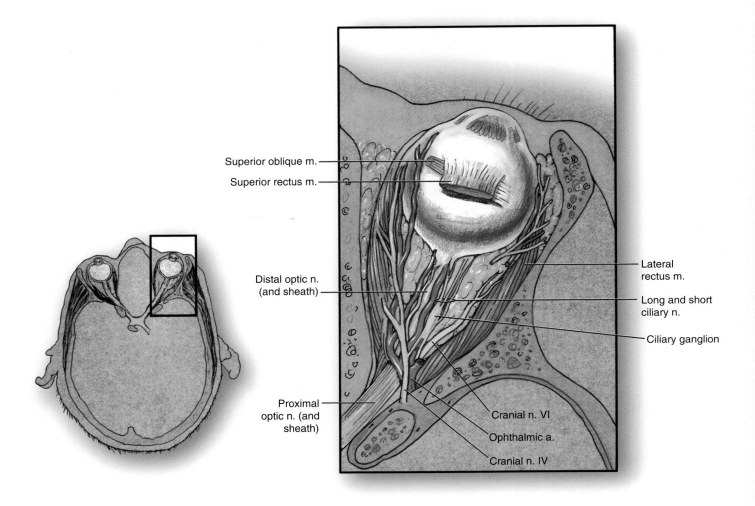

Superior oblique m.
Superior rectus m.
Distal optic n. (and sheath)
Proximal optic n. (and sheath)
Lateral rectus m.
Long and short ciliary n.
Ciliary ganglion
Cranial n. VI
Ophthalmic a.
Cranial n. IV

Figure 24-5. Orbital functional anatomy.

POTENTIAL PROBLEMS

The most common complication with retrobulbar block is hematoma formation. This can be minimized by using a needle shorter than 31 mm. Hematoma formation is more likely if a longer needle is used and the needle tip rests in the vicinity of the ophthalmic artery as it crosses the optic nerve. Hematoma can also be minimized by using a peri-bulbar approach. Other complications that can accompany retrobulbar block include local anesthetic toxicity, development of the oculocardiac reflex, and cases of sudden apnea and obtundation after retrobulbar injection. The latter two results are probably related to injection within the optic nerve sheath, resulting in unexpected spinal anesthesia, or intravascular injection affecting the respiratory centers in the midbrain, as illustrated in Figure 24-5.

PEARLS

If anesthesiologists carry out retrobulbar anesthesia, they must work with ophthalmologists who are supportive and willing to share this part of their practice. Theoretically, many of the complications of retrobulbar anesthesia can be avoided if peribulbar block is carried out. This can be produced by placing the needle along the muscular cone of extraocular muscles rather than within the muscular cone. Although slightly larger volumes of local anesthetic are required with this technique, most of the major complications can be avoided.

Cervical Plexus Block

25

PERSPECTIVE

Cervical plexus blocks are used to carry out both superficial and deep operations in the region of the neck and supraclavicular fossa. The choice of deep or superficial block depends on the surgical procedure.

Patient Selection. This block can be performed easily in a supine patient; thus, almost any patient is a candidate. Bilateral deep cervical plexus block should be avoided because the phrenic nerve may be partially blocked with this technique. Examples of procedures that are suitable for this technique are carotid endarterectomy, lymph node biopsy, and plastic surgical procedures.

Pharmacologic Choice. Most procedures carried out with cervical plexus block do not demand significant motor relaxation. Thus, lower concentrations of local anesthetics, such as 0.75% to 1% lidocaine or mepivacaine, 0.25% bupivacaine, or 0.2% ropivacaine, are appropriate with these techniques.

PLACEMENT

Anatomy. Cervical plexus block can be divided into superficial and deep techniques. The cutaneous innervation of the cervical nerves is schematically illustrated in Figure 25-1. The cervical nerves have both dorsal and ventral

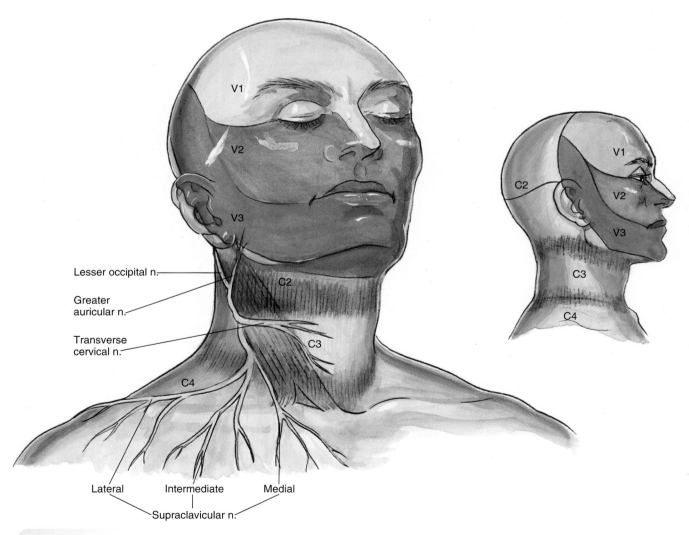

Figure 25-1. Cervical plexus: anatomy and cutaneous innervation.

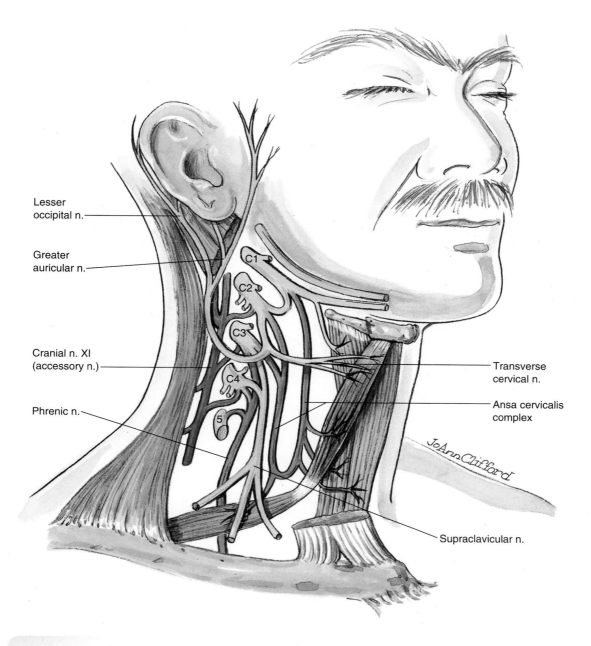

Figure 25-2. Cervical plexus: functional anatomy of the ventral rami of C1-C4.

Lesser
occipital n.

Greater
auricular n.

Cranial n. XI
(accessory n.)

Phrenic n.

Transverse
cervical n.

Ansa cervicalis
complex

Supraclavicular n.

C1
C2
C3
C4
5

JoAnn Clifford

rami, and those illustrated in Figure 25-2 represent the ventral rami of C1-C4. In addition, there are both sensory and motor branches from the dorsal rami of C1-C4 that are not shown. Before regrouping to form the cervical plexus, the cervical nerves exit from the cervical vertebrae through a gutter in the transverse process in an anterocaudolateral direction, immediately posterior to the vertebral artery.

To simplify understanding the cervical plexus, it can be divided into (1) cutaneous branches of the plexus, (2) the ansa cervicalis complex, (3) the phrenic nerve, (4) contributions to the accessory nerve, and (5) direct muscular branches (see Fig. 25-2). The *cutaneous branches of the plexus* are the lesser occipital, greater auricular, transverse cervical, and supraclavicular nerves (see Fig. 25-1). The first three arise from the second and third cervical nerves, and the supraclavicular nerves arise from the third and fourth cervical nerves. The *ansa cervicalis complex* provides innervation to the infrahyoid and geniohyoid muscles. The *phrenic nerve* is the sole motor nerve to the diaphragm and also provides sensation to its central portion. The nerve arises by a large root from the fourth cervical nerve, reinforced by smaller contributions from the third and fifth nerves. Its course takes it to the lateral border of the anterior scalene muscle before it descends vertically over the ventral surface of this muscle and enters the chest along its medial border. The *accessory nerve* (cranial nerve XI) receives contributions from the cervical plexus at several points and provides innervation to the sternocleidomastoid muscle as well as the trapezius muscles. The *direct muscular branches* of the plexus supply prevertebral muscles in the neck. The superficial plexus becomes subcutaneous at the midpoint of the posterior border of the sternocleidomastoid muscle (Fig. 25-3, and see Fig. 25-5).

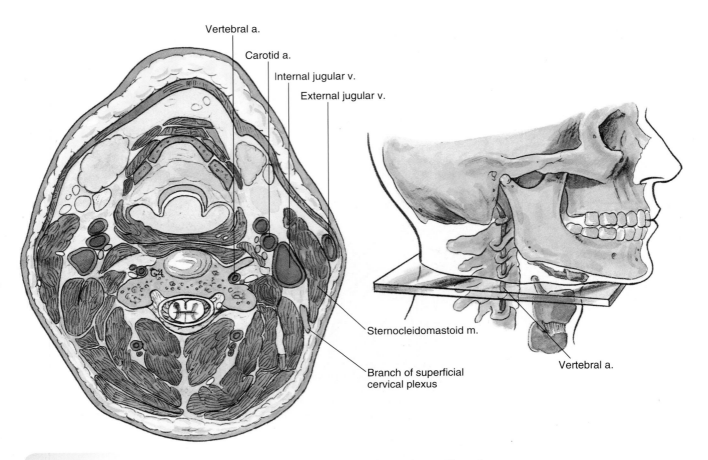

Vertebral a.

Carotid a.

Internal jugular v.

External jugular v.

Sternocleidomastoid m.

Vertebral a.

Branch of superficial cervical plexus

Figure 25-3. Cervical plexus: cross-sectional anatomy at the midpoint of the sternocleidomastoid muscle.

Position. The patient is placed in the supine position, with the head and neck turned opposite the side to be blocked. The anesthesiologist should stand at the patient's side, approximately at the level of the shoulder.

Needle Puncture: Deep Cervical Plexus Block. The patient should be positioned with the neck slightly extended and the head turned away from the side to be blocked. A line should be drawn on the skin between the tip of the mastoid process and Chassaignac's tubercle (i.e., the most easily palpable transverse process of the cervical vertebra, C6). A second line should be drawn parallel and 1 cm posterior to the first line, as illustrated in blue in Figure 25-4. The C4 transverse process should be located by first finding the C2 transverse process 1 to 2 cm caudal to the mastoid process and then identifying C3 and subsequently C4. Each of these transverse processes is palpable approximately 1.5 cm caudal to the immediately more cephalad process. Ultrasonographic guidance can also assist in locating the C4 transverse process. Once the C4 transverse process is identified, a 22-gauge, 5-cm needle is inserted immediately over the C4 transverse process so that it will contact that process at a depth of approximately 1.5 to 3 cm. If a par-

esthesia is obtained, 10 to 12 mL of local anesthetic is injected at this site. It is helpful to obtain a paresthesia with this technique before injection because one is relying on the continuity of the paravertebral space in the neck to facilitate local anesthetic spread. If a paresthesia is not elicited on the first pass, the needle should be withdrawn and "walked" in a stepwise fashion in an anteroposterior manner. Again, ultrasonographic guidance will also allow you to observe the spread of local anesthetic in the paravertebral space.

Needle Placement: Superficial Cervical Plexus Block. The superficial cervical plexus block, as illustrated in Figure 25-5, relies on local anesthetic "volume" to be effective. At the midpoint on the posterior border of the sternocleidomastoid muscle, the superficial cervical plexus is arranged such that infiltration deep to the posterior border of the sternocleidomastoid muscle will produce a block. To perform the block, a 22-gauge, 4-cm needle is inserted subcutaneously posterior and immediately deep to the sternocleidomastoid muscle, and 5 mL of local anesthetic is injected. The needle is then redirected both superiorly and inferiorly along the posterior border of the sterno-

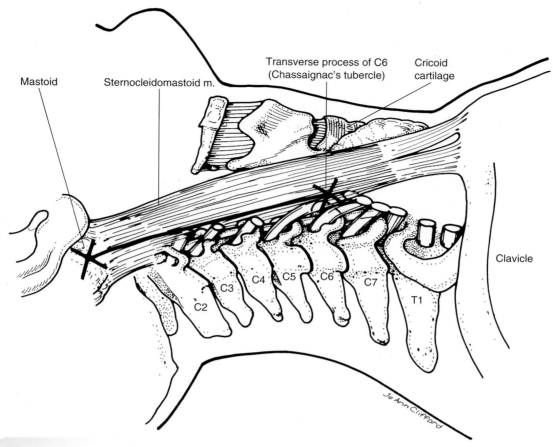

Figure 25-4. Deep cervical plexus block: technique.

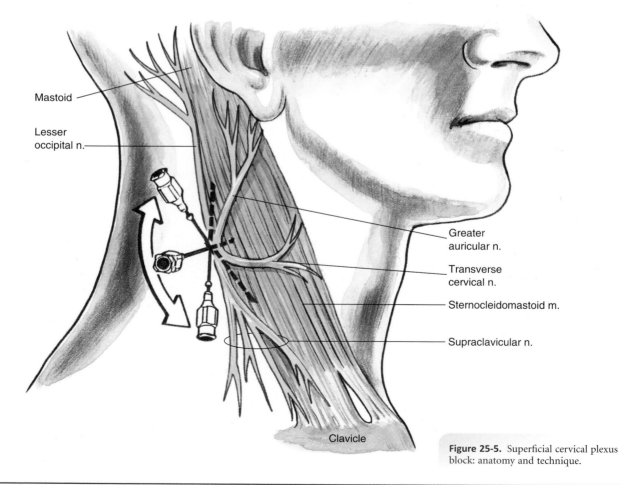

Figure 25-5. Superficial cervical plexus block: anatomy and technique.

cleidomastoid, and 5 mL of solution is injected along each of these sites. In this fashion, a field block of the superficial plexus is created.

POTENTIAL PROBLEMS

Deep cervical plexus block is often accompanied by at least partial phrenic nerve block, so bilateral blocks should be used with caution. The block also places the needles near the vertebral artery and other neuraxial structures. When carrying out the superficial block, one should simply avoid the external jugular vein, which often overlies the block site. Likewise, intravascular injection through the internal jugular vein can occur if the needle is inserted too deeply during performance of the field block.

PEARLS

If patients are properly positioned for this block, the superficial block should rarely result in problems. If the deep block is carried out and proper palpation is used to limit the amount of tissue between the anesthesiologist's fingertips and the transverse process, very short needles can help minimize the occurrence of errant deep injections. If a deep cervical plexus block is to be carried out for carotid endarterectomy, the anesthesiologist should consult with his or her surgical colleagues to learn their expectations so that anesthesia is adequate. Superficial cervical plexus block can be used effectively in addition to interscalene block during shoulder surgery to ensure the presence of cutaneous anesthesia when the surgical procedure is started soon after the block.

Stellate Block

26

PERSPECTIVE

The primary use of stellate block is in the diagnosis and treatment of complex regional pain syndromes of the upper extremity. It may also be used in clinical situations when increased perfusion to the upper extremity is desired, although this can also be accomplished with the brachial plexus blocks.

Patient Selection. Patients for this block are primarily those with complex regional pain syndromes of the upper extremity or those with impaired perfusion to the upper extremity after trauma.

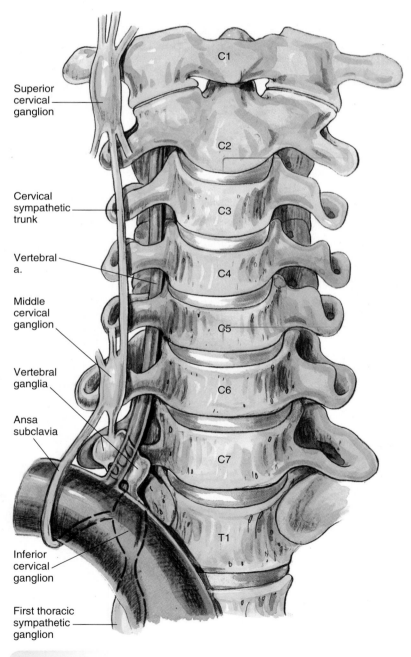

Superior cervical ganglion

C1

C2

Cervical sympathetic trunk

C3

Vertebral a.

C4

Middle cervical ganglion

C5

Vertebral ganglia

C6

Ansa subclavia

C7

Inferior cervical ganglion

T1

First thoracic sympathetic ganglion

Figure 26-1. Stellate ganglion block: simplified sympathetic chain anatomy.

Pharmacologic Choice. Even during diagnostic use of stellate ganglion block, it is often desirable to produce a long-lasting block. Therefore, a solution of 0.25% bupivacaine, or 0.2% ropivacaine with 1:200,000 epinephrine is often my first choice.

PLACEMENT

Anatomy. The cervical sympathetic trunk is a cephalad continuation of the thoracic sympathetic trunk. It is composed of three ganglia: the superior cervical ganglion, gen-

erally opposite the first cervical vertebra; the middle cervical ganglion, usually opposite the sixth cervical vertebra; and the stellate (cervicothoracic) ganglion, generally opposite the seventh cervical and first thoracic vertebrae near the head of the first rib. The stellate ganglion is a fusion of the inferior cervical ganglion and the first thoracic ganglion—hence the name *cervicothoracic ganglion* (Fig. 26-1). The cervical part of the sympathetic chain and ganglion lies on the anterior surface of, and is separated from, the transverse processes of the cervical vertebrae by the thin prevertebral musculature (primarily the longus colli muscle), as illustrated in Figure 26-2. Because the anterior approach to

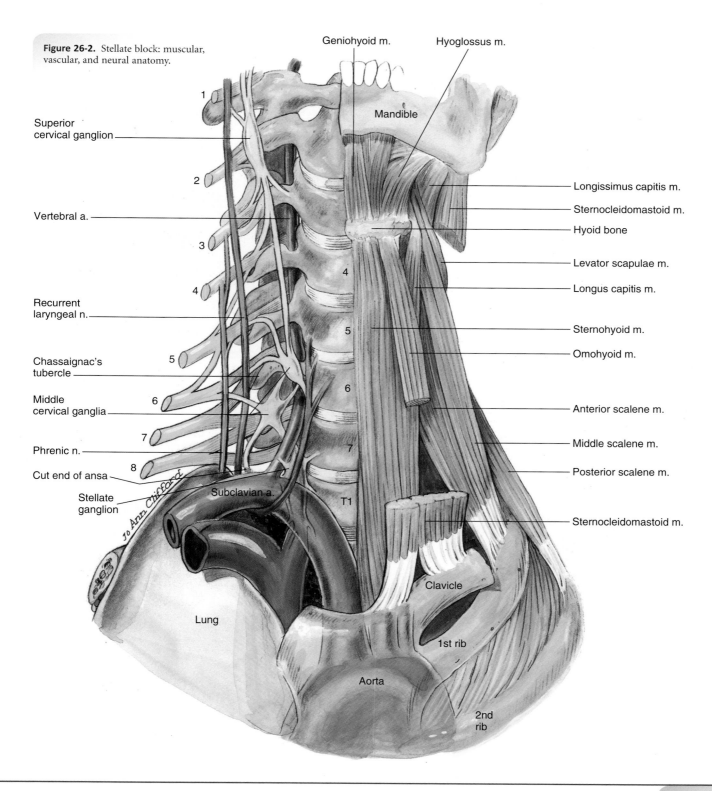

Figure 26-2. Stellate block: muscular, vascular, and neural anatomy.

Superior cervical ganglion

Vertebral a.

Recurrent laryngeal n.

Chassaignac's tubercle

Middle cervical ganglia

Phrenic n.

Cut end of ansa

Stellate ganglion

Subclavian a.

Lung

Aorta

Geniohyoid m.

Hyoglossus m.

Mandible

Longissimus capitis m.

Sternocleidomastoid m.

Hyoid bone

Levator scapulae m.

Longus capitis m.

Sternohyoid m.

Omohyoid m.

Anterior scalene m.

Middle scalene m.

Posterior scalene m.

Sternocleidomastoid m.

Clavicle

1st rib

2nd rib

the stellate ganglion is often made at the level of the sixth cervical vertebral (Chassaignac's) tubercle, it can be seen that the term *stellate block* is really a misnomer. To produce stellate (cervicothoracic) ganglion block, the anesthesiologist must rely on spread of the local anesthetic solution along the prevertebral muscles, or place the needle at the level of the seventh cervical vertebra with the use of ultrasonography or fluoroscopy.

Position. The patient should be in the supine position, with the neck in slight extension (Fig. 26-3). This is often facilitated by removing the patient's pillow before positioning. The anesthesiologist should stand beside the patient's neck and identify the sixth cervical vertebral

tubercle with palpation. This can be accomplished by locating the cricoid cartilage and moving the fingers laterally until they contact this easily palpable vertebral tubercle.

Needle Puncture. Once the sixth cervical vertebral tubercle is identified as shown in Figure 26-3, the anesthesiologist should place the index and third fingers between the carotid artery laterally and the trachea medially at the level of C6. A short, 22- or 25-gauge needle is inserted until it contacts the transverse process of C6. The needle is then withdrawn approximately 1 to 2 mm, and 5 to 10 mL of local anesthetic is injected (Fig. 26-4).

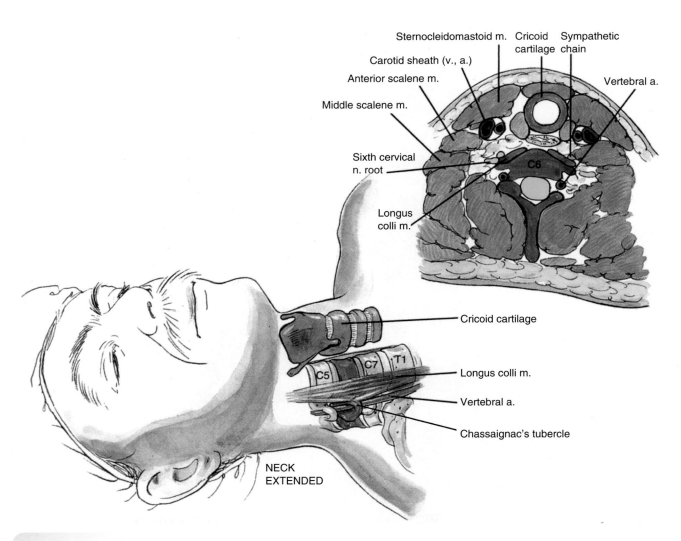

Figure 26-3. Stellate block: surface and cross-sectional anatomy.

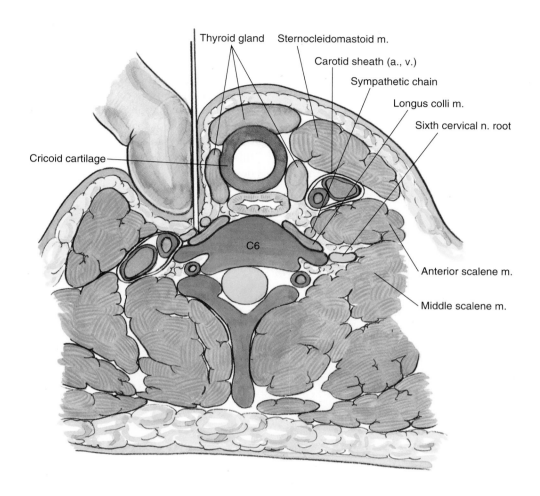

Thyroid gland Sternocleidomastoid m.

Carotid sheath (a., v.)

Sympathetic chain

Longus colli m.

Sixth cervical n. root

Cricoid cartilage

C6

Anterior scalene m.

Middle scalene m.

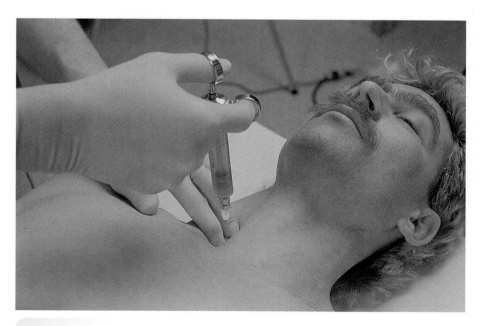

Figure 26-4. Stellate block: anatomy and technique.

POTENTIAL PROBLEMS

As illustrated in Figure 26-2, the vertebral artery runs close to the transverse process of C6, and intravascular injection must be avoided. The recurrent laryngeal and phrenic nerves may also be blocked if the needle position is not ideal. Patients should be cautioned that they may experience a lump in the throat or a sense of dyspnea. Reassurance is usually all that is necessary.

PEARLS

The most useful maneuver to facilitate this block is to use the index and third fingers of the palpating hand to compress the tissues overlying the sixth cervical vertebral tubercle. The patient will experience some deep pressure discomfort from this maneuver, but clear identification of the tubercle will make this block efficient, and most patients are willing to accept the deep discomfort if the block is carried out efficiently. In a small number of patients (<5%), a motor block of the ipsilateral upper extremity may develop after a stellate block performed without imaging guidance. Most likely this is because a prominent posterior tubercle at the posterior aspect of the transverse process is mistaken on palpation for the typically more prominent anterior portion of the sixth cervical vertebra. It is important to inform patients undergoing a stellate block about this possibility to minimize disappointment if it does develop.

SECTION V:
Airway Blocks

Airway Block Anatomy

27

If there is one set of regional blocks that an anesthesiologist should master, it is airway blocks. Even those anesthesiologists who prefer to use general anesthesia for the majority of their cases will be faced with the need to provide airway blocks before anesthetic induction in patients who may have airway compromise, trauma to the upper airway, or unstable cervical vertebrae. As illustrated in Figure 27-1, innervation of the airway can be separated into three principal neural pathways: trigeminal, glossopharyngeal, and vagus. If nasal intubation is planned, some method of anesthetizing the maxillary branches from the trigeminal nerve will need to be carried out. As our manipulations involve the pharynx and posterior third of the tongue, glossopharyngeal block will be required. Structures more distal in the airway to the epiglottis will require block of vagal branches.

Specific glossopharyngeal nerves that are of interest to anesthesiologists who undertake airway anesthesia are the pharyngeal nerves, which are primarily sensory to the pharyngeal mucosa; the tonsillar nerves, which provide sensation to the mucosa overlying the palatine tonsil and contiguous parts of the soft palate; and sensory branches to the posterior third of the tongue. The glossopharyngeal nerve exits the skull through the jugular foramen in close contact with the spinal accessory nerve. As the glossopharyngeal nerve exits the jugular foramen, it is also in close contact with the vagus nerve, which likewise travels within the carotid sheath in the upper portion of the neck.

The vagus nerve supplies innervation to the mucosa of the airway from the level of the epiglottis to the distal airways, through both the superior and the recurrent

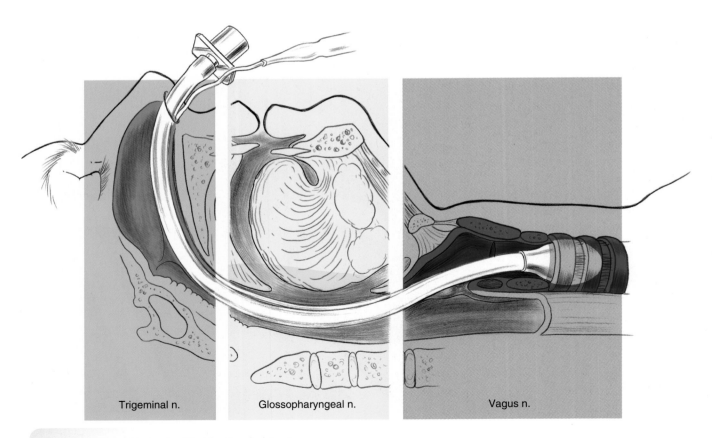

| Trigeminal n. | Glossopharyngeal n. | Vagus n. |

Figure 27-1. Airway blocks: simplified functional anatomy.

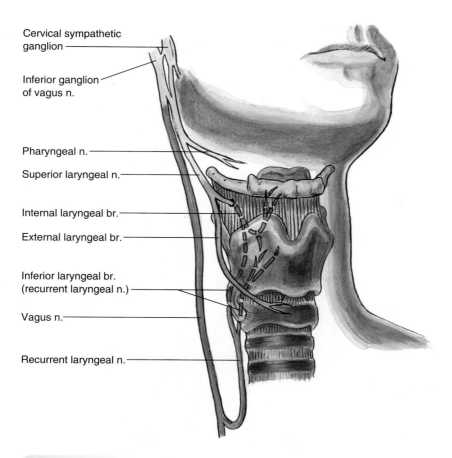

Cervical sympathetic
ganglion

Inferior ganglion
of vagus n.

Pharyngeal n.

Superior laryngeal n.

Internal laryngeal br.

External laryngeal br.

Inferior laryngeal br.
(recurrent laryngeal n.)

Vagus n.

Recurrent laryngeal n.

Figure 27-2. Airway blocks: anatomy of laryngeal innervation.

laryngeal nerves, as illustrated in Figures 27-2 and 27-3. Although the vagus is primarily a parasympathetic nerve, it also contains some fibers from the cervical sympathetic chain, as well as motor fibers to laryngeal muscles. The superior laryngeal nerve provides sensation to the surfaces of the epiglottis and to the airway mucosa to the level of the vocal cords. It provides innervation to the mucosa after entering the thyrohyoid membrane just inferior to the hyoid bone between the greater and the lesser cornua of the hyoid. This mucosal innervation is carried out through the internal laryngeal nerve, a branch of the superior laryngeal nerve. The superior laryngeal nerve also continues as the external laryngeal nerve along the exterior of the larynx; it provides motor innervation to the cricothyroid muscle.

The recurrent laryngeal nerve is a branch of the vagus nerve that ascends along the posterolateral margin of the trachea after looping under the right subclavian artery as it leaves the vagus nerve on the right, or around the left side of the arch of the aorta, lateral to the ligamentum arteriosum, on the left. The recurrent nerves ascend and innervate the larynx and the trachea caudal to the vocal cords. This anatomy is illustrated in Figures 27-2, 27-3, and 27-4. Figure 27-5 shows a sagittal magnetic resonance image with an interpretive illustration of airway innervation keyed to the colors used in Figure 27-1.

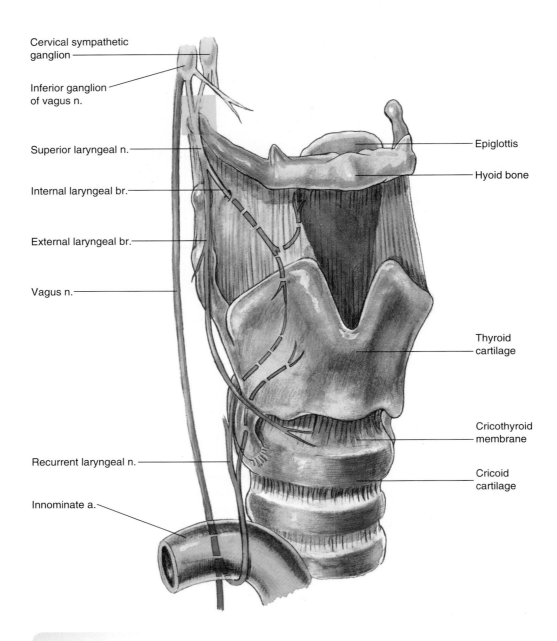

Cervical sympathetic
ganglion

Inferior ganglion
of vagus n.

Superior laryngeal n.

Internal laryngeal br.

External laryngeal br.

Vagus n.

Recurrent laryngeal n.

Innominate a.

Epiglottis

Hyoid bone

Thyroid
cartilage

Cricothyroid
membrane

Cricoid
cartilage

Figure 27-3. Airway blocks: anatomy of laryngeal, vagal, and sympathetic connections.

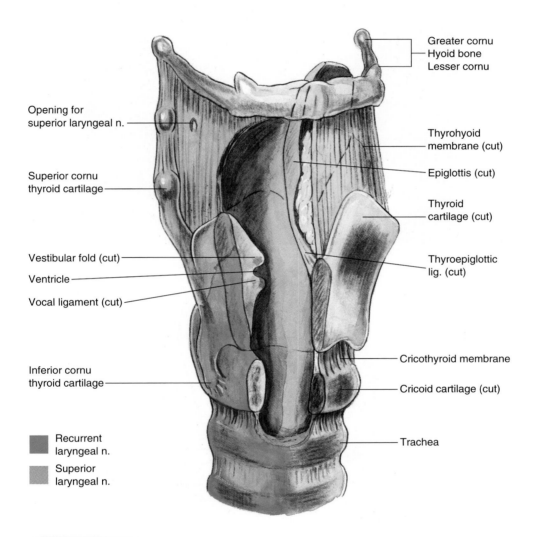

Greater cornu
Hyoid bone
Lesser cornu

Opening for
superior laryngeal n.

Thyrohyoid
membrane (cut)

Epiglottis (cut)

Superior cornu
thyroid cartilage

Thyroid
cartilage (cut)

Vestibular fold (cut)

Thyroepiglottic
lig. (cut)

Ventricle

Vocal ligament (cut)

Inferior cornu
thyroid cartilage

Cricothyroid membrane

Cricoid cartilage (cut)

Recurrent
laryngeal n.

Trachea

Superior
laryngeal n.

Figure 27-4. Airway blocks: anatomy of laryngeal structures and simplified innervation.

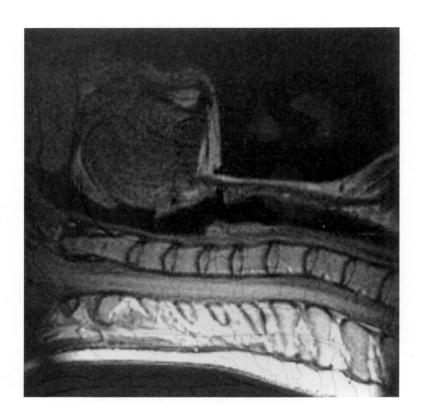

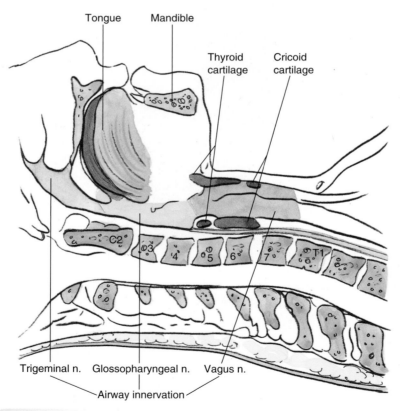

Tongue Mandible

Thyroid
cartilage

Cricoid
cartilage

C2

3

4

5

6

7

T1

Trigeminal n.   Glossopharyngeal n.   Vagus n.

Airway innervation

Figure 27-5. Airway blocks: sagittal anatomy on magnetic resonance imaging and an interpretive line drawing.

Glossopharyngeal Block

28

PERSPECTIVE

Glossopharyngeal block is useful for anesthesia of the mucosa of the pharynx and soft palate as well as for eliminating the gag reflex that results when pressure is applied to the posterior third of the tongue.

Patient Selection. Glossopharyngeal block can be used in most patients who need atraumatic, sedated, spontaneously ventilating, "awake" tracheal intubation.

Pharmacologic Choice. The local anesthetic chosen for glossopharyngeal block does not need to provide motor blockade. Lidocaine (0.5%) is an appropriate choice of local anesthetic.

PLACEMENT

Anatomy. The glossopharyngeal nerve exits from the jugular foramen at the base of the skull, as illustrated in Figure 28-1, in close association with other structures of the carotid sheath, vagus nerve, and styloid process. The glossopharyngeal nerve descends in the neck, passes between the internal carotid and the external carotid arteries, and then divides into pharyngeal branches and motor branches to the stylopharyngeus muscle as well as branches innervating the area of the palatine tonsil and the posterior third of the tongue. These distal branches of the glossopharyngeal nerve are located submucosally immediately posterior to the palatine tonsil, deep to the posterior tonsillar pillar.

Position. Glossopharyngeal block can be carried out intraorally or in a peristyloid manner. If the block is to be carried out intraorally, the patient must be able to open the mouth, and sufficient topical anesthesia of the tongue must be provided to allow needle placement at the base of the posterior tonsillar pillar. If the block is to be carried out in a peristyloid manner, the patient does not need to be able to open the mouth.

Needle Puncture: Intraoral Glossopharyngeal Block. After topical anesthesia of the tongue, the patient's mouth is opened widely and the posterior tonsillar pillar (palatopharyngeal fold) is identified by using a no. 3 Macintosh laryngoscope blade. An angled 22-gauge, 9-cm needle (see comment in Pearls section) is inserted in the caudad portion of the posterior tonsillar pillar. The needle tip is inserted submucosally and then, after careful aspiration for blood, 5 mL of local anesthetic is injected. The block is repeated on the contralateral side (Fig. 28-2).

Needle Puncture: Peristyloid Approach. The patient lies supine with the head in a neutral position. Marks are placed on the mastoid process and the angle of the mandible, as illustrated in Figure 28-3. A line is drawn between these two marks, and at the midpoint of that line the needle is inserted to contact the styloid process. To facilitate styloid identification, a finger palpates the styloid process with deep pressure and, although this can be uncomfortable for the patient, the short 22-gauge needle is then inserted until it impinges on the styloid process. This needle is then withdrawn and redirected off the styloid process posteriorly. As soon as bony contact is lost and aspiration for blood is negative, 5 to 7 mL of local anesthetic is injected. The block can then be repeated on the contralateral side.

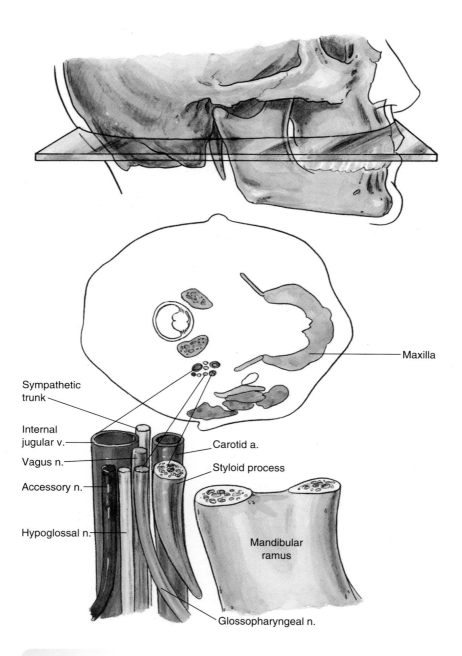

Figure 28-1. Glossopharyngeal block: cross-sectional view of peristyloid anatomy with detail.

Maxilla

Sympathetic trunk

Internal jugular v.

Vagus n.

Accessory n.

Hypoglossal n.

Carotid a.

Styloid process

Mandibular ramus

Glossopharyngeal n.

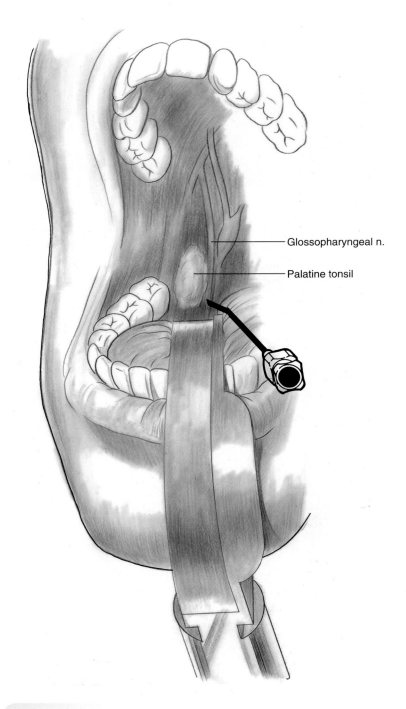

Glossopharyngeal n.

Palatine tonsil

Figure 28-2. Glossopharyngeal block: intraoral anatomy and technique.

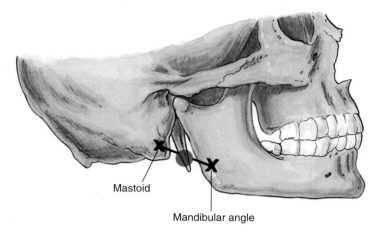

Mastoid

Mandibular angle

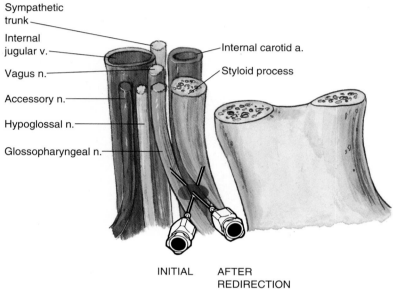

Sympathetic trunk

Internal jugular v.

Vagus n.

Accessory n.

Hypoglossal n.

Glossopharyngeal n.

Internal carotid a.

Styloid process

INITIAL

AFTER REDIRECTION

Figure 28-3. Glossopharyngeal block: peristyloid technique.

POTENTIAL PROBLEMS

Both the intraoral and the peristyloid blocks have few complications if careful aspiration for blood is carried out. In the peristyloid approach, the glossopharyngeal nerve is closely related to both the internal jugular vein and the internal carotid artery. In the intraoral approach, the terminal branches of the glossopharyngeal nerves are closely related to the internal carotid arteries, which lie immediately lateral to the needle tips if they are correctly positioned.

PEARLS

A frequent problem with the intraoral glossopharyngeal block is finding a needle to use for the block. This problem can be easily overcome by using a 22-gauge disposable spinal needle. In an aseptic manner, the stylet should be removed from the disposable spinal needle and discarded. Subsequently, using the sterile container in which the 22-gauge spinal needle was packaged, the distal 1 cm of the needle is bent to allow more control during submucosal insertion.

This block is underused when airway anesthesia is needed for sedated, spontaneously ventilating, "awake" patients requiring tracheal intubation. I believe that the block is effective in further reducing the gag reflex that results from pressure on the posterior third of the tongue, even after adequate topical mucosal anesthesia has been obtained.

Superior Laryngeal Block

29

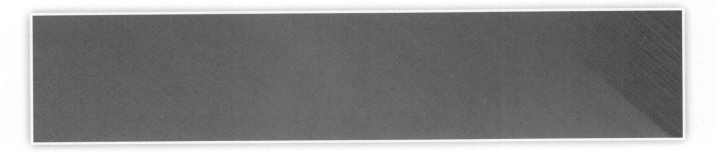

PERSPECTIVE

The superior laryngeal nerve block is one of the methods of providing airway anesthesia. Block of the superior laryngeal nerve provides anesthesia of the larynx from the epiglottis to the level of the vocal cords.

Patient Selection. This block may be appropriate for any patient requiring tracheal intubation before anesthetic induction.

Pharmacologic Choice. Lidocaine (0.5%) is an appropriate local anesthetic for this block.

PLACEMENT

Anatomy. The superior laryngeal nerve is a branch of the vagus nerve. After it leaves the main vagal trunk, it courses through the neck and passes medially, caudal to the greater cornu of the hyoid bone, at which point it divides into an internal branch and an external branch. The internal branch is the nerve of interest in superior laryngeal nerve block, and it is blocked where it enters the thyrohyoid membrane just inferior to the caudal aspect of the hyoid bone (Fig. 29-1).

Position. The patient is placed supine with the neck extended. The anesthesiologist should displace the hyoid

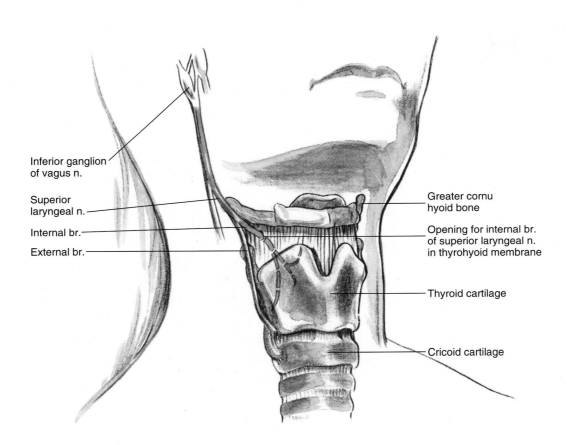

Inferior ganglion of vagus n.

Superior laryngeal n.

Internal br.

External br.

Greater cornu hyoid bone

Opening for internal br. of superior laryngeal n. in thyrohyoid membrane

Thyroid cartilage

Cricoid cartilage

Figure 29-1. Superior laryngeal nerve block: anatomy.

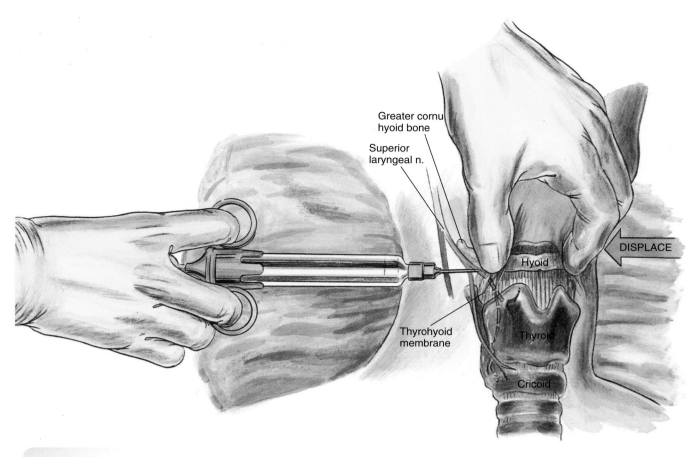

Greater cornu
hyoid bone

Superior
laryngeal n.

DISPLACE

Hyoid

Thyrohyoid
membrane

Thyroid

Cricoid

Figure 29-2. Superior laryngeal nerve block: technique.

bone toward the side to be blocked by grasping it between the index finger and the thumb (Fig. 29-2). A 25-gauge, short needle is then inserted to make contact with the greater cornu of the hyoid. The needle is "walked off" the caudal edge of the hyoid and advanced 2 to 3 mm so that the needle tip rests between the thyrohyoid membrane laterally and the laryngeal mucosa medially. Two to 3 mL of the drug is then injected; an additional 1 mL is injected while the needle is withdrawn.

POTENTIAL PROBLEMS

It is possible to place the needle into the interior of the larynx with this approach, although that should not result in long-term problems. If the block is carried out as described, intravascular injection should be infrequent despite the presence of the superior laryngeal artery and vein, which pierce the thyrohyoid membrane with the internal laryngeal nerve.

PEARLS

One helpful maneuver when performing this block is to firmly displace the hyoid bone toward the side to be blocked, even if it causes the patient some minor discomfort. The discomfort usually can be minimized by using appropriate amounts of sedation. If a three-ring syringe is used, the sedation, coupled with an efficient block, provides an acceptable experience for both patient and anesthesiologist.

Translaryngeal Block

30

PERSPECTIVE

This block, like all airway blocks, can be useful in sedated, spontaneously ventilating, "awake" patients requiring tracheal intubation.

Patient Selection. Any patient is a candidate in whom it is desirable to avoid the Valsalva-like straining that may follow awake tracheal intubation (in which the patient is sedated and spontaneously ventilating).

Pharmacologic Choice. The local anesthetic most often chosen for this block is 3 to 4 mL of 4% lidocaine. When multiple airway blocks are administered, the anesthesiologist should be aware of the total dose of local anesthetic used.

PLACEMENT

Anatomy. Translaryngeal block is most useful in providing topical anesthesia to the laryngotracheal mucosa innervated by branches of the vagus nerve. Both surfaces of the epiglottis and laryngeal structures to the level of the vocal cords receive innervation through the internal branch of the superior laryngeal nerve, a branch of the vagus. The distal airway mucosa also receives innervation through the vagus nerve but through the recurrent laryngeal nerve. Translaryngeal injection of local anesthetic is helpful in providing topical anesthesia for both of these vagal branches because injection below the cords through the cricothyroid membrane results in solution's being spread onto the tracheal structures and coughed onto the more superior laryngeal structures (Fig. 30-1).

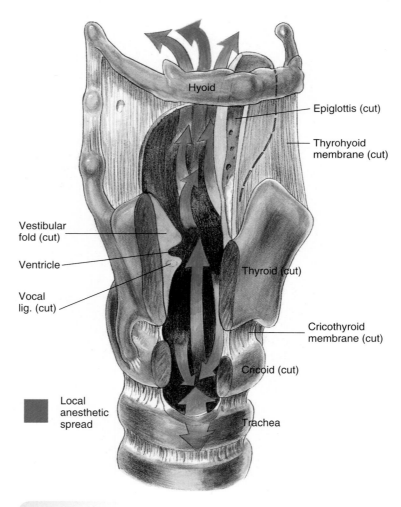

Figure 30-1. Translaryngeal block: anatomy and local anesthetic spread.

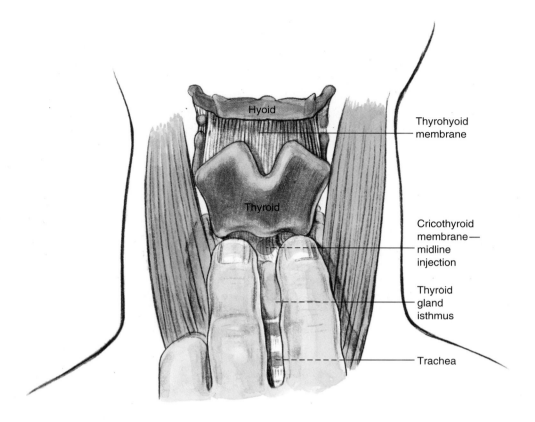

Figure 30-2. Translaryngeal block: anatomy and technique.

Position. The patient should be in a supine position, with the pillow removed and the neck slightly extended. As illustrated in Figure 30-2, the anesthesiologist should be in position to place the index and third fingers in the space between the thyroid and the cricoid cartilages (cricothyroid membrane).

Needle Puncture. The cricothyroid membrane should be localized, the midline identified, and the needle, 22-gauge or smaller, inserted into the midline until air can be freely aspirated. When air can be freely aspirated, 3 mL of local anesthetic is rapidly injected. The needle should be removed immediately because it is almost inevitable that the patient will cough at this point. Conversely, a needle-over-the-catheter assembly (intravenous catheter) can be used for the block. Once air has been aspirated, the inner needle is removed and the injection is performed through the catheter.

POTENTIAL PROBLEMS

This block can result in coughing, which should be considered in patients in whom coughing is clearly undesirable. The midline should be used for needle insertion because the area is nearly devoid of major vascular structures. The needle does not need to be misplaced far off the midline to encounter significant arterial and venous vessels.

PEARLS

This block is most effective after the patient has been appropriately sedated. There has long been a belief that this block should be used cautiously, if at all, in patients at high risk for gastric aspiration. My belief is that the block is more frequently misused by not being applied in appropriate situations than by being applied when the patient is at risk for gastric aspiration.

Another hint is to perform the local anesthetic injection after asking the patient to forcefully exhale. This forces the patient to initially inspire before coughing, making distal airway anesthesia predictable.

SECTION VI:
Truncal Blocks

Truncal Block Anatomy

31

A number of regional anesthetic techniques rely on block of the thoracic or lumbar somatic (paravertebral) nerves. As illustrated in Figure 31-1, thoracic and lumbar somatic innervation extends from the chest and axilla to the toes. Although few major surgical procedures can be carried out under somatic block alone, appropriate use of somatic block with long-acting local anesthetics provides unique and useful analgesia. Also, when even longer-acting local anesthetics become available, possibly some form of thoracic or lumbar somatic nerve block, such as intercostal or paravertebral nerve block, will be able to provide even more useful postoperative analgesia. This is approaching clinical relevance with thoracic paravertebral use during care of patients undergoing breast surgery.

One of the advantages that somatic (paravertebral) block has over neuraxial blocks is the ability to avoid wide-spread interruption of the sympathetic nervous system. As shown in Figure 31-2, the major somatic nerves are the ventral rami of the thoracic and lumbar nerves. In addition, as shown in the inset in Figure 31-2, the nerves contribute preganglionic sympathetic fibers to the sympathetic chain through the white rami communicantes and receive postganglionic neurons from the sympathetic chain through gray rami communicantes. These rami from the sympathetic system connect to the spinal nerves near their exit from the intervertebral foramina. The dorsal rami of these spinal nerves provide innervation to dorsal midline structures. The medial branch of the dorsal primary ramus supplies the dorsal vertebral structures, including the supraspinous and intraspinous ligaments, the periosteum, and the fibrous capsule of the facet joint.

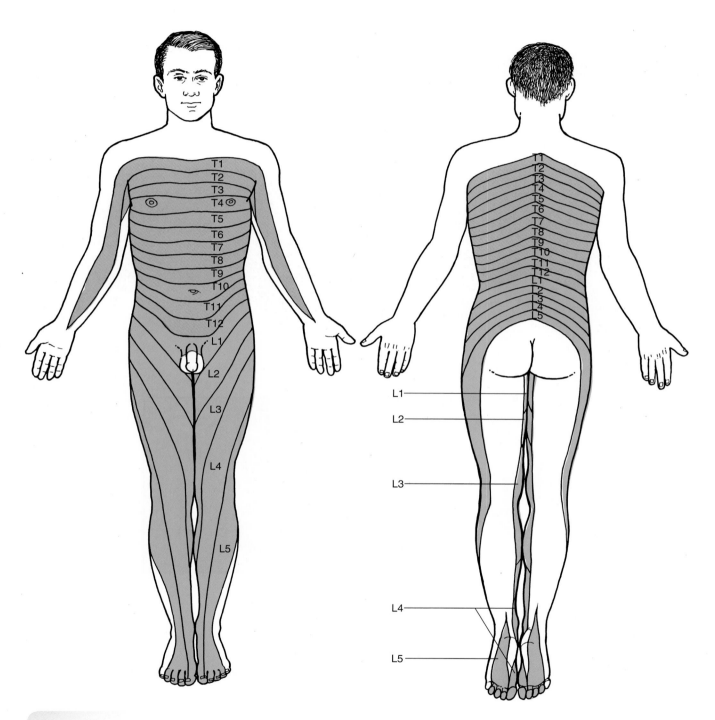

Figure 31-1. Truncal anatomy: dermatomes.

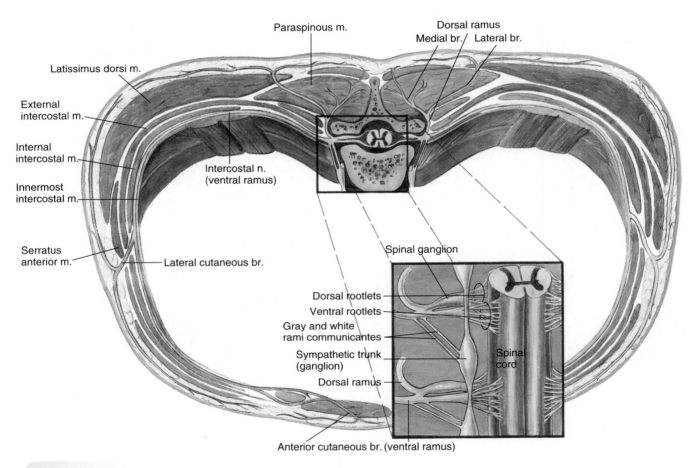

Paraspinous m.

Dorsal ramus
Medial br. / Lateral br.

Latissimus dorsi m.

External
intercostal m.

Internal
intercostal m.

Innermost
intercostal m.

Intercostal n.
(ventral ramus)

Spinal ganglion

Serratus
anterior m.

Lateral cutaneous br.

Dorsal rootlets

Ventral rootlets

Gray and white
rami communicantes

Sympathetic trunk
(ganglion)

Dorsal ramus

Spinal
cord

Anterior cutaneous br. (ventral ramus)

Figure 31-2. Truncal anatomy: cross-sectional view.

Breast Block

32

PERSPECTIVE

There is increasing emphasis on carrying out "lesser" surgical procedures for breast cancer. These lesser procedures often consist of lumpectomy or simple mastectomy and avoid extensive chest wall procedures that in the past also involved shoulder structures. For this reason, breast blocks may become more appropriate for women undergoing operations for breast cancer.

Patient Selection. Any individual requiring a breast surgical procedure is a candidate for breast block, although appropriate sedation for the block and procedure must be kept in mind.

Pharmacologic Choice. This block is designed to provide sensory block rather than motor block. For this reason, lower concentrations of local anesthetic are possible. For example, 0.75% to 1% lidocaine or mepivacaine is appropriate, as is 0.25% bupivacaine or 0.2% ropivacaine if longer duration of postoperative analgesia is the goal.

PLACEMENT

Anatomy. The nerves that must be blocked to carry out the breast block are the second through seventh intercostal (ventral rami for paravertebral) nerves and some terminal branches from the superficial cervical plexus (Fig. 32-1).

Position. This block can be carried out with the patient in the supine position if block of the intercostal nerves is undertaken in the mid-axillary line. Conversely, the same somatic nerves can be blocked from a posterior approach if the patient is placed in the prone position.

Needle Puncture. This block can be carried out with the patient in the supine position by performing intercostal nerve block from T2 to T7 in the patient's mid-axillary line, as shown in Figure 32-2A. Fewer intercostal nerves may be blocked if a limited breast procedure is planned, allowing a more tailored approach. In any event, the patient's arm should be abducted at the shoulder and placed on an arm board or "tucked under" the head, as shown in Figure 32-2A. The intercostal nerve block can be carried out by using a 22-gauge, short-beveled, 3-cm needle and placing 4 to 5 mL of local anesthetic solution inferior to each rib, after "walking" the needle tip off each rib's inferior border. If insufficient analgesia is produced, subcutaneous infiltration may have to be added because the lateral cutaneous branches of the intercostal nerve may have been missed. This is possible because the lateral cutaneous nerve may branch more posteriorly in some patients. In addition to the intercostal nerve block, subcutaneous infiltration of local anesthetic must be performed in an "upside-down L" pattern, as shown in Figure 32-2C. This infraclavicular infiltration must be added to interrupt those branches of the superficial cervical plexus that provide sensation to portions of the upper chest wall. Subcutaneous infiltration is also required in the midline to block those intercostal nerve fibers that cross the midline from the contralateral side. Subcutaneous infiltration is facilitated by using a 10- to 12-cm needle.

If a posterior approach to the intercostal nerves (or paravertebral block) is used, the patient must be placed in the prone position and intercostal nerve block carried out by "walking" the needle off, and immediately inferior to, the ribs from T2 through T7 (see Fig. 32-2B). This technique is described in Chapter 33, Intercostal Block. If a paravertebral block is planned, the technique is described in Chapter 37, Paravertebral Block. In any event, if the posterior approach is chosen, the subcutaneous infiltration, as previously outlined, must also be added.

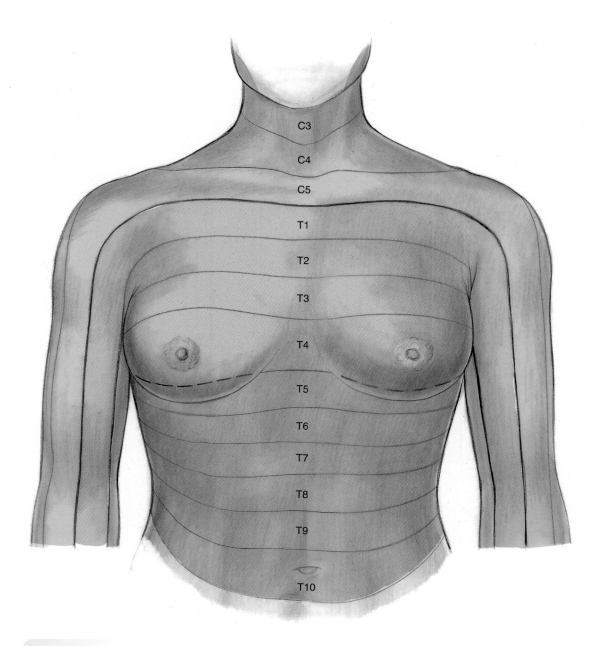

Figure 32-1. Breast block anatomy: dermatomes.

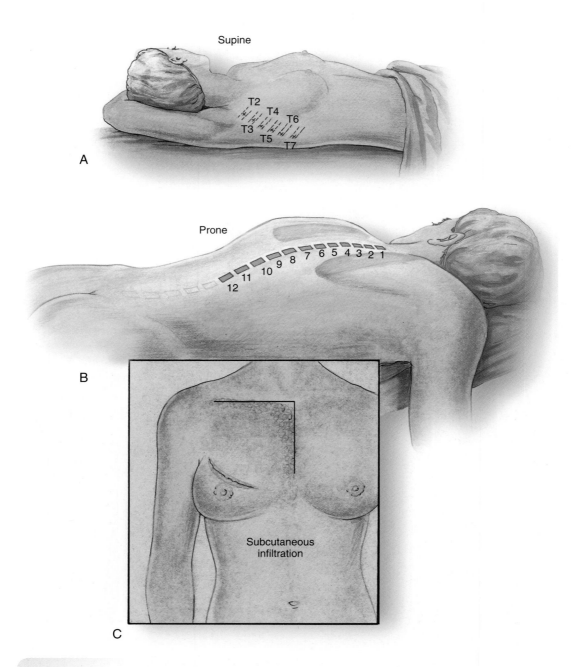

Figure 32-2. Breast block: positioning and technique.

POTENTIAL PROBLEMS

Pneumothorax can occur with this technique (or with paravertebral block), although it should be infrequent.

PEARLS

Owing to the understandable anxiety that often accompanies breast surgery, patients should understand before undergoing this anesthetic approach that heavy sedation or light general anesthesia (TIVA: total intravenous anesthesia) is most often appropriate in combination with the breast block. Patients who desire to maintain a sense of control during reconstructive or augmentation breast surgery are ideal candidates for a technique in which the loss of control accompanying general anesthesia is avoided. Finally, an emerging trend, thoracic paravertebral blocks (see Chapter 37, Paravertebral Block), are often used effectively in place of the intercostal portion of this nerve block.

Intercostal Block

33

PERSPECTIVE

Intercostal nerve blocks provide unexcelled analgesia of the body wall. Thus, it is appropriate to use the technique for analgesia after upper abdominal and thoracic surgery or for rib fracture analgesia. It is possible to perform minor surgical procedures on the chest or abdominal wall using only intercostal blocks, but most often some supplementation is appropriate. This block can also be used when chest tubes (thoracostomy tubes) are placed or when feeding gastrostomy tubes are inserted.

Patient Selection. All patients are candidates for this block, although as patients become more obese the blocks are technically more difficult to carry out.

Pharmacologic Choice. As with any decision about local anesthetic choice, it must be decided whether motor blockade will be required for a successful block. If intercostal nerve block is combined with light general anesthesia for intra-abdominal surgery and the intercostal block is prescribed to provide abdominal muscle relaxation, a higher concentration of local anesthetic will be needed. In this setting, 0.5% bupivacaine or ropivacaine, 1.5% lidocaine, or 1.5% mepivacaine is an appropriate choice. Conversely, if sensory analgesia is all that is necessary from the block, then 0.25% bupivacaine, 0.2% ropivacaine, 1% lidocaine, or 1% mepivacaine is appropriate.

PLACEMENT

Anatomy. The intercostal nerves are the ventral rami of T1 through T11. The 12th thoracic nerve travels a subcostal course and is technically not an intercostal nerve. The subcostal nerve can provide branches to the ilioinguinal and iliohypogastric nerves. Some fibers from the first thoracic nerve also unite with fibers from C8 to form the lowest trunk of the brachial plexus. The other notable variation in intercostal nerve anatomy is the contribution of some fibers from T2 and T3 to the formation of the intercostobrachial nerve. The terminal distribution of this nerve is to the skin of the medial aspect of the upper arm.

Examination of an individual intercostal nerve shows that there are five principal branches (Fig. 33-1). The intercostal nerve contributes preganglionic sympathetic fibers to the sympathetic chain through the white rami communicantes *(branch 1)* and receives postganglionic neurons from the sympathetic chain ganglion through the gray rami communicantes *(branch 2)*. These rami are joined to the spinal nerves near their exit from the intervertebral foram-

ina. Also, shortly after exiting from the intervertebral foramina, the dorsal rami carrying posterior cutaneous and motor fibers *(branch 3)* supply skin and muscles in the paravertebral region. The lateral cutaneous branch of the intercostal nerve arises just anterior to the mid-axillary line before sending subcutaneous fibers posteriorly and anteriorly *(branch 4)*. The termination of the intercostal nerve is known as the anterior cutaneous branch *(branch 5)*. Medial to the angle of the rib, the intercostal nerve lies between the pleura and the internal intercostal fascia. In the paravertebral region, there is loose areolar and fatty tissue between the nerve and the pleura. At the rib's posterior angle, the area most commonly used during intercostal nerve block, the nerve lies between the internal intercostal muscles and the intercostalis intimus muscle. Throughout the intercostal nerve's course, it traverses the intercostal spaces inferior to the intercostal artery and vein of the same space.

Position. To block the intercostal nerve in its preferred location (i.e., just lateral to the paraspinous muscles at the angle of the ribs), the patient ideally is placed in the prone position. A pillow should be placed under the patient's mid-abdomen to reduce the lumbar lordosis and to accentuate the intercostal spaces posteriorly. The arms should be allowed to hang down from the edge of the block table (or gurney) to permit the scapula to rotate as far laterally as possible.

Needle Puncture. It is advisable to use a marking pen to outline the pertinent anatomy for most regional blocks, and in no block is this more important than in the intercostal nerve block. The midline should be marked from T1 to L5, then two paramedian lines should be drawn at the posterior angle of the ribs. These lines should angle medially in the upper thoracic region so that they parallel the medial edge of the scapula. By successfully palpating and marking the inferior edge of each rib along these two paramedian lines, a diagram like that shown in Figure 33-2 is created. Before needle puncture, appropriate intravenous sedation should be administered to produce amnesia and analgesia during the multiple injections needed for the block. Barbiturates, benzodiazepines, ketamine, or short-acting opioids can be combined. Skin wheals are raised with a 30-gauge needle at each of the previously marked sites of injection, and then intercostal block is carried out bilaterally. As illustrated in Figure 33-3, a 22-gauge, short-beveled, 3- to 4-cm needle is attached to a 10-mL control syringe. It is important that the anesthesiologist adhere to the hand and finger positions illustrated in Figure 33-3 and incorporate them into his or her systematic technique.

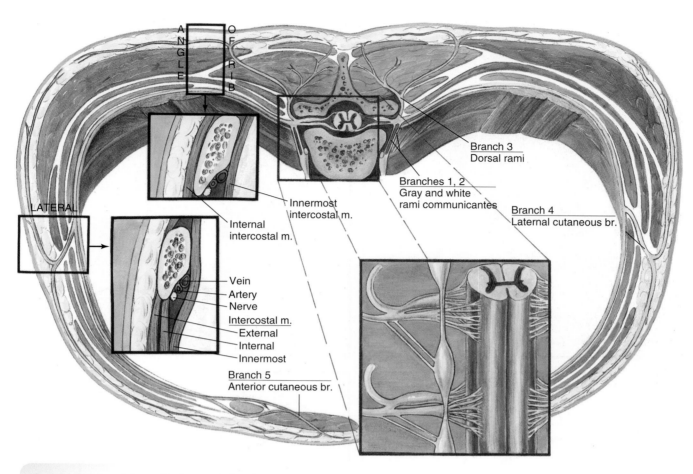

Figure 33-1. Intercostal nerve block: cross-sectional anatomy.

ANGLE OF RIB

LATERAL

Innermost intercostal m.

Internal intercostal m.

Branch 3
Dorsal rami

Branches 1, 2
Gray and white rami communicantes

Branch 4
Lateral cutaneous br.

Vein
Artery
Nerve
Intercostal m.
External
Internal
Innermost

Branch 5
Anterior cutaneous br.

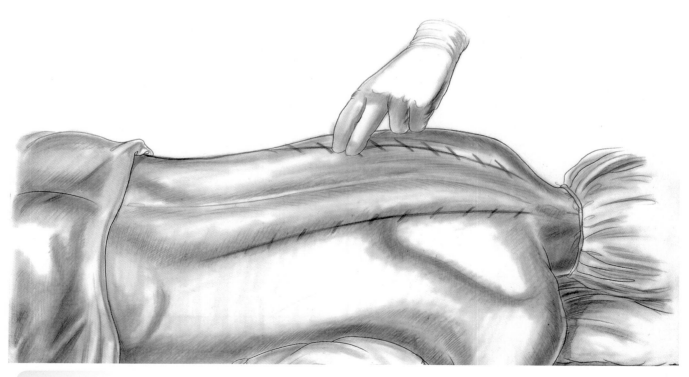

Figure 33-2. Intercostal block: position and technique.

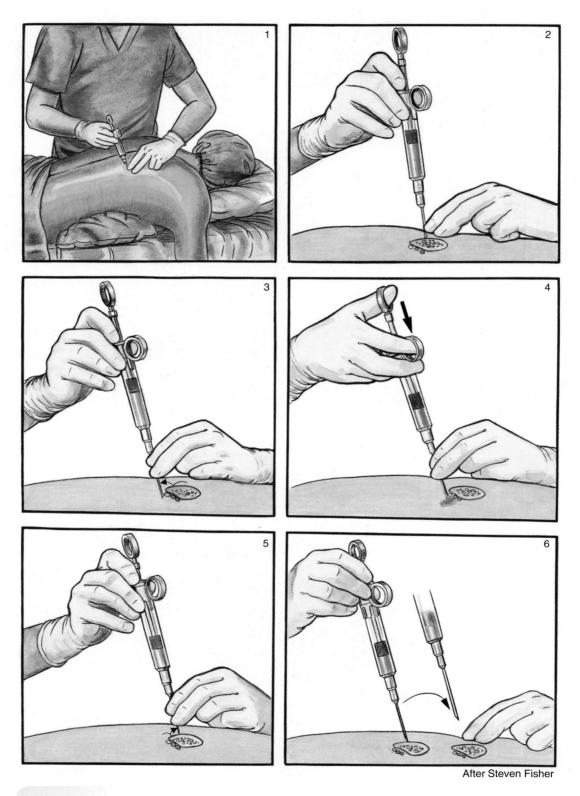

After Steven Fisher

Figure 33-3. Intercostal block: stepwise technique (1 to 6).

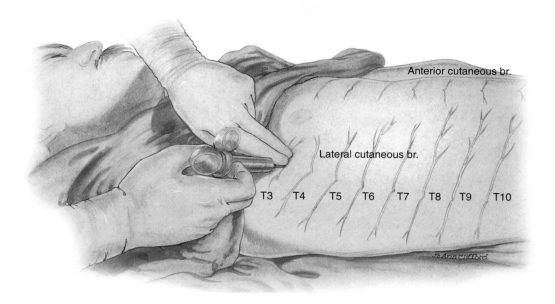

Figure 33-4. Intercostal block: lateral technique.

Beginning at the most caudal rib to be blocked, the index and third fingers of the left hand are used to retract the skin up and over the rib. The needle should be introduced through the skin between the tips of the retracting fingers and advanced until it contacts rib. It is important not to allow the needle to enter to a depth greater than the depth that the palpating fingers define as rib. Once the needle contacts the rib, the right hand firmly maintains this contact while the left hand is shifted to hold the needle's hub and shaft between the thumb, the index finger, and the middle finger. The left hand's hypothenar eminence should be firmly placed against the patient's back. This hand placement allows maximal control of the needle depth as the left hand "walks" the needle off the inferior margin of the rib and into the intercostal groove (i.e., a distance of 2 to 4 mm past the edge of the rib). With the needle in position, 3 to 5 mL of local anesthetic solution is injected. The process is then repeated for each of the nerves to be blocked. In certain patients with cachexia or a severe barrel chest deformity, the intercostal injection can be most effectively carried out with an even shorter 23- or 25-gauge needle.

Intercostal block at the posterior angle of the rib is not the only method applicable to clinical regional anesthesia. As outlined in Chapter 32, Breast Block, intercostal block also can be effectively carried out at the mid-axillary line while the patient is in a supine position (Fig. 33-4). This position is clinically more convenient in many situations and probably underused. Some anesthesiologists are concerned that the lateral approach to the intercostal nerve may miss the lateral cutaneous branch of the intercostal nerve. This does not seem to be the case clinically, and computed tomographic studies show that injected solutions spread readily along the subcostal groove for a distance of many centimeters. Therefore, even when lateral intercostal block is carried out, the lateral branch should most often be bathed with local anesthetic solution.

POTENTIAL PROBLEMS

The principal concern with intercostal nerve block is pneumothorax. Although the incidence of this complication is extremely low, many physicians avoid this block because of the imagined high frequency and seriousness of complications. Data suggest that the incidence of pneumothorax is less than 0.5% and, even when it occurs, careful clinical observation is usually all that is necessary. The incidence of symptomatic pneumothorax after intercostal block is even lower—approximately 1 in 1000. If treatment is deemed necessary, often needle aspiration can produce reexpansion of the lung. Chest tube drainage should be performed only if the lung fails to reexpand after observation or percutaneous aspiration.

Because of the vascularity of the intercostal space, blood levels of local anesthetic are higher for multiple-level intercostal block than for any other standard regional anesthetic technique. Because these peak blood levels may be delayed for 15 to 20 minutes, patients should be closely monitored after the completion of a block for at least that interval.

PEARLS

Effective intercostal nerve block requires adequate sedation so that patients are able to lie comfortably on the table during the block. Combinations of sedatives seem to be the most effective, and patients find a combination of benzodiazepine with a short-acting narcotic or ketamine acceptable. The anesthesiologist should develop a recipe for sedation; likewise, the anesthesiologist should develop a consistent method of maintaining hand and needle control for the block.

Interpleural Anesthesia

34

PERSPECTIVE

Interpleural anesthesia is a technique developed in an attempt to simplify body wall and visceral anesthesia after upper abdominal or thoracic surgery. Although considerable research has been carried out on the technique, accurate stratification of the risks and benefits of interpleural anesthesia remains elusive, and it is primarily a technique of historical interest.

Patient Selection. Patients undergoing upper abdominal or flank surgery or those recovering from fractured ribs have been most frequently selected for interpleural anesthesia. The appropriate selection of these patients remains ill defined.

Pharmacologic Choice. Most commonly, 20 to 30 mL of local anesthetic solution is injected through the interpleural needle or catheter. The most common local anesthetic concentrations used have been 0.25% to 0.5% bupivacaine or 0.2% to 0.5% ropivacaine.

PLACEMENT

Anatomy. The pleural space extends from the apex of the lung to the inferior reflection of the pleura at approximately L1. The pleural space also relates to the posterior and anterior mediastinal structures, as illustrated in Figure 34-1.

Position. The patient is most often turned to an oblique position with the side to be blocked uppermost, as illustrated in Figure 34-2. The anesthesiologist stands facing the patient's back.

Needle Puncture. Once the patient is positioned properly and supported by a pillow, a skin wheal is raised immediately superior to the eighth rib in the seventh intercostal space, approximately 10 cm lateral to the midline. If a continuous technique is selected, a needle allowing passage of a catheter (often epidural) is selected. If a single-injection technique is chosen, a short, beveled needle of sufficient length to reach the pleural space can be used. (The propo-

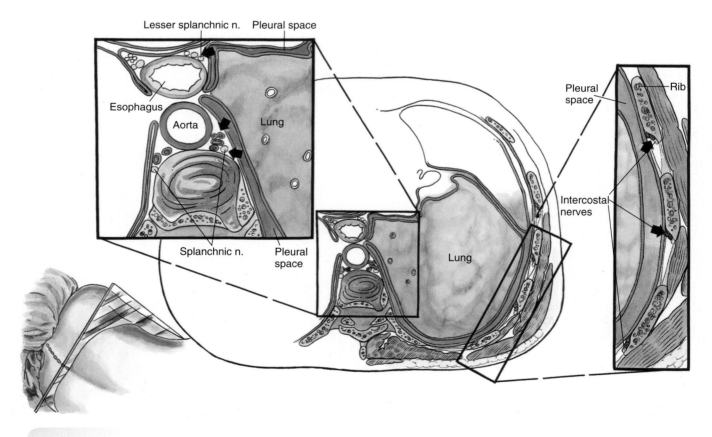

Figure 34-1. Interpleural block: anatomy.

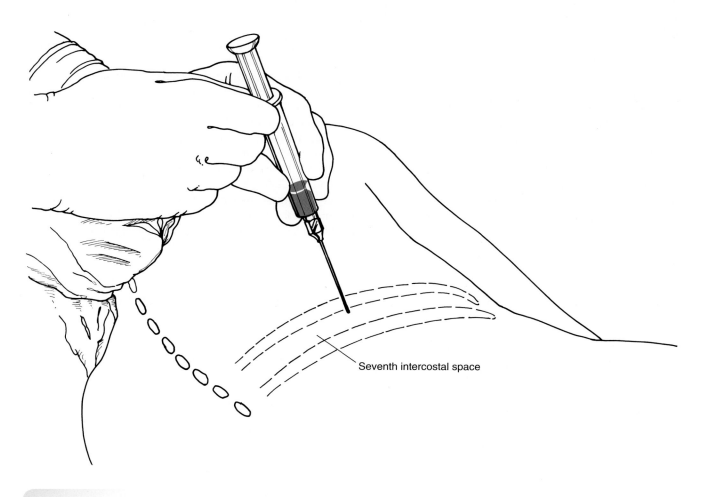

Seventh intercostal space

Figure 34-2. Interpleural block: position and technique.

nents of this block most often advocate intermittent injections by catheter; thus, a single-injection technique is unusual.) Before inserting the needle, a syringe containing approximately 2 mL of saline solution is inserted immediately superior to the eighth rib, using a loss-of-resistance technique much like that used during epidural anesthesia. When the needle tip is in the pleural space, it is very easy to inject local anesthetic solution.

Conversely, some clinicians are proponents of a modified hanging-drop technique to identify entry into the pleural space. These anesthesiologists suggest a new term, *falling column*, to describe this technique. If the syringe plunger shown in Figure 34-2 is removed and the column of solution in the syringe barrel is observed, entry of the needle tip into the pleural space is identified by a falling column of saline solution. The needle is then secured and the procedure continues as it does with the loss-of-resistance method.

Once the needle is in position, either the local anesthetic is injected, if it is to be a single-injection technique, or a catheter is threaded through the needle. If a catheter is used, it should be threaded approximately 10 cm into the pleural space, taking care to minimize the volume of air entrained through the needle. The catheter is then taped in a position that will not interfere with the surgical procedure and local anesthetic is injected. Typically, 20 to 30 mL of local anesthetic is injected, after which the patient is rolled into the supine position to allow distribution of the anesthetic.

POTENTIAL PROBLEMS

Although pneumothorax might seem to be associated with any technique that violates the pleural space, this complication is apparently infrequent with interpleural anesthesia. A second problem with interpleural anesthesia is the unpredictable nature of the analgesia accompanying what seems to be an otherwise acceptable technique. This may be a result of anesthesiologists' varying levels of experience with the technique, or perhaps it is the result of overzealous promotion of the technique.

PEARLS

The mechanism behind interpleural anesthesia remains uncertain. As illustrated in Figure 34-1, one mechanism proposed is that the local anesthetic diffuses from the pleural space through the intercostal membrane to reach the intercostal nerves along the chest wall. A second mechanism is that the local anesthetic is distributed through the pleura and into the region of the posterior mediastinum, at which point the local anesthetic provides visceral analgesia by contacting the greater, lesser, and least splanchnic nerves. When more data are available, we will probably find that interpleural anesthesia results from a combination of these two mechanisms, plus the absorption of enough local anesthetic from the pleural space to produce blood levels that promote systemic analgesia.

Lumbar Somatic Block

35

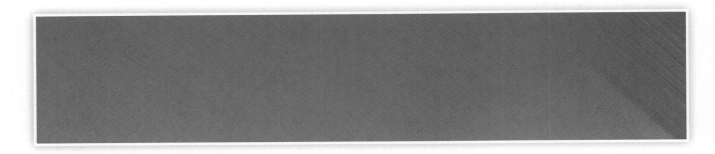

PERSPECTIVE

Lumbar somatic block is often used to complement multiple intercostal nerve blocks, thus allowing anesthesia for lower abdominal and even upper leg surgery. For example, lumbar somatic block of T12, L1, and L2 will cover most of the requirements for inguinal herniorrhaphy. Likewise, individual blocks of lumbar nerves (including block of T12 off the L1 spine) may allow differentiation of lower abdominal and post-herniorrhaphy pain syndromes. Because this nerve block is carried out in a paravertebral location, it can be considered a form of paravertebral nerve block. The paravertebral block described in Chapter 37, Paravertebral Block, is a large-volume, single-injection method.

Patient Selection. Lumbar somatic block is often used in a pain clinic setting. In addition, some surgical patients, such as those undergoing herniorrhaphy, benefit from appropriate use of the block. Also, although the frequency of flank incision for renal surgical procedures has decreased since the advent of lithotripsy, patients undergoing flank incisions are well managed with a combination of lower intercostal and lumbar somatic block and light general anesthesia.

Pharmacologic Selection. The local anesthetic choice for lumbar somatic block is limited only by the extent of additional blockade and concerns over systemic toxicity. If pinpoint diagnostic accuracy is essential for chronic pain syndromes, local anesthetic volumes as small as 1 to 2 mL are appropriate; if surgical anesthesia is desired, volumes of 5 to 7 mL per lumbar root are appropriate.

PLACEMENT

Anatomy. It is useful to conceptualize paravertebral lumbar somatic block as an intercostal block in miniature. Using this concept, the short vertebral transverse process (a "rudimentary rib") becomes the principal focus and landmark for needle position. Lumbar somatic nerves leave the vertebral foramina slightly caudad and ventral to the transverse process of its respective vertebral level (Fig. 35-1).

As Figure 35-2 illustrates, from the intervertebral foramina the lumbar somatic nerves angle caudad and anteriorly and hence pass anterior to the lateral extent of the transverse process of the next-lower vertebral body (see Fig. 35-1). For example, as the L1 somatic root leaves its intervertebral foramen, its route places it immediately anterior at the lateral border of the L2 transverse process. Similarly,

the T12 somatic root (a subcostal nerve) is found immediately anterior at the lateral extent of the L1 transverse process.

Returning to the intercostal nerve analogy, each lumbar nerve gives off an immediate posterior branch to the paravertebral muscles and skin of the back. Again, as with intercostal nerve anatomy, the lumbar somatic nerve also receives white rami communicantes from the upper two or three lumbar nerves and gives rise to gray rami communicantes to all lumbar somatic nerves. After these connections to the sympathetic nervous system, the main somatic nerve passes directly into the psoas major muscle or comes to lie in a plane between the psoas and the quadratus lumborum muscles. Here the nerves intertwine to form the lumbar plexus. Figure 35-3 highlights this cross-sectional anatomy. Figure 35-4 illustrates the cutaneous distribution of the lumbar somatic nerves.

Position. The conceptual similarity of this block to an intercostal nerve block carries through to the actual performance of the technique. The most advantageous position is to have the patient prone with a pillow under the lower abdomen to reduce lumbar lordosis. Skin markings are made as illustrated in Figure 35-5 (i.e., the lumbar spinous process of each vertebra corresponding to the roots to be blocked is identified and marked). Then, from the cephalad edge of each of these lumbar posterior spines, lines are drawn horizontally, and marks are placed on the lines 2.5 to 3 cm from the midline (paravertebral in location). The anatomic rationale behind these markings is that the cephalad edge of each lumbar posterior spine is approximately on the same horizontal plane as its own vertebral transverse process. Skin wheals are made at the site 2.5 to 3 cm from the midline on the lines overlying the lower edge of the transverse process. Through the skin wheals an 8-cm, 22-gauge needle is inserted in a vertical plane without a syringe attached (Fig. 35-6). As the needle is advanced, it will contact the transverse process at a depth of 3 to 5 cm in the average adult (*needle position 1*). Failure to contact the transverse process at that depth implies that the needle has passed between the two transverse processes.

To contact bone, a repeat insertion is made through the same skin wheal, but with a slight cephalad angulation of the needle. Once the transverse process has been identified, the needle tip is withdrawn to a subcutaneous location before being reinserted to pass just caudad to the previously identified transverse process. This allows block of the lumbar root corresponding to the same lumbar vertebra. The needle is reinserted just cephalad to the corresponding transverse process in order to block the lumbar root one segment more cephalad. As the needle slides off and past the

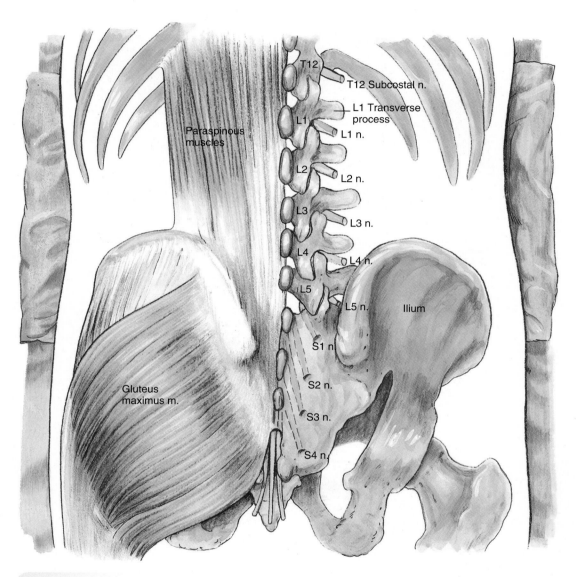

Figure 35-1. Lumbar somatic block: anatomy.

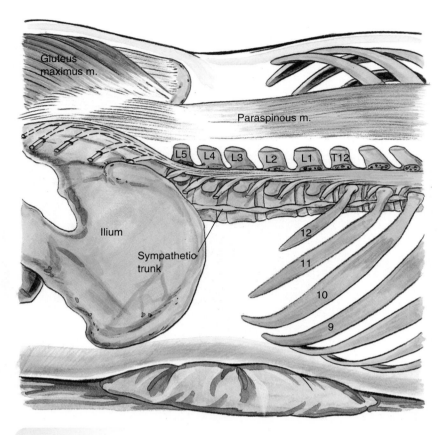

Figure 35-2. Lumbar somatic block: anatomy.

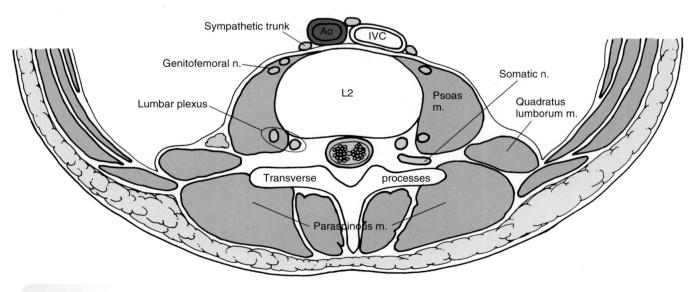

Figure 35-3. Lumbar somatic block: cross-sectional anatomy. Ao, aorta; IVC, inferior vena cava.

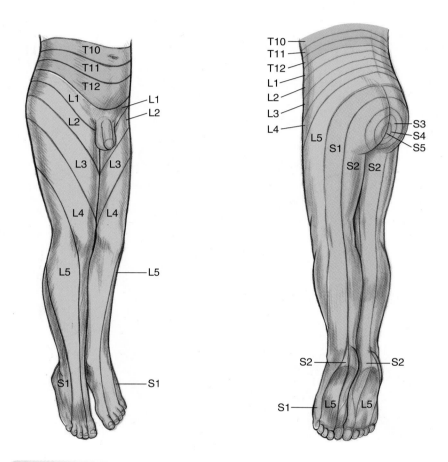

Figure 35-4. Lumbar somatic block: dermatomal anatomy.

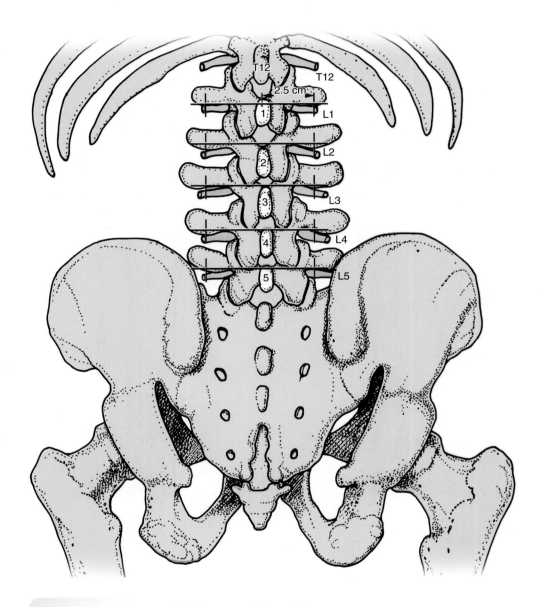

Figure 35-5. Lumbar somatic block: placement of skin markings.

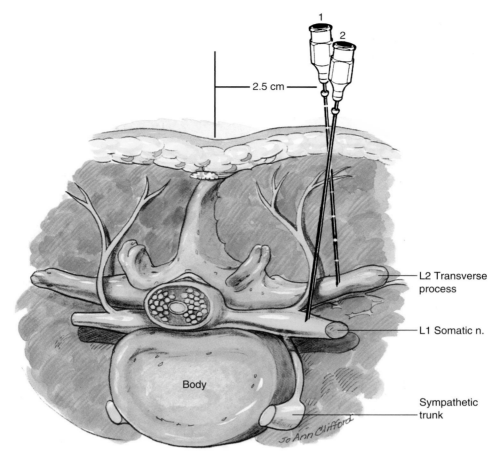

2.5 cm

1
2

L2 Transverse process

L1 Somatic n.

Body

Sympathetic trunk

Jo Ann Clifford

Figure 35-6. Lumbar somatic block: technique.

transverse process, it should be advanced approximately the thickness of the transverse process, or approximately 1 to 2 cm, after contact with bone is lost (*needle position 2*). This will place the tip in the plane immediately anterior to the transverse process. When final needle position has been established, approximately 5 mL of local anesthetic solution is injected. The process should be repeated at each site at which local anesthetic block is desired.

POTENTIAL PROBLEMS

Because the lumbar roots are close to other neuraxial structures, epidural and subarachnoid anesthesia can be inadvertently produced with lumbar somatic block. It is most likely that in these cases the needle was angled medially during insertion rather than being maintained in a parasagittal plane. Likewise, because of the proximity of the sympathetic ganglion to the lumbar roots, if the needles are inserted too deeply, the volume of local anesthetic solution

injected is often enough to cause lumbar sympathetic blockade. That may result in a decrease in blood pressure similar to that seen during low spinal anesthesia.

PEARLS

Blockade of the 12th thoracic nerve is effectively carried out by blocking the root immediately superior to the L1 transverse process. This method is often preferable to attempts to block it like an intercostal nerve at the angle of the ribs. If these blocks are used for herniorrhaphy procedures, use of a long-acting local anesthetic of sufficient concentration to produce motor blockade may limit patients from walking normally for a number of hours, because some weakness of the hip flexors may be produced with blockade of the L1 and L2 roots. If this technique is chosen for pain clinic diagnostic evaluation, fluoroscopy is advised to minimize confusion over the vertebral level injected.

Inguinal Block

36

PERSPECTIVE

Inguinal block is primarily a technique of peripheral block for inguinal herniorrhaphy.

Patient Selection. Increasing numbers of patients are undergoing inguinal herniorrhaphy as outpatients; thus, this block may be incorporated in most practices.

Pharmacologic Choice. As with many of the peripheral regional blocks, motor blockade is not essential for success with inguinal block. Therefore, lower concentrations of intermediate- to long-acting local anesthetics can be chosen. For example, 1% lidocaine or mepivacaine is appropriate, as is 0.25% bupivacaine or 0.2% ropivacaine.

Often the surgeon must supplement inguinal block intra-operatively by injecting near the spermatic cord, so the volume of local anesthetic used during the initial block should not preclude additional intraoperative injection.

PLACEMENT

Anatomy. Innervation of the inguinal region arises from the distal extensions of the more cephalad lumbar plexus nerves: the iliohypogastric and ilioinguinal nerves, which have their origin from the first lumbar nerve, and the geni-tofemoral nerve, which has its origin from the first and second lumbar nerves (Fig. 36-1). These peripheral exten-sions of the lumbar plexus and the 12th thoracic nerve

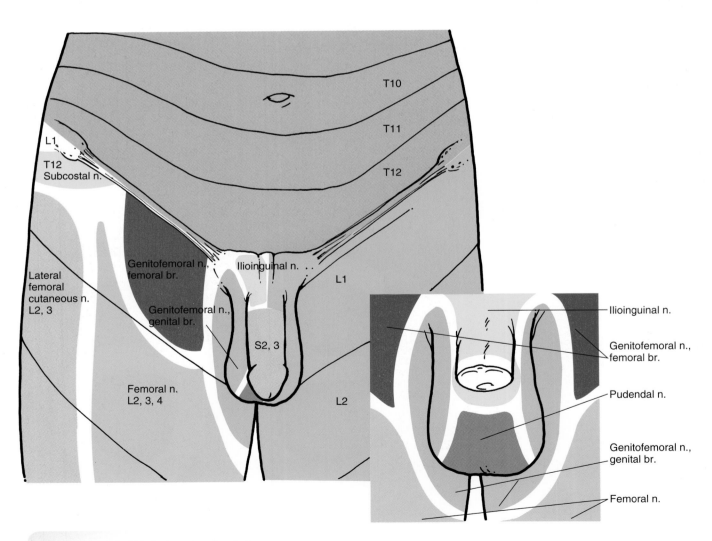

Figure 36-1. Inguinal block: dermatomal anatomy.

follow a circular course that is influenced by the bowl-like shape of the ilium. As these nerves course anteriorly, as illustrated in Figure 36-2, they pass near an important landmark for the block, the anterior superior iliac spine. Near the anterior superior iliac spine, the 12th thoracic and iliohypogastric nerves lie between the internal and the external oblique muscles. The ilioinguinal nerve lies between the transversus abdominis muscle and the internal oblique muscle initially and then penetrates the internal oblique muscle some distance medial to the anterior superior iliac spine. All these nerves continue anteriorly in a medial orientation and become superficial as they terminate in the skin and muscles of the inguinal region (Fig. 36-3). As also shown in Figure 36-3, the genitofemoral nerve follows a different course, and it is this nerve that must often be supplemented intraoperatively to make this regional block effective for inguinal herniorrhaphy.

Position. This block can be carried out with the patient in the supine position and the anesthesiologist at the patient's side in a position to use the anterior superior iliac spine as a landmark.

Needle Puncture. The anterior superior iliac spine should be marked while the patient is supine. Another mark should be made approximately 3 cm medial and inferior to the anterior superior iliac spine (see Fig. 36-3). A skin wheal is created, and an 8-cm, 22-gauge needle is inserted in a cephalolateral direction (*needle position 1*) to contact the inner surface of the ilium, as illustrated in Figure 36-4. Ten milliliters of local anesthetic solution is injected as the needle is slowly withdrawn through the layers of the abdominal wall. The needle should then be reinserted at a steeper angle to ensure penetration of all three abdominal muscle layers (*needle position 2*). Again, the injection is repeated as the needle is withdrawn. In patients who are heavily muscled or obese, a third injection may be necessary at an even steeper angle. From the previously placed skin wheal, the injection is extended toward the umbilicus, creating a subcutaneous field block. This process is repeated from umbilicus to pubis (Fig. 36-5). Because the surgeon may need to inject additional local anesthetic into the cord, the anesthesiologist should allow for it to be added intraoperatively without concern over local anesthetic systemic toxicity.

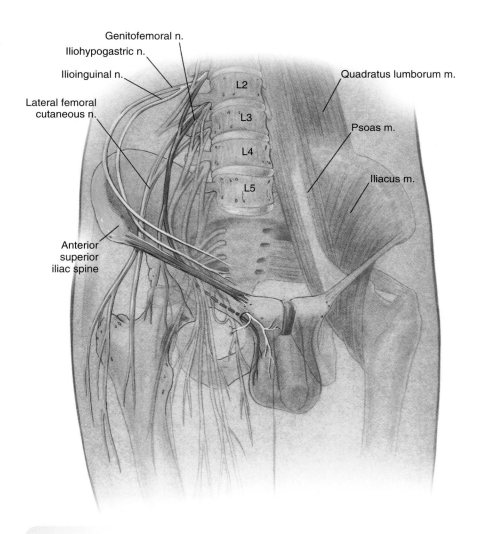

Figure 36-2. Inguinal block: anatomy.

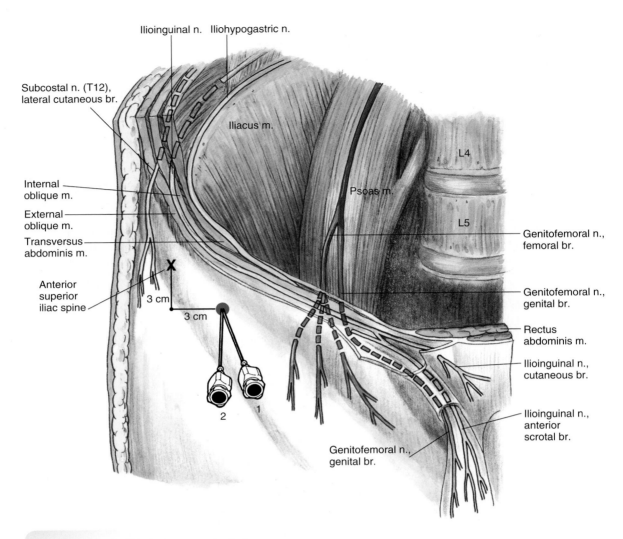

Figure 36-3. Inguinal block: anatomy and technique.

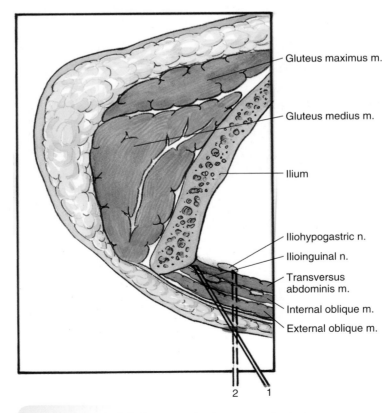

Figure 36-4. Inguinal block: cross-sectional anatomy and technique.

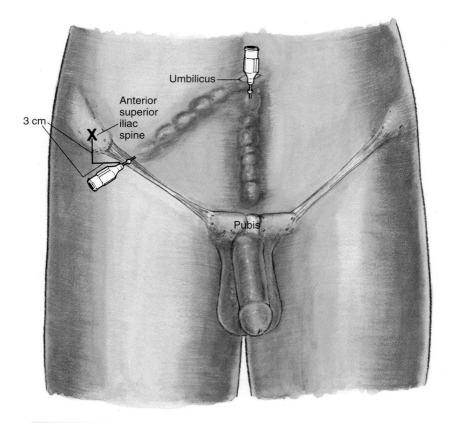

Figure 36-5. Inguinal block: infiltration technique.

POTENTIAL PROBLEMS

This block is primarily a superficial block and is associated with few major complications. Some proponents of this technique advocate making a preoperative injection in the region of the inguinal canal and spermatic cord. However, this additional injection may cause hematoma formation in the region of the cord. While this does not harm the patient, it may make it difficult for the surgeon to perform an adequate surgical dissection.

PEARLS

The key to using this block successfully is to combine adequate sedation with a systematic method of injecting local anesthetic near the iliac crest. The system should be established to ensure that the anesthetic has been deposited at all body wall levels.

Paravertebral Block

André P. Boezaart and Richard W. Rosenquist

37

Continuous Cervical Paravertebral Block

PERSPECTIVE

The cervical paravertebral brachial plexus block is a brachial root block with the same indications as continuous interscalene block; however, the classic interscalene block popularized by Winnie describes a trunk-level block. This difference has significant clinical implications. After interscalene block, patients frequently complain of an uncomfortable "dead" feeling of the arm because of dense sensory, motor, and proprioceptive block. This is generally not the case with cervical paravertebral block (PVB) because the catheter ends on the posterior root, which consists of sensory fibers. The desire to provide a pure sensory block with motor sparing, enabling patients to participate in physical therapy (especially patients with "frozen shoulder"), was the primary concern in designing the continuous cervical paravertebral block (CCPVB). In the paravertebral space, the posterior sensory and anterior motor fibers join to become the individual nerve roots. This may be the reason that more electrical current is often required to elicit a motor response when performing a cervical PVB through the posterior approach (sensory

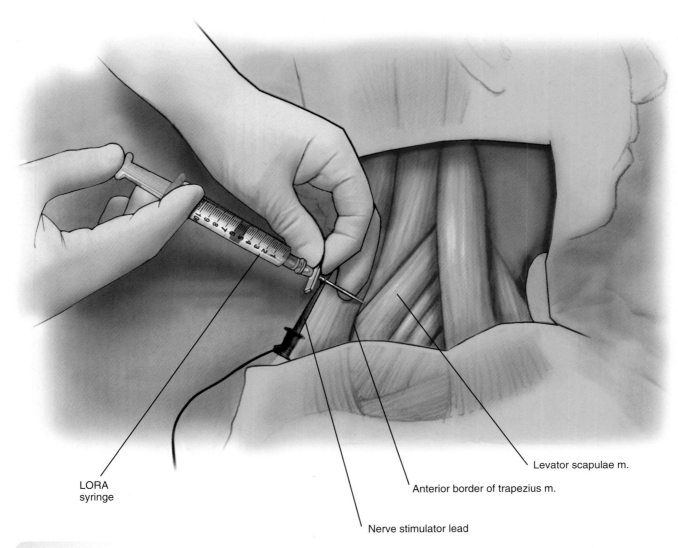

LORA
syringe

Nerve stimulator lead

Anterior border of trapezius m.

Levator scapulae m.

Figure 37-1. Cervical paravertebral block: landmarks for needle puncture in right oblique view. Note needle insertion in "V" of junction of anterior border of trapezius and posterior border of levator scapulae muscles. LORA, loss of resistance to air.

part) than with the anterior interscalene approach, and why the cervical PVB is more sensory.

The first true cervical PVB was originally described by Kappis in the 1920s. The modification later described by Pippa in 1990 was actually a posterior approach to the interscalene block because it does not "walk off the posterior tubercle of the transverse process of the vertebra" and therefore places the local anesthetic not in the paravertebral space but more laterally, in the interscalene space with the aid of nerve stimulation. Although this differentiation can become a matter of semantics, clinical experience has demonstrated the clinical relevance of this difference over the past decade.

As originally described, this block was painful because it required multiple injections and penetrated the often-tender paraspinal extensor muscles of the neck. Recently, a modification was described that avoids penetration of the extensor cervical muscles. This technique minimizes the pain associated with this approach to the brachial plexus by inserting the needle in the window between the levator scapulae and trapezius muscles at the level of the sixth cervical vertebra (Fig. 37-1).

Patient Selection. CCPVB is indicated for anesthesia and postoperative analgesia after upper extremity surgery or for prolonged continuous catheter analgesia in other clinical settings involving the upper limb. It has recently proved to be valuable in the management of pain due to conditions such as lung tumors infiltrating the brachial plexus (Pancoast tumors) and complex regional pain syndromes. CCPVB is especially suitable for patients scheduled for major shoulder surgery when preservation of motor function is desirable. Because ultrasonography, nerve stimulation, and loss-of-resistance techniques may be used for placement of this block, it is well suited for postoperative placement or for placement in patients with painful upper extremity conditions, in whom motor activation by nerve stimulator may be poorly tolerated.

Pharmacologic Choice. An initial bolus of 20 to 30 mL of 0.5% bupivacaine, 0.5% to 0.75% ropivacaine, or 0.5% to 0.75% levobupivacaine is usually used. When used for postoperative analgesia, this is usually followed by a continuous infusion of a lower concentration of the same drug (i.e., 0.25% bupivacaine, 0.2% ropivacaine, or 0.25% levobupivacaine) at an infusion rate of 3 to 15 mL/hr with or without the addition of patient-controlled boluses. Local anesthetic systemic toxic blood levels should be avoided when selecting an infusion rate and method.

PLACEMENT

Anatomy. The brachial plexus is situated between the anterior and middle scalene muscles (Fig. 37-2). The phrenic nerve is anterior to the anterior scalene muscle and lateral to the superior cervical plexus. The vertebral artery and vein are situated anterior to the pars intervertebralis (articular column of the vertebrae) and typically travel through the transverse foramen in the center of the transverse processes of the first to sixth cervical vertebrae. The

vertebral artery lies anterior to the interarticular parts of the vertebrae, so there is minimal risk of arterial injury with a posterior needle approach.

Position. The patient is positioned in either the sitting or the lateral decubitus position (the levator scapulae muscle is usually easier to identify if the patient is sitting, but effective sedation is easier when the patient is in the lateral decubitus position). The patient's neck is slightly flexed forward. The anesthesiologist stands behind the patient.

Needle Puncture. After preparation of the skin with an appropriate disinfectant and placement of sterile drapes, local anesthetic infiltration of the skin and subcutaneous tissue is performed to the level of the pars intervertebralis (which is easily seen with ultrasonography) and along the intended catheter tunneling site. The transverse process of C6 is distinctly different from that of other cervical vertebrae on ultrasonography because of the larger anterior tubercle of Chassaignac.

Next, an insulated 17- or 18-gauge Tuohy needle is inserted at the apex of the "V" formed by the trapezius and levator scapulae muscles at the level of the sixth cervical vertebra (see Fig. 37-1). The negative lead of the nerve stimulator, set to a current of 1.5 to 3 mA, a frequency of 2 Hz, and a pulse width of 100 to 300 μsec, is attached to the needle. If the block is intended for the management of pain associated with shoulder surgery, the needle is advanced anteromedially and is angled approximately 30 degrees caudad, aiming toward the suprasternal notch or cricoid cartilage until the transverse process of C6 or the pars intervertebralis of C6 is encountered. If the block is intended for wrist or elbow surgery, the needle is directed toward C7. This block is readily performed with ultrasonographic guidance, which avoids bony contact. However, close proximity to the bone is necessary if a true root-level block is intended. If the needle is directed too far laterally, the procedure will become no different from a traditional interscalene block except that the needle approach is posterior and not lateral.

The stylet of the needle is removed after bone is encountered, and a loss-of-resistance syringe is attached to the needle. While continuously testing for loss of resistance, the needle is laterally "walked off" this bony structure and advanced anteriorly. Its course may be followed with ultrasonography, if available. Usually a distinct loss of resistance to air occurs simultaneously with a motor response observed in the biceps muscle (C5-C6) as the cervical paravertebral space is entered approximately 0.5 to 1 cm beyond the transverse process. At this level, the motor (anterior) and sensory (posterior) fibers have joined to become the roots of the brachial plexus, and more current is typically required to elicit a motor response than with an anterior interscalene technique (Fig. 37-3). If more distal surgery is planned (i.e., elbow, wrist, or hand), it is necessary to place the needle (and catheter) on the C7-C8 root, and a triceps motor response should be sought.

Catheter Placement. When the tip of the needle nears the roots of the brachial plexus (indicated either by a motor response or by patient report of sensory pulsation at a nerve stimulator output setting of approximately 0.5 mA),

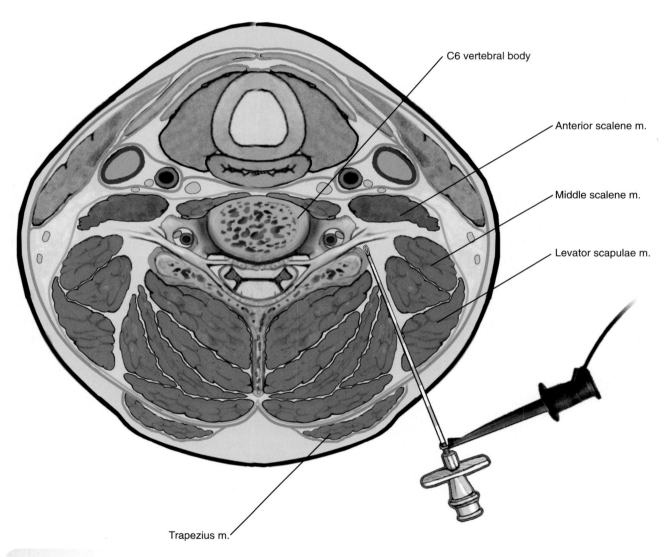

C6 vertebral body

Anterior scalene m.

Middle scalene m.

Levator scapulae m.

Trapezius m.

Figure 37-2. Cervical paravertebral block: cross-sectional view.

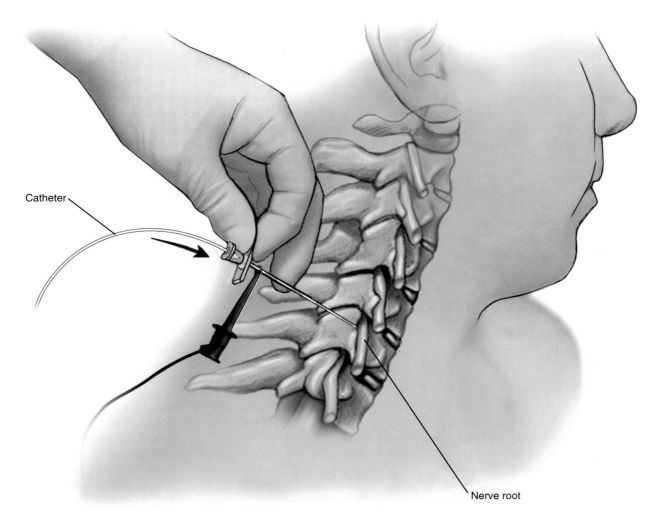

Catheter

Nerve root

Figure 37-3. Cervical paravertebral block: catheter insertion after stimulation.

the needle is held steady while the loss-of-resistance syringe is removed. If ultrasonography is being used, a few milliliters of 5% dextrose and water can be injected through the needle to confirm correct needle placement. The nerve stimulator lead is now attached to the proximal end of a 19- or 20-gauge stimulating catheter and its distal end is inserted into the needle shaft. If a nonstimulating technique is used, a bolus injection is performed through the needle followed by advancement of a standard epidural catheter, but the stimulation technique is highly recommended for all needle placements because it clearly indicates the specific nerve root being blocked. For example, a C5-C6 block will be of minimal value for wrist or elbow surgery, whereas a C7-C8 root block will be of limited value for shoulder surgery.

As the stimulating catheter is advanced, nerve stimulator output should be kept constant at a current that provides brisk muscle twitches of the shoulder or upper extremity muscles but is not uncomfortable to the patient. The cath-

eter tip should be advanced 3 to 5 cm beyond the tip of the needle, as described in Chapter 2, Continuous Peripheral Nerve Blocks. After catheter advancement, the catheter is tunneled approximately 5 cm away from the insertion site to a convenient position and covered with a transparent dressing.

POTENTIAL PROBLEMS

Horner's syndrome occurs frequently with this block, whereas phrenic nerve paralysis is relatively rare. Both of these problems and recurrent laryngeal nerve palsy and hoarseness seem to be dose dependent and are rarely seen if initial bolus injections of less than 20 mL are used. Posterior neck pain most likely indicates that some of the extensor muscles of the neck have been penetrated with resultant muscular irritation and, in some cases, pain related to muscular spasm.

Patients should be advised of the possible "crunching" sound they may hear as the Tuohy needle enters the skin and advances through the subcutaneous tissues. Appropriate sedation addresses this problem. In addition, it is sometimes necessary to block the superficial cervical plexus to alleviate the pain associated with the anterior and posterior skin incisions of shoulder surgery or arthroscopy. This is especially true for the posterior portal made for arthroscopic shoulder surgery or the incision made for a posterior Bankart repair. Because the nerve roots are surrounded by the dural sleeve at the level of the paravertebral space, all paravertebral blocks (cervical, thoracic, and lumbar) should be regarded as paraspinal (paraneuraxial) epidural blocks and given the same consideration as spinal (neuraxial) epidural blocks.

Thoracic Paravertebral Block: Single Injection or Continuous Infusion

PERSPECTIVE

Thoracic paravertebral block of the intercostal nerve roots as they exit the neural foramina provides unilateral block of the ipsilateral chest wall. The number of levels blocked depends both on the number of thoracic levels injected and on the volume of the injectate. Spread of the block (segments up or down, or laterally following the intercostal nerves) probably depends on the relation of the injectate to the endothoracic fascia and is a function of the volume injected.

Patient Selection. This block is effective for superficial surgical procedures of the chest wall (e.g., mastectomy), insertion of chest tubes, and analgesia after thoracotomy or rib fractures. It may also be performed through a catheter to produce prolonged analgesia after unilateral thoracic surgery, such as thoracotomy or unilateral upper abdominal surgery (e.g., nephrectomy or rib fractures). This block is especially indicated for patients with unilateral or bilateral pain when avoidance of hypotension related to the sympathectomy often associated with epidural block is desirable. However, hypotension may still occur with epidural spread in patients receiving larger volumes of local anesthetic in the paravertebral space.

Pharmacologic Choice. The total volume of local anesthetic injected should be considered. Each level injected with the single-injection technique requires 5 mL of local anesthetic; total volumes can easily range from 30 mL with unilateral injections to 60 mL with bilateral injections. A continuous infusion of a lower concentration of the same drug at 5 to 15 mL/hr is commonly used for continuous analgesia. Any of the amino amide local anesthetics can be used for single-injection blocks or continuous infusions.

Anatomy. Figure 37-4 identifies the nerves in the thoracic paravertebral region that are anesthetized after injection of local anesthetic in the paravertebral space. The paravertebral space is immediately anterior to the transverse process and is bordered medially by the pedicle and vertebral body, anteriorly by the costovertebral joint, laterally by the rib and costotransverse joint, and posteriorly by the costotransverse ligament and transverse process. The endothoracic fascia bisects this space.

Position. The patient can be placed in the lateral or sitting position for this procedure. The anesthesiologist stands behind the patient in a position similar to that for a thoracic epidural insertion.

Needle Puncture. The midline of the back is identified, and the thoracic levels to be blocked are identified. A point 2 to 2.5 cm lateral to the midline and at the level of the superior border of the vertebral spinous process is marked at each level (Fig. 37-5). It is important not to choose an entry point too far lateral to minimize needle entry into the pleural cavity. The skin overlying the proposed needle insertion sites is cleaned with an appropriate disinfectant. Local anesthesia of the skin and subcutaneous tissues is produced using 1% lidocaine.

An 18-gauge Tuohy needle attached to a loss-of-resistance syringe is advanced anteriorly and slightly medially toward the transverse process. The transverse process can easily be identified on ultrasonography and the needle can be followed in-plane or out-of-plane until it contacts the transverse process, usually 3 to 5 cm from the skin in most patients. After the needle contacts the transverse process and the depth is marked, the needle should be withdrawn, redirected slightly caudad and laterally, and advanced 1 to 1.5 cm deeper than the depth at which the transverse process was encountered. Using a needle with 1-cm markings along the shaft facilitates placement, but this advancement can also be guided by ultrasonography. It is important not to advance more than 1 to 1.5 cm beyond the transverse process to limit entry into the pleural space (see Fig. 37-5). Entry of the needle into the paravertebral space should be associated with a typical loss of resistance to air (or 5% dextrose in water) as the needle penetrates the costotransverse ligament. Aspiration for air, blood, or cerebrospinal fluid should be negative, and the subsequent injection should flow easily. A total volume of 5 mL of local anesthetic is injected at each level.

A catheter can be placed through the needle using the same procedure previously described for CCPVB. Nerve stimulation for catheter placement is useful but not essential for this block. If the catheter feeds too easily, it may be an indication of intrapleural catheter placement. More than one catheter may be required if the pain originates from multiple sites, such as multiple unilateral rib fractures, thoracotomy with placement of a chest tube, and bilateral surgery or trauma.

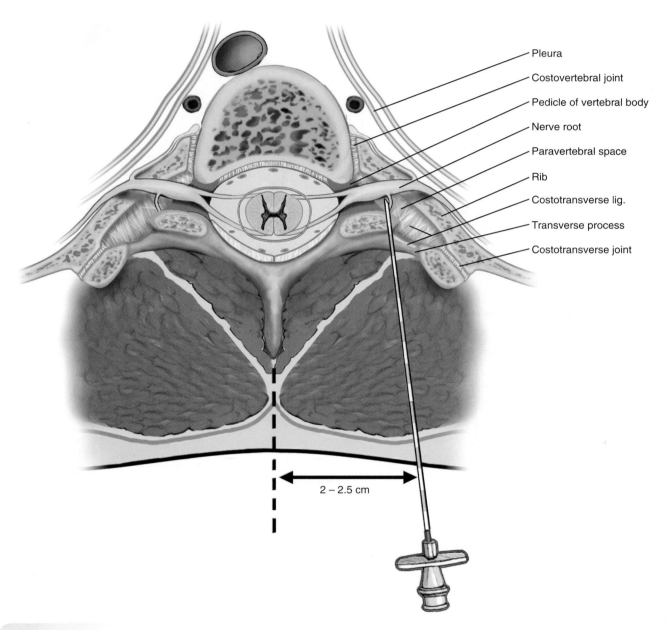

Pleura

Costovertebral joint

Pedicle of vertebral body

Nerve root

Paravertebral space

Rib

Costotransverse lig.

Transverse process

Costotransverse joint

2 – 2.5 cm

Figure 37-4. Thoracic paravertebral block: cross-sectional view.

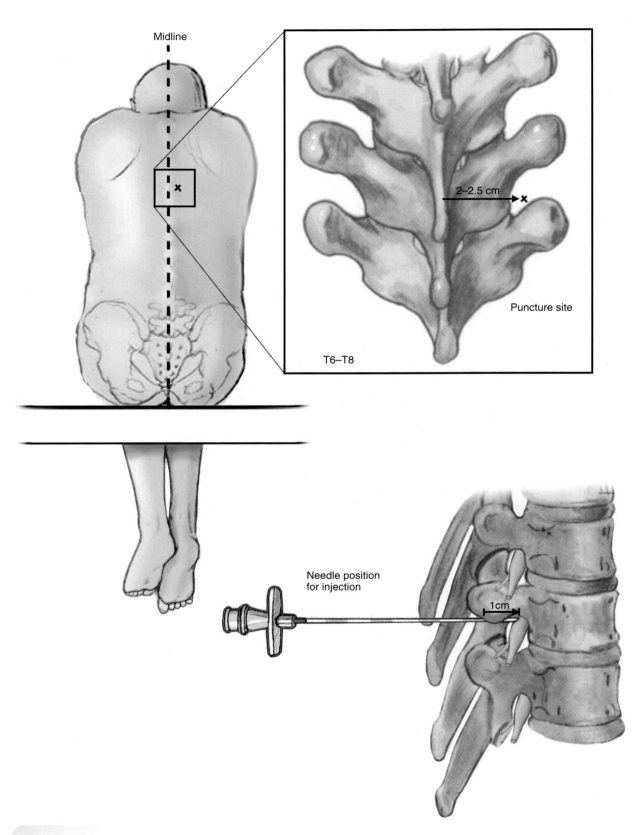

Midline

2–2.5 cm

Puncture site

T6–T8

Needle position
for injection

1cm

Figure 37-5. Thoracic paravertebral block: landmarks for block.

Sedation to make the patient comfortable during the procedure is essential. Although similar anesthesia and analgesia may be accomplished with a thoracic epidural approach, there are advantages to the paravertebral technique in settings where prolonged analgesia after a unilateral procedure and limited sympathetic blockade are desired.

Lumbar Paravertebral Block (Psoas Compartment Block): Single Injection or Continuous Infusion

PERSPECTIVE

Ideally, the lumbar paravertebral block will block all lumbar plexus nerve roots and potentially some sacral nerve roots to produce anesthesia or analgesia of the anterior, lateral, and medial thigh and the medial aspect of the lower leg. If anesthesia or analgesia of the lateral lower leg, foot, ankle, or posterior thigh is required, a sciatic nerve block must be added.

Patient Selection. This block is indicated for postoperative analgesia after lower limb surgery and trauma involving the hip or thigh. Its most common use is for pain associated with hip arthroplasty, but procedures like surgery to the femur and acetabulum of the hip are also appropriate indications. This block is typically used when it is not practical or possible to place a femoral nerve block.

Pharmacologic Choice. When selecting a local anesthetic, the degree of motor and sensory block desired must be considered, taking into account that a total of 20 to 40 mL of local anesthetic is suggested for the block and that this block may need to be combined with an additional block of the sciatic nerve. A continuous infusion of a lower concentration of a long-acting local anesthetic drug at 5 to 15 mL/hr is commonly used for continuous analgesia. Any of the amino amide local anesthetics can be used effectively for single-injection blocks or continuous infusions.

PLACEMENT

Anatomy. The nerves of the lumbar plexus are anesthetized by injecting a local anesthetic solution near the lumbar plexus, which is situated in the psoas compartment, anterior to the transverse process of the lumbar vertebral body (Fig. 37-6).

Position. Patients are placed in the lateral decubitus position with the thighs flexed. Alternatively, they may be

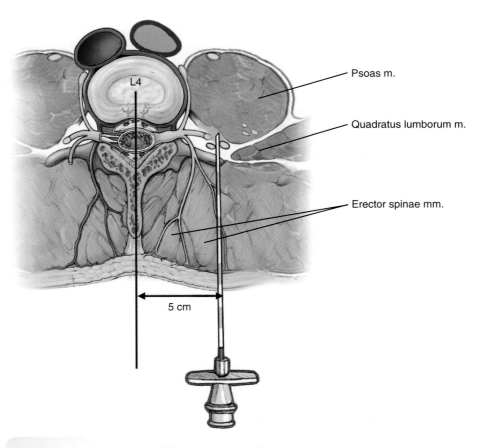

Figure 37-6. Lumbar paravertebral block: cross-sectional view.

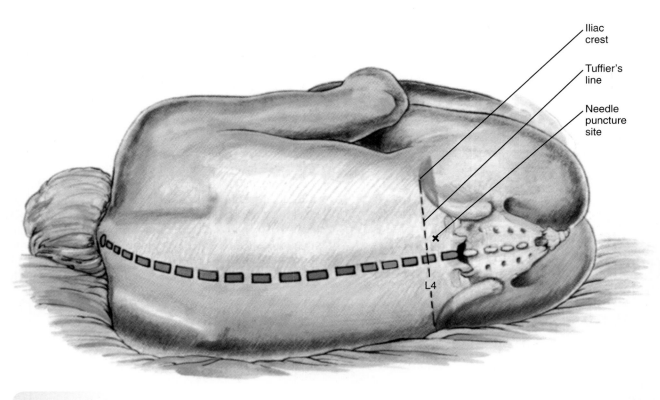

Iliac
crest

Tuffier's
line

Needle
puncture
site

L4

Figure 37-7. Lumbar paravertebral block: landmarks for block.

placed in the sitting or prone position. The anesthesiologist's position is similar to that for a neuraxial puncture.

Needle Puncture. After the patient is positioned, a line is drawn between the superior margins of the iliac crests (i.e., Tuffier's line). The vertebral spine palpable on this line in the midline is most often the fourth lumbar vertebra. The midline is marked and a second line, parallel to the midline, is drawn from the posterior superior iliac spine cephalad on the side being anesthetized. The needle insertion site is marked at a point on Tuffier's line two thirds of the distance between the midline and the second, more laterally placed line originating from the posterior superior iliac spine (Fig. 37-7). Alternatively, the needle insertion site may be determined by identifying the L4-L5 interspace with ultrasonography. The skin overlying the proposed needle insertion site is then prepared aseptically and sterile drapes applied. The skin and subcutaneous tissues are anesthetized with 1% lidocaine.

An insulated 17- or 18-gauge needle is attached to a loss-of-resistance syringe, and a nerve stimulator is set to a current output of 1.5 mA, a frequency of 2 Hz, and a pulse width of 100 to 300 μsec. The needle is then advanced in a parasagittal or slightly medial fashion until it makes contact with the transverse process. The needle's progress can be guided by ultrasonography. Bony contact typically occurs at a depth of 5 to 8 cm. The needle is then withdrawn and redirected caudad until it just slides past the transverse process. As the needle enters the psoas compartment, a loss of resistance will occur. Slightly deeper, and sometimes as much as 2 cm deeper, the lumbar plexus will be encountered and a motor response of the quadriceps muscle

observed during nerve stimulation. If it is not observed immediately after the loss of resistance is encountered and the needle is advanced a maximum of 2 cm, it may require increased current or redirection of the needle.

After the lumbar plexus is identified, a total of 20 to 30 mL of the local anesthetic solution is injected in divided doses. Because the nerve roots are covered with a dura mater sleeve, this block and the other paravertebral blocks (cervical and thoracic) should be regarded as paraspinal (or paraneuraxial) epidural blocks and should be in many ways similar to spinal or neuraxial epidural blocks. A catheter may be placed through the needle using the same procedure previously described for CCPVB. Nerve stimulation for catheter placement is useful for this block.

PEARLS

This block is technically uncomplicated. The patient will be more comfortable with an appropriate level of sedation. It is important to identify the transverse process before advancing too deeply, and ultrasonography is playing an increasingly important role in this necessary step. In the absence of an appropriate landmark to limit and guide subsequent anterior advancement, it is possible to enter the abdominal cavity. Similar to neuraxial (spinal) epidural block, this paraspinal paraneuraxial block should not be performed in the presence of significant anticoagulation or with thin, sharp needles. Although this block may be used for primary anesthesia, there are few clinical indications for this, and it is more commonly used to provide postoperative analgesia.

Transversus Abdominis Plane Block

Ursula Galway

38

PERSPECTIVE

The transversus abdominis plane (TAP) block is used for patients undergoing surgeries involving anterior abdominal wall incisions. The TAP block provides analgesia to the anterior abdominal wall. The lateral abdominal wall comprises three layers of muscle and their associated fascia: the most superficial muscle is the external oblique; deep to this is the internal oblique; and still deeper is the transversus abdominis. The anterior rami of the lower six thoracic and first lumbar nerves provide sensation to the skin, muscles, and parietal peritoneum of the anterior abdominal wall. After exiting the vertebral column's foramina, these nerves pass through the lateral abdominal wall within the fascial plane between the internal oblique and transversus abdominis muscles (the transversus abdominis neurofascial plane; Fig. 38-1). Injecting local anesthetic into the fascial plane between the internal oblique and transversus abdominis muscles produces the TAP block.

The TAP block may be placed without imaging guidance by approach through the triangle of Petit or with use of ultrasonography. The block may be performed unilaterally for lateral incisions or bilaterally if a midline incision is planned.

Patient Selection. The TAP block may be performed on any patient undergoing a procedure that involves an incision to the abdominal wall, such as open colectomy, kidney transplant, and abdominal hysterectomy. The block is generally placed after the induction of general anesthesia but may be placed at any point in the perioperative period.

Pharmacologic Choice. The most commonly used local anesthetic is ropivacaine 0.2% to 0.5%, although bupivacaine 0.25% is also an option. It is unusual to use shorter-acting agents—mepivacaine or lidocaine—for this block because the rationale for the block is prolonged postoperative analgesia. For midline incisions, a maximum of 20 mL per side is used. If a unilateral TAP block is planned, a local anesthetic volume of 20 mL is used on the side to be blocked.

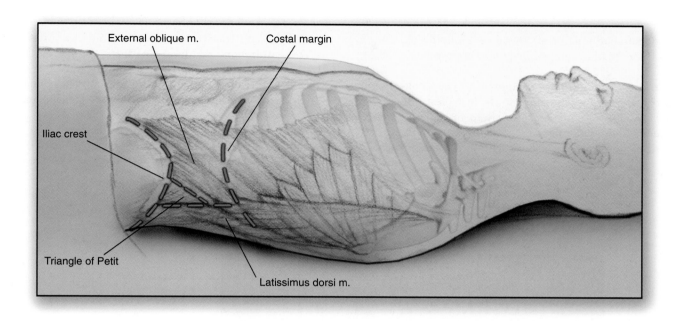

External oblique m.

Costal margin

Iliac crest

Triangle of Petit

Latissimus dorsi m.

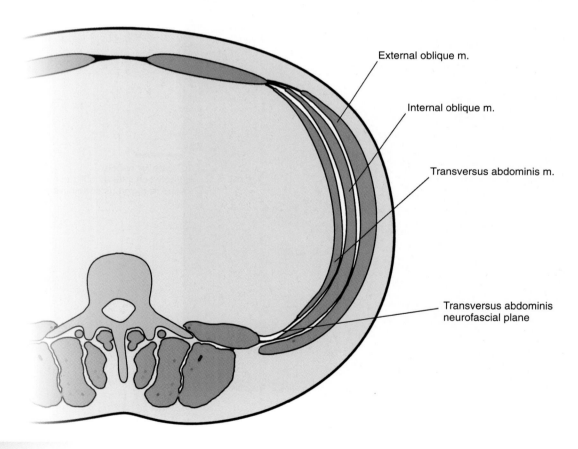

External oblique m.

Internal oblique m.

Transversus abdominis m.

Transversus abdominis
neurofascial plane

Figure 38-1. Transversus abdominis plane block: anatomy of abdominal wall.

PLACEMENT

The TAP block is generally placed in a supine patient after the induction of anesthesia and before the surgical incision. After aseptic skin preparation and draping, a 2-inch, 24-gauge, blunt regional anesthesia needle is used for the *triangle of Petit* approach. A 2-inch, 24-gauge, blunt regional anesthesia or an 18-gauge Tuohy needle can be used for the ultrasonography-guided approach (Fig. 38-2).

Ultrasonography-Guided Approach. The ultrasound probe is placed just superior to the iliac crest in the mid-axillary line, oriented transversely to the abdomen (see *Video 12: Transversus Abdominis Plane Block* on the Expert Consult Website) (Fig. 38-3). The three abdominal wall muscle layers are identified: the external oblique muscle superiorly, the internal oblique in the middle, and the transversus abdominis inferiorly. The peritoneum lies deep to the transversus abdominis muscle. The needle is introduced within the plane of the ultrasound probe and maneuvered until it is easily viewed sonographically. The needle is then advanced until the tip lies between the internal oblique and transversus abdominis muscles. After a negative aspiration, the local anesthetic is injected in divided aliquots. The transversus abdominis muscle layer will bulge inferiorly and away from the internal oblique muscle as the local anesthetic expands in the fascial plane.

Triangle of Petit Approach. The lumbar triangle of Petit is an anatomic space between the posterior attachment of the

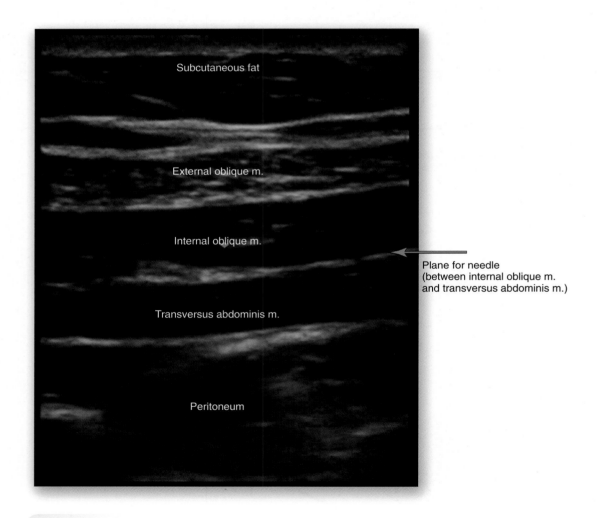

Figure 38-2. Transversus abdominis plane block: sonographic anatomy, showing plane of needle insertion.

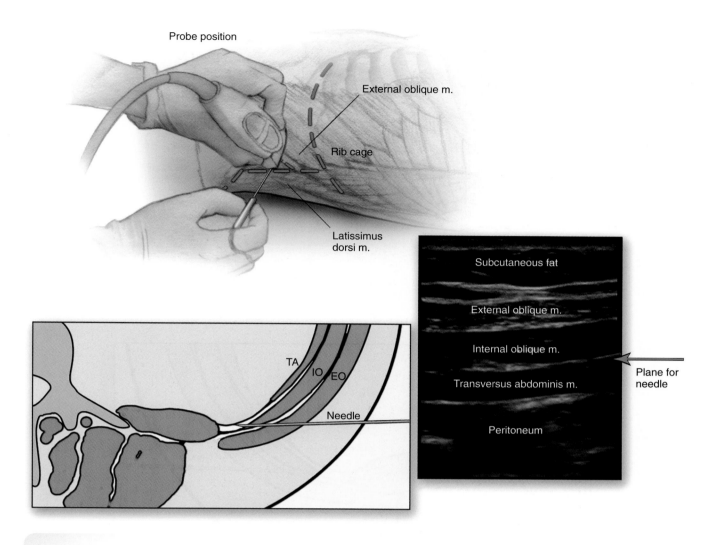

Figure 38-3. Transversus abdominis plane block: ultrasonography-guided block. EO, external oblique muscle; IO, internal oblique muscle; TA, transversus abdominis muscle.

external oblique muscle and the anterior attachment of the latissimus dorsi muscle to the iliac crest. It consists of three walls: the iliac crest forms the inferior wall, the external oblique forms the anterior wall, and the latissimus dorsi provides the posterior wall. The floor of the triangle is formed by the external oblique fascia; deep to this is the internal oblique fascia and deeper still is the transversus abdominis fascia. After aseptic skin preparation in a supine patient, the operator's finger palpates along the cephalad iliac crest from anterior to posterior until a slight irregularity is identified; this marks the attachments of the external oblique and latissimus dorsi muscles. On further posterior

movement of the finger, the edge of a muscle is palpated. This is the lateral border of the latissimus dorsi muscle. The area just anterior to the lateral border of the latissimus dorsi muscle is the triangle of Petit. At this point, a blunt regional anesthetic needle is advanced perpendicular to the plane of the triangle of Petit (Fig. 38-4). The needle is advanced until two fascial "pops" are felt. The first pop is felt as the needle penetrates the external oblique fascia, and the second is felt as the needle penetrates the internal oblique fascial layer and enters the plane just external to the transversus abdominis muscle. Local anesthetic is injected after negative aspiration.

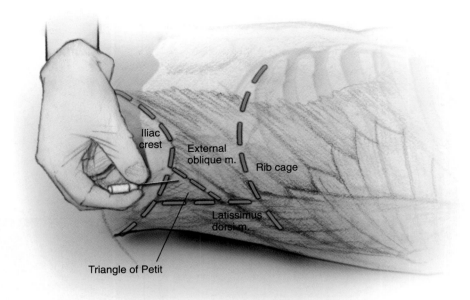

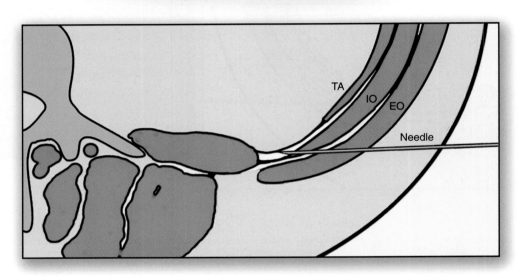

Figure 38-4. Transversus abdominis plane block: triangle of Petit approach to block. EO, external oblique muscle; IO, internal oblique muscle; TA, transversus abdominis muscle.

POTENTIAL PROBLEMS

Potential problems with the TAP block include intravascular injection of local anesthetic, allergy to the local anesthetic, and, if the needle is inserted too deeply, perforation of the peritoneum or even an intra-abdominal structure. Because of the relatively low risk associated with this technique, problems are few.

PEARLS

The TAP block is straightforward and has few associated complications. The TAP block provides analgesia to the parietal peritoneum and abdominal wall; however, it does not block visceral pain and therefore cannot be used as the sole method of analgesia for intra-abdominal surgery. The TAP block is typically used in conjunction with other analgesics in an attempt to limit the amount of opioid needed for postoperative pain relief.

SECTION VII:
Neuraxial Blocks

Neuraxial Block Anatomy

39

Neuraxial blocks—spinal, epidural, and caudal—are the most widely used regional blocks. The main reasons for their popularity are that neuraxial blocks have well-defined end points and the anesthesiologist can produce the blocks reliably with a single injection. The first step in being able to use neuraxial blocks effectively is to gain an understanding of neuraxial anatomy.

To understand the neuraxial anatomy it is necessary to develop a concept of the relationship between surface and bony anatomy pertinent to the neuraxial structures (Fig. 39-1). Beginning cephalad, the spinous process of the seventh cervical vertebra, the vertebral prominence, is the most prominent midline structure at the base of the neck. A line drawn between the lower borders of the scapula crosses the vertebral axis at approximately the spinous process of T7. The lower extent of the spinal cord, the conus medullaris, ends in the adult at approximately L1. (In the infant the conus medullaris may extend to L3.) The line between the iliac crests (Tuffier's or the intercrestal line) most often crosses through the spinous process of L4. A line drawn between the posterior superior iliac spines identifies the level of the second sacral vertebra and the caudal extent of the dural sac containing cerebrospinal fluid (CSF).

The 33 vertebrae from C1 to the tip of the coccyx have a number of common features as well as differences that should be highlighted. Each vertebra contains a spinous process joined to the lamina, from which a transverse process extends laterally into both lamina and pedicle. The

pedicle joins this posterior assembly to the vertebral body, which relates to the neighboring vertebral bodies through both superior and inferior facet joints (Fig. 39-2). Figure 39-3 outlines the general relationship of these structures at levels that correspond to common sites for cervical, thoracic, and lumbar punctures of the neuraxis.

The lateral, oblique, and posterior views highlight two features of the bony anatomy that need emphasis. First, in the cervical and lumbar vertebrae, the spinous process assumes a more horizontal orientation than in the mid-thoracic region. The caudal angulation of the spinous process in the mid-thoracic region highlights why needle puncture of the neuraxial structures in this area requires a more cephalad needle angulation. Conversely, in both the cervical and lumbar regions, it is possible to use a more direct (perpendicular) needle angle to reach the neuraxial structures. The second feature is the angulation of the lamina immediately lateral to the spinous process in the three regions. As illustrated by the black line in the lateral view of the vertebral bodies, from cephalad to caudad the vertebral laminae become more vertical. Both of these features are important for understanding the technique of "walking" needles off the lamina into the desired neuraxial locations.

In addition to the bony relationships of the vertebral bodies, there are important ligamentous relationships. As illustrated in Figure 39-4, defining the posterior limit of the epidural space is the ligamentum flavum, or "yellow ligament." This ligament extends from the foramen magnum

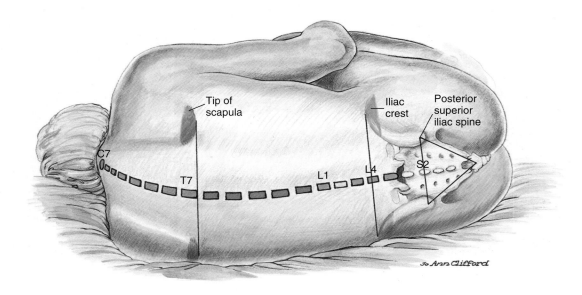

Figure 39-1. Neuraxial anatomy: surface relationships.

LUMBAR VERTEBRA

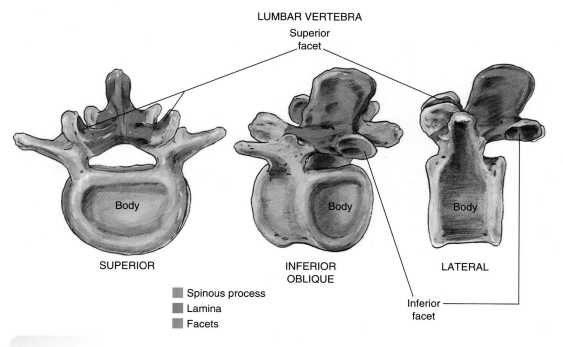

Superior
facet

Body

Body

Body

SUPERIOR

INFERIOR
OBLIQUE

LATERAL

Spinous process
Lamina
Facets

Inferior
facet

Figure 39-2. Neuraxial anatomy: lumbar vertebra.

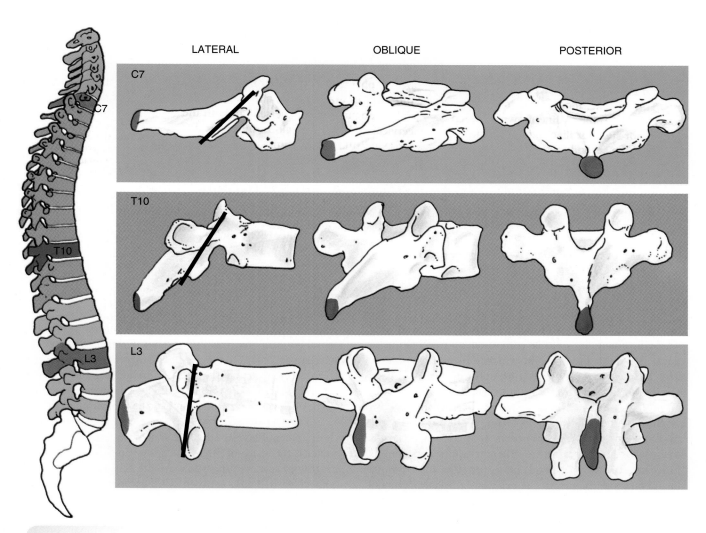

LATERAL

OBLIQUE

POSTERIOR

C7

T10

L3

Figure 39-3. Neuraxial anatomy: vertebral column relationships.

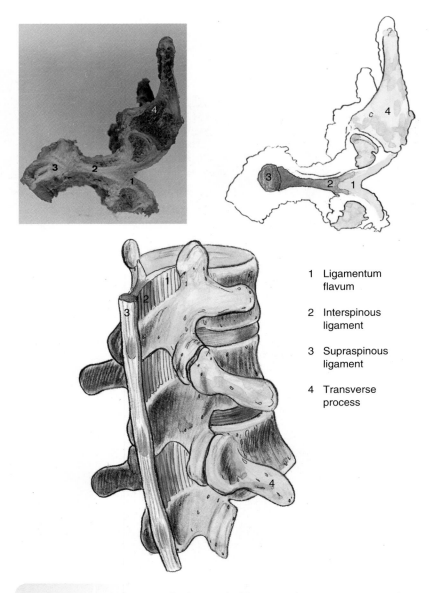

1 Ligamentum
flavum

2 Interspinous
ligament

3 Supraspinous
ligament

4 Transverse
process

Figure 39-4. Neuraxial anatomy: lumbar vertebral ligaments. *(From Zarzur E. Anatomic studies of the human lumbar ligamentum flavum. Anesth Analg. 1984;63:499-502, with permission.)*

to the sacral hiatus. Although classically portrayed as a single ligament, it is really composed of two ligamenta flava, the right and the left, which join in the midline. The ligamentum flavum is not uniform from skull to sacrum or even within an intervertebral space. Within an individual intervertebral space, the ligamentum flavum is thicker caudally than cephalad and thicker in the midline than on its lateral borders. Immediately posterior to the ligamentum flavum are either the lamina and spinous processes of the vertebral body, or the interspinous ligament. Extending from the external occipital protuberance to the coccyx posterior to these structures is the supraspinous ligament, which joins the vertebral spinous processes.

Most neuraxial blocks are performed in the lumbar region. Figures 39-5, 39-6, and 39-7 illustrate the lumbar anatomy in the posterior, lateral, and horizontal planes,

respectively. Surrounding the spinal cord in the bony vertebral column are three membranes. From the immediate overlay of the cord to the periphery, these are the pia mater, the arachnoid mater, and the dura mater. The *pia mater* is a highly vascular membrane that closely invests the spinal cord. The *arachnoid mater* is a delicate, nonvascular membrane that is closely attached to the outermost layer, the dura mater. Between the pia mater and the arachnoid mater is the space of interest in spinal anesthesia, the subarachnoid space. In this space are the CSF, spinal nerves, a trabecular network between the two membranes, blood vessels that supply the spinal cord, and the lateral extensions of the pia mater, the dentate ligaments. These dentate ligaments supply lateral support from the spinal cord to the dura mater and may become important conceptually when unilateral or patchy spinal anesthesia results from what appears to be a technically adequate block. The third

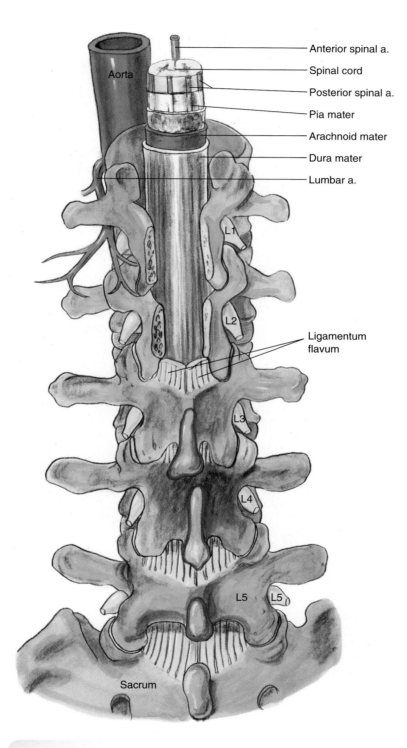

Anterior spinal a.

Spinal cord

Posterior spinal a.

Pia mater

Arachnoid mater

Dura mater

Lumbar a.

Aorta

L1

L2

Ligamentum flavum

L3

L4

L5   L5

Sacrum

Figure 39-5. Neuraxial anatomy: posterior lumbar details.

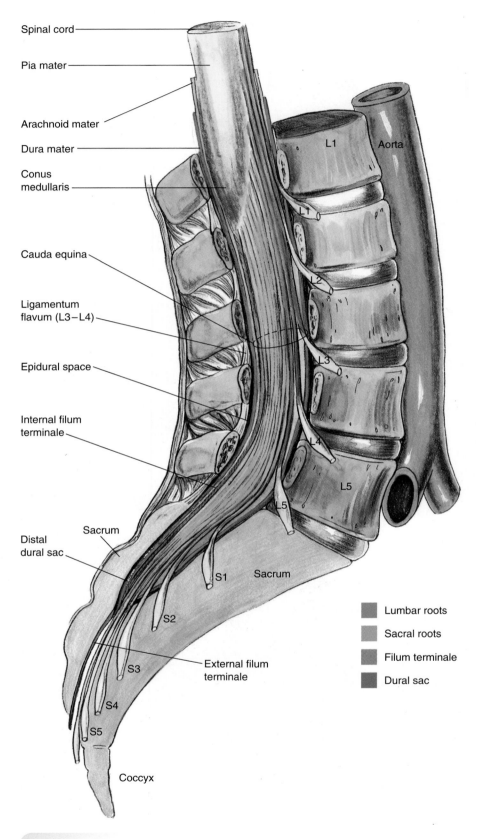

Spinal cord

Pia mater

Arachnoid mater

Dura mater

Conus
medullaris

Cauda equina

Ligamentum
flavum (L3–L4)

Epidural space

Internal filum
terminale

Distal
dural sac

Sacrum

Coccyx

L1

Aorta

L1

L2

L3

L4

L5

L5

Sacrum

S1

S2

S3

S4

S5

External filum
terminale

Lumbar roots

Sacral roots

Filum terminale

Dural sac

Figure 39-6. Neuraxial anatomy: lateral lumbar details.

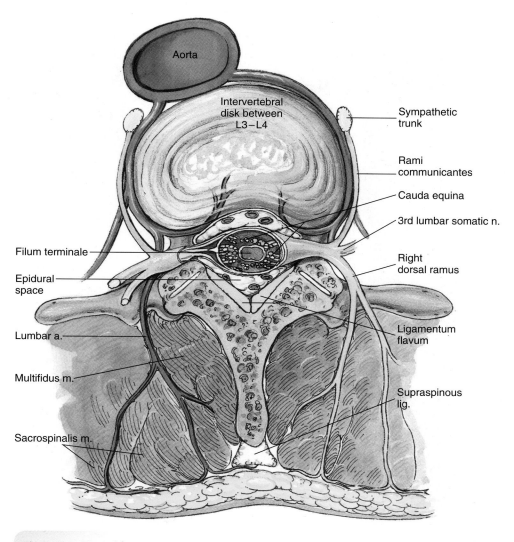

Figure 39-7. Neuraxial anatomy: cross-sectional (horizontal) lumbar details.

and outermost membrane in the spinal canal is the longitudinally organized fibroelastic membrane called the *dura mater* (or theca). This layer is the direct extension of the cranial dura mater and extends as spinal dura mater from the foramen magnum to S2, where the filum terminale (an extension of the pia mater beginning at the conus medullaris) blends with the periosteum on the coccyx (see Fig. 39-6). There is a potential space between the dura mater and the arachnoid, the subdural space, which contains only small amounts of serous fluid to allow the dura and arachnoid to move over each other. This space is not intentionally used by anesthesiologists, although injection into it during spinal anesthesia may explain the occasional failed spinal anesthetic and the rare "total spinal" after epidural anesthesia, when there was no indication of errant injection of the local anesthetic into the CSF.

Surrounding the dura mater, and in its posterior extent immediately anterior to the ligamentum flavum, is another space effectively used by anesthesiologists, the epidural space. The spinal epidural space extends from the foramen magnum to the sacral hiatus and surrounds the dura mater anteriorly, laterally, and, more usefully, posteriorly. Contents of the epidural space include the nerve roots that traverse it from the intervertebral foramina to peripheral locations, as well as fat, areolar tissue, lymphatics, and blood vessels, which include the well-organized venous plexus of Batson.

Advances in epiduroscopy and epidurography provide an anatomic explanation for the occasional unilateral anesthesia that may follow an apparently adequate epidural technique. The almost universal appearance of a dorsomedian connective tissue band in the midline of the epidural space has been noted with these invasive imaging techniques as well as with some anatomic dissection specimens. This explanation for the occurrence of unilateral epidural block must be considered in view of microscopic thin-section anatomic evidence suggesting that the structure called the "dorsomedian connective tissue band" is really a midline posterior fat pedicle.

The anatomy important during caudal anesthesia is an extension of the epidural anatomy, although the frequent variations in sacral anatomy deserve emphasis. The sacrum results from the fusion of the five sacral vertebrae, whereas the sacral hiatus results from the failure of the laminae of S5 and usually part of S4 to fuse in the midline. The sacral hiatus results in a variably shaped and sized, inverted "V"-

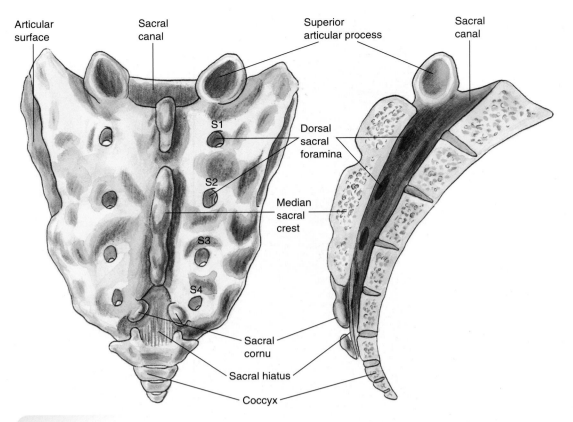

Figure 39-8. Neuraxial anatomy: sacrum.

shaped bony defect, covered by the posterior sacrococcygeal ligament, which is a functional counterpart to the ligamentum flavum (Fig. 39-8). The hiatus may be identified by locating the sacral cornu (remnants of the S5 articular processes). This bony defect allows percutaneous access to the sacral canal, although the frequent anatomic variation of the sacral hiatus can make caudal block confusing. The sacral canal is functionally the distal extent of the epidural space, and from this canal the pelvic sacral foramina open ventrally toward the ischial rectal fossa, whereas the dorsal sacral foramina open in a posterior direction (see Fig. 39-8). In the sacral canal, the nerves of the cauda equina continue until they exit through their respective vertebral foramina. Once again, the dural sac continues to the level of S2, or the line joining the posterior superior iliac spines.

Spinal Block

40

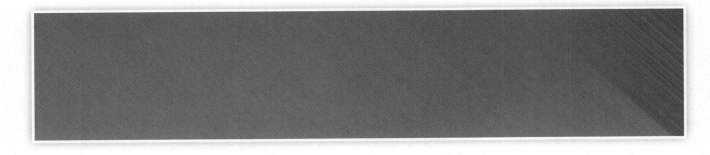

PERSPECTIVE

Spinal anesthesia is unparalleled in that a small mass of drug, virtually devoid of systemic pharmacologic effect, can produce profound, reproducible surgical anesthesia. Further, by altering the small mass of drug, very different types of spinal anesthesia can be produced. Low spinal anesthesia, a block below T10, has a different physiologic impact than does a block performed to produce higher spinal anesthesia (above T5). The block is unexcelled for lower abdominal or lower extremity surgical procedures. However, for operations in the mid- to upper abdomen, light general anesthesia may have to supplement the spinal block because stimulation of the diaphragm during upper abdominal procedures often causes some discomfort. This area is difficult to block completely through high spinal anesthesia because to do so requires blockade of the phrenic nerve.

Patient Selection. Patient selection for spinal anesthesia often places too much emphasis on a side effect of the technique—namely, spinal headache—than on the applicability of the technique in a given patient. It is clear that the incidence of spinal headache increases with decreasing age and female sex; however, with proper technique and selection of needle size and tip configuration, the incidence of headache should not preclude the use of spinal anesthesia in young, healthy patients if the block has advantages over epidural anesthesia. Almost any patient who is to have a lower extremity operation is a candidate for spinal anesthesia, as are most patients scheduled for lower abdominal surgery, such as inguinal herniorrhaphy and gynecologic, urologic, and obstetric procedures.

Pharmacologic Choice. In the United States, three local anesthetics are commonly used to produce spinal anesthesia: lidocaine, tetracaine, and bupivacaine. Lidocaine is a short- to intermediate-acting spinal drug; tetracaine and bupivacaine provide intermediate- to long-acting block. Lidocaine, without epinephrine, is often chosen for procedures that can be completed in 1 hour or less. It is likely that the lidocaine mixture most commonly used is still a 5% solution in 7.5% dextrose, although increasingly anesthesiologists are using 1.5% to 2% concentrations of lidocaine without dextrose as alternatives. When epinephrine (0.2 mg) is added to lidocaine, the useful length of clinical anesthesia in the lower abdomen and lower extremities is approximately 90 minutes. Tetracaine is packaged both as niphanoid crystals (20 mg) and as a 1% solution (2 mL total). When dextrose is added to make tetracaine hyper-

baric, the drug generally produces effective clinical anesthesia for procedures of up to 1.5 to 2 hours in the plain form, for up to 2 to 3 hours when epinephrine (0.2 mg) is added, and for up to 5 hours for lower extremity procedures when phenylephrine (5 mg) is added as a vasoconstrictor. Bupivacaine spinal anesthesia is commonly carried out with 0.5% or 0.75% solution, either plain or in 8.25% dextrose. My impression is that the clinical difference between 0.5% tetracaine and 0.75% bupivacaine as hyperbaric solutions is minimal. Bupivacaine is appropriate for procedures lasting up to 2 or 3 hours.

In addition to hyperbaric technique, local anesthetics can be mixed to produce hypobaric spinal anesthesia. A common method of formulating a hypobaric solution is to mix tetracaine in a 0.1% to 0.33% solution with sterile water. Also, lidocaine can be mixed to provide useful hypobaric spinal anesthesia. This drug is diluted from a 2% solution with sterile water to make a 0.5% solution, using a total of 30 to 40 mg.

Many anesthesiologists avoid vasoconstrictors for fear of somehow increasing the risk in spinal anesthesia. These anesthesiologists believe that phenylephrine or epinephrine has such potent vasoconstrictive action that it puts the blood supply of the spinal cord at risk. There are no human data supporting this theory. In fact, because most local anesthetics are vasodilators, the addition of these vasoconstrictors does little more than maintain spinal cord blood flow at a basal level. Commonly used doses of vasoconstrictors are 0.2 to 0.3 mg of epinephrine and 5 mg of phenylephrine added to the spinal anesthetic.

PLACEMENT

Anatomy. As outlined in Chapter 39, Neuraxial Block Anatomy, the spinous processes of the lumbar vertebrae have an almost horizontal orientation in relation to the long axis of their respective vertebral bodies (Fig. 40-1). When a midline needle is inserted between the lumbar vertebral spinous processes, it is most effective if it is placed almost perpendicularly in relation to the long axis of the back. To facilitate spinal anesthesia, the anesthesiologist must constantly keep in mind the midline of the patient's body and the neuraxis in relation to the needle. As illustrated in Figure 40-1, as a midline needle is inserted into the cerebrospinal fluid (CSF), it logically must puncture the skin, subcutaneous tissue, supraspinous ligament, interspinous ligament, ligamentum flavum, epidural space, and finally the dura mater and arachnoid mater to reach the CSF.

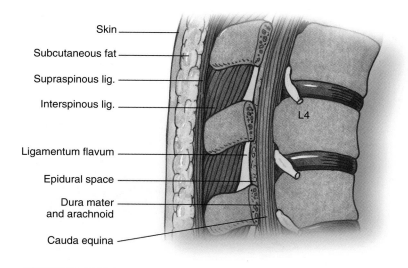

Skin

Subcutaneous fat

Supraspinous lig.

Interspinous lig.

Ligamentum flavum

Epidural space

Dura mater
and arachnoid

Cauda equina

L4

Figure 40-1. Spinal block: functional lumbar anatomy.

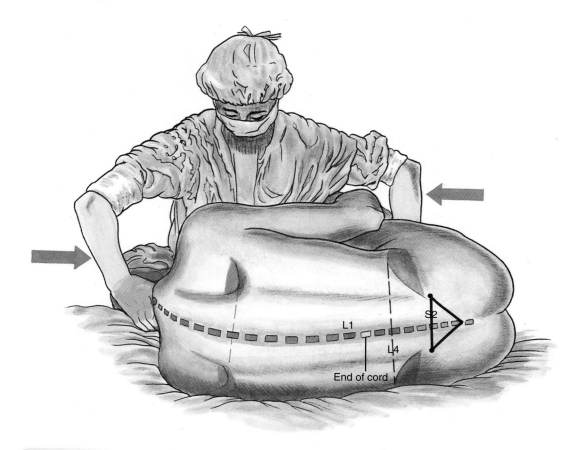

L1

L4

End of cord

S2

Figure 40-2. Spinal block: lateral decubitus position.

Position. Spinal anesthesia is carried out in three principal positions: lateral decubitus (Fig. 40-2), sitting (Fig. 40-3), and prone jackknife (Fig. 40-4). In both the lateral decubitus and sitting positions, a well-trained assistant is essential if the block is to be easily and efficiently administered by the anesthesiologist. As illustrated in Figure 40-2, the assistant can help the patient assume the position of legs flexed on the abdomen and chin flexed on the chest. This is most easily accomplished by having the assistant pull the head toward the chest, place an arm behind the patient's knees, and push the head and knees together. The position can also be facilitated by using an appropriate amount of sedation that allows the patient to be relaxed yet cooperative.

In some patients, the sitting position can facilitate location of the midline, especially in obese patients or in those with some scoliosis that makes midline identification more difficult. As illustrated in Figure 40-3A, the patient should assume a comfortable sitting position, with the legs placed

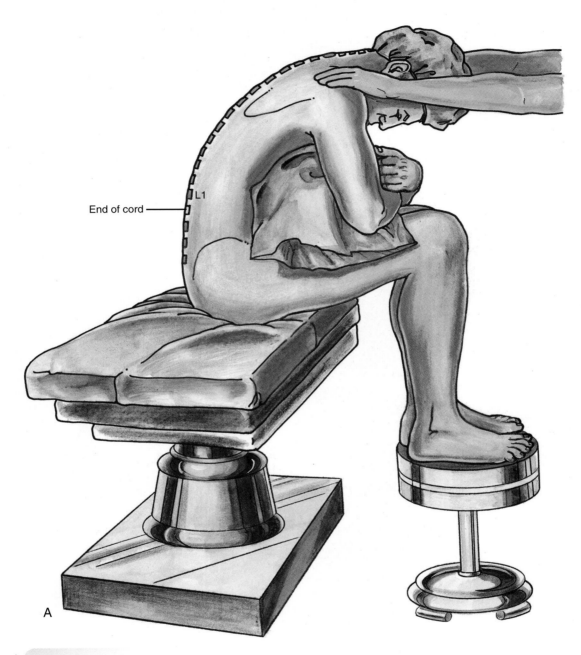

End of cord —— L1

A

Figure 40-3. Spinal block: sitting position. **A,** Lateral view.

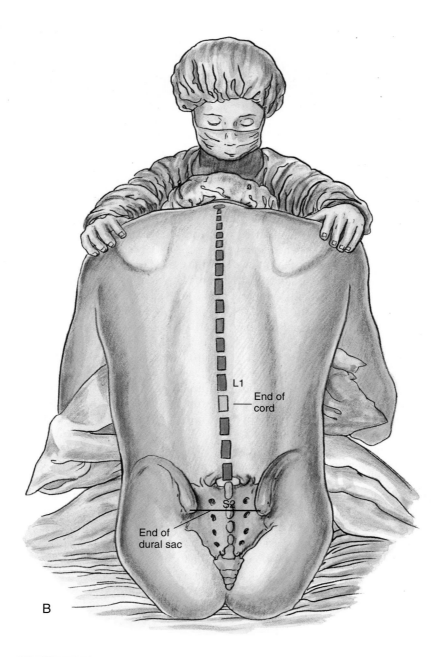

L1

End of
cord

S2

End of
dural sac

B

Figure 40-3, cont'd. **B,** Posterior view.

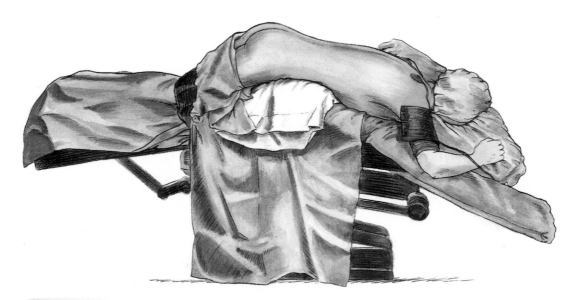

Figure 40-4. Spinal block: prone jackknife position.

over the edge of the operating table and the feet supported by a stool. A pillow should be placed in the patient's lap and the patient's arms allowed to drape over the pillow, resting on the flexed lower extremities. The assistant should be positioned immediately in front of the patient, supporting the shoulders and allowing the patient to minimize lumbar lordosis while ensuring that the vertebral midline remains in a vertical position (see Fig. 40-3B).

Sometimes it is more efficient to place the patient in a prone jackknife position before administering the spinal anesthetic (see Fig. 40-4). An assistant is not as essential for this technique as for the lateral decubitus and sitting positions, although to make the most efficient use of operating room block time, it is often helpful for the assistant to position the patient in the prone jackknife position while the anesthesiologist readies the spinal anesthesia tray and drugs.

In all three positions, the goal is to place the patient so that the midline is readily identifiable and lumbar lordosis is reduced. Figure 40-5 shows what the lumbar anatomy looks like when the patient's lumbar lordosis has been ineffectively reduced by poor positioning. As illustrated, the intralaminar space is small and difficult to enter with a needle in the midline. In contrast, Figure 40-6 illustrates how effective positioning can open the intralaminar space to allow easy access for subarachnoid puncture.

Needle Puncture. One of the first decisions to be made in considering spinal anesthesia is what kind of needle to use. Although there are many eponyms for spinal needles, they fall into two main categories: those that cut the dura sharply and those that disrupt the dural fibers by spreading with a cone-shaped tip. The former category includes the traditional disposable spinal needle, the Quincke-Babcock needle; the latter category comprises the Greene, Whitacre, and Sprotte needles. If a continuous spinal technique is chosen, the use of a Tuohy or other thin-walled, curve-tipped needle will facilitate passage of the catheter. To make a logical choice of a spinal needle, the risks and benefits of each must be understood. The use of small needles reduces the incidence of post–dural puncture headache; the use of larger needles improves the tactile sense of needle placement, thus increasing operator confidence.

Probably the risk–benefit calculation is not as simple as this. For example, the use of a small needle, such as a 27-gauge needle, will not decrease the incidence of headache in younger patients if a number of "passes" through the dura are required before CSF flow is recognized. Likewise, a larger needle, such as a 22-gauge Whitacre needle, may result in a lower incidence of post–dural puncture headache if the subarachnoid needle location is recognized on the first pass. Different needle tip designs result in differences in the incidence of post–dural puncture headache even when needle sizes are comparable.

With the patient in the proper position, the anesthesiologist uses the palpating hand to clearly identify the patient's intervertebral space and midline. As illustrated in Figure 40-7, *Step 1*, the anesthesiologist can effectively carry out this important maneuver by moving the fingers of the palpating hand alternately cephalocaudad and rolling them from side to side. When the appropriate intervertebral space has been clearly identified, a skin wheal is raised over the space. Next, an introducer is inserted into the substance of the interspinous ligament, taking care to firmly seat it in the midline (Fig. 40-7, *Step 2*). The introducer is grasped with the palpating fingers and steadied while the other hand holds the spinal needle, somewhat like a dart, as illustrated in Figure 40-7, *Step 3*. With the fifth finger of the needle hand used as a tripod against the patient's back, the needle, with bevel (if present) parallel to the long axis of the spine, is advanced slowly to heighten the sense of tissue planes traversed as well as to avoid skewing the nerve roots, until a characteristic change in resistance is noted as the needle passes through the ligamentum flavum and dura. The stylet is then removed, and CSF should appear at the needle hub. If it does not, the needle is rotated in 90-degree increments until CSF appears. If CSF does not appear in any quadrant, the needle should

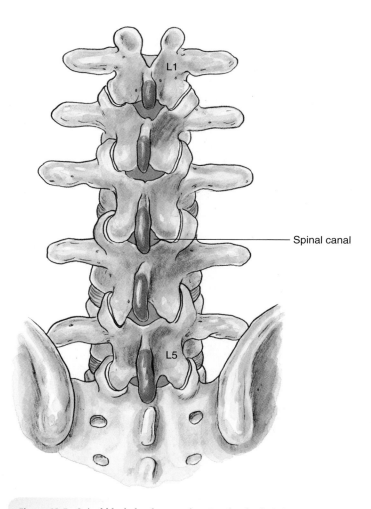

Figure 40-5. Spinal block: lumbar vertebra. Lumbar lordosis is present because the positioning is inadequate.

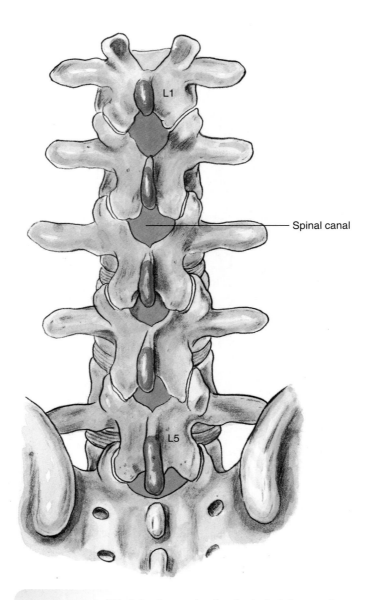

Figure 40-6. Spinal block: lumbar vertebra. Lumbar lordosis is reversed with ideal spinal positioning.

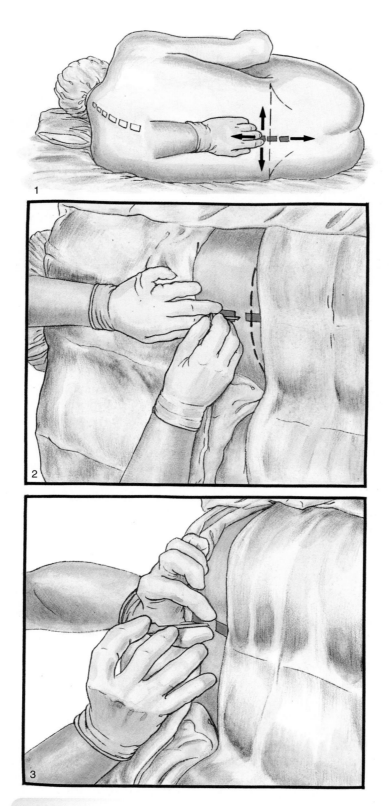

Figure 40-7. Spinal block: technique.

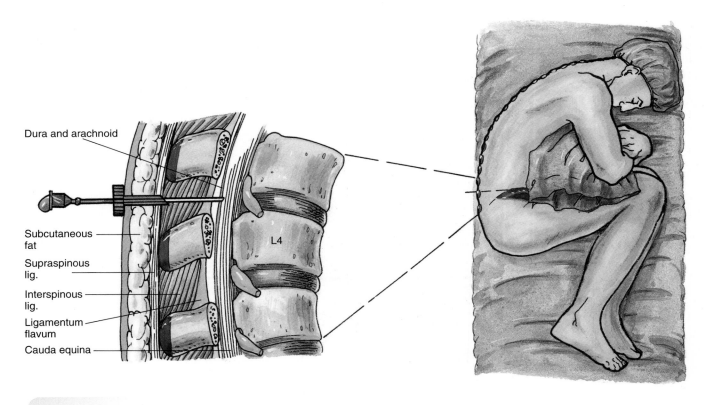

Dura and arachnoid

Subcutaneous fat

Supraspinous lig.

Interspinous lig.

Ligamentum flavum

Cauda equina

L4

Figure 40-8. Spinal block: avoiding too large a cephalad angle on insertion.

be advanced a few millimeters and rechecked in all four quadrants. If CSF still has not appeared and the needle is at a depth appropriate for the patient, the needle and introducer should be withdrawn and the insertion steps repeated, because the most common reason for lack of CSF return is that the needle was inserted off the midline. Another common error preventing subarachnoid placement is insertion of the needle with too great a cephalad angle on the initial insertion (Fig. 40-8).

Once CSF is freely obtained, the dorsum of the anesthesiologist's nondominant hand steadies the spinal needle against the patient's back while the syringe containing the therapeutic dose is attached to the needle. CSF is again freely aspirated into the syringe, and the dose is injected. Sometimes, when the syringe has been attached to a needle from which CSF was clearly previously dripping, aspiration of additional CSF becomes impossible. As illustrated in Figure 40-9, one technique that can be used to facilitate CSF aspiration is to "unscrew" the syringe plunger (see Fig. 40-9A) rather than providing constant steady pressure (see Fig. 40-9B).

After the local anesthetic has been injected, the patient and the operating table should be placed in the position appropriate for the surgical procedure and the drugs being used. The midline approach to subarachnoid block is the technique of first choice because it requires anatomic projection in only two planes, and the needle insertion plane is a relatively avascular one. When difficulties with needle insertion are encountered with the midline approach, an option is to use the paramedian route, which does not require the same level of patient cooperation or reversal of lumbar lordosis to be successful. As illustrated in Figure 40-10, the paramedian approach exploits the

larger "subarachnoid target" that exists if a needle is inserted slightly lateral to the midline. In the paramedian approach, the palpating fingers should identify the caudal edge of the cephalad spinous process of the intervertebral space chosen, and a skin wheal should be raised 1 cm lateral and 1 cm caudal to this point. A longer needle, such as a 4-cm, 22-gauge, short-beveled needle, is then used to infiltrate the deeper tissues in a cephalomedial plane. The spinal introducer and needle are then inserted 10 to 15 degrees off the sagittal plane in a cephalomedial plane, as noted in Figure 40-10. As with the midline approach, the most common error made with this technique is to angle the needle too far cephalad in its initial insertion. Once the needle contacts bone with this approach, it is redirected in slightly cephalad. If bone is again contacted after the needle has been redirected, but at a deeper level, this needle redirection is continued because it is likely that the needle is being "walked up" the lamina toward the intervertebral space. After CSF is obtained, the block continues in the same way as that described for the midline approach.

A variation of the paramedian approach is the lumbosacral approach of Taylor. The technique is carried out at the L5-S1 interspace, the largest interlaminar interspace of the vertebral column. As illustrated in Figure 40-11, the skin insertion site is 1 cm medial and 1 cm caudal to the ipsilateral posterior superior iliac spine. Through this point, a 12- to 15-cm spinal needle is inserted in a cephalomedial direction toward the midline. If bone is encountered on the first needle insertion, the needle is "walked off" the sacrum into the subarachnoid space, as in the method used for a lumbar paramedian approach. Once CSF is obtained, the steps are similar to those previously outlined.

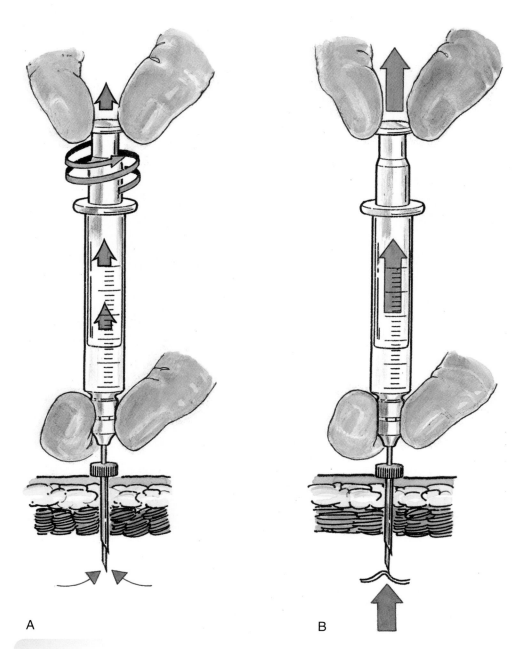

A   B

Figure 40-9. Spinal block: syringe technique to facilitate aspiration of cerebrospinal fluid.

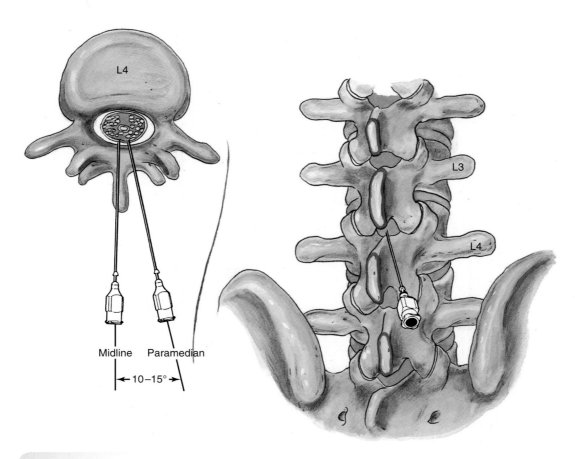

Figure 40-10. Spinal block: paramedian technique.

L4

L3

L4

Midline   Paramedian

10–15°

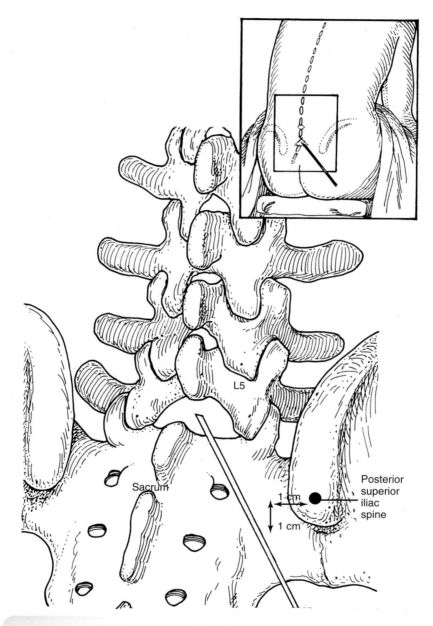

Figure 40-11. Spinal block: L5-S1 paramedian technique (Taylor's approach).

POTENTIAL PROBLEMS

The complication most feared by patients and many anesthesiologists after spinal anesthesia is neurologic injury. However, the risk–benefit calculation of neurologic injury after anesthesia must include those cases of neurologic injury that are possible after general anesthesia. These comparisons may show that the incidence of neurologic injury after spinal anesthesia is in fact lower than that after general anesthesia. However, this statement must remain speculative.

In patients in whom the spinal block level has to be precisely controlled or in whom the operation is expected to outlast the usual duration of the anesthetic drugs, a continuous spinal catheter may be used. However, when using a continuous spinal technique one should be cautious about repeating local anesthetic injections if the block height does not reach the predicted levels. Neurotoxicity (cauda equina syndrome) is hypothetically possible when the spinal catheter position allows local anesthetic concentrations to reach higher-than-expected levels.

A more common complication of spinal anesthesia is postoperative headache. Factors that influence the incidence of post–dural puncture headache are age (more frequent in younger patients), sex (more likely in female patients), needle size (more frequent with larger needles), needle bevel orientation (increased incidence when dural fibers are cut transversely), pregnancy (incidence increased), and number of dural punctures necessary to obtain CSF (more likely with multiple punctures). Perhaps more important to physicians than knowing the factors resulting in an increased incidence of post–dural puncture headache is the knowledge of how and when to carry out definitive therapy—that is, an epidural blood patch. To use spinal anesthesia effectively, epidural blood patching, when indicated, must be used early. The success rate from a single epidural blood patch should be in the 90% to 95% range and, if a second patch is required, a similar percentage should be obtainable.

One other common side effect of spinal anesthesia is the appearance of a backache in approximately 25% of patients. Patients often blame "the spinal" for backache, but, when looked at systematically, it appears that just as many patients have backaches after general anesthesia as after spinal anesthesia. Thus, backache after neuraxial block should not be attributed immediately to "needling" of the back.

PEARLS

Probably the most important factor contributing to success with spinal anesthesia in the day-to-day life of an anesthesiologist is the efficiency of the technique. If nurses and surgeons are to be advocates of spinal anesthesia, its use cannot measurably add time to the surgical day. Thus, one should plan ahead to maximize efficiency. Often overlooked in this maxim is the fact that patient preparation for operation can begin almost as soon as the block is administered if the patient is properly sedated.

Intraoperatively, during high spinal anesthesia (often during cesarean section), patients occasionally complain of dyspnea. This often appears to be a result of loss of chest wall sensation rather than of significantly decreased inspiratory capacity. The loss of chest wall sensation does not allow the patient to experience the reassurance of a deep breath. This impediment to patient acceptance can often be overcome simply by asking the patient to raise a hand in front of his or her mouth and exhale forcefully. The tactile appreciation of a deep exhalation often seems to provide the needed reassurance.

If spinal anesthesia has been used and a neurologic complication is noted after surgery, it is essential to obtain neurologic consultation early. In this way, an unbiased consultant can examine the patient and determine whether the "new" neurologic finding preexisted, is related to a peripheral neuropathy, or, more rarely, is potentially related to the spinal anesthetic. Latent electromyographic alterations associated with denervation due to neurologic injury take time to develop in the lower extremities (14 to 21 days). Therefore, after a potentially spinal anesthesia–related lesion has been identified, electromyographic studies should be obtained early to establish a preblock baseline and allow serial comparison.

It is also useful to consider adding fentanyl (15 to 25 μg) rather than epinephrine to some shorter-acting spinal local anesthetic mixtures (e.g., lidocaine) because they prolong the effective sensory block without measurably prolonging the motor block or the time to voiding. This is especially useful in selected surgical outpatients.

Another way to titrate spinal anesthesia for outpatients or any surgical procedure in which the length of surgery is difficult to predict is to use a combined spinal–epidural technique. In this technique an epidural needle is placed in the epidural space in a standard fashion, and then a small-gauge spinal needle is advanced through the epidural needle into the CSF. A spinal local anesthetic mixture is then injected and matched to the projected length of the shortest surgical procedure planned. After removal of the spinal needle, an epidural catheter is inserted into the epidural space. At this point, if the surgical procedure lasts longer than anticipated, the epidural catheter can be injected with a local anesthetic appropriate for the anticipated surgical needs. This combined spinal–epidural technique provides the flexibility for both spinal and epidural anesthesia in selected patients.

Epidural Block

41

PERSPECTIVE

Epidural anesthesia is the second primary method of neuraxial block. In contrast to spinal anesthesia, epidural block requires pharmacologic doses of local anesthetics, making systemic toxicity a concern. In skilled hands, the incidence of post–dural puncture headache should be lower with epidural anesthesia than with spinal anesthesia. Nevertheless, as outlined in Chapter 40, Spinal Block, I do not believe this should be the major differentiating point between the two techniques. Spinal anesthesia is typically a single-shot technique, whereas frequently intermittent injections are given through an epidural catheter, thus allowing reinjection and prolongation of epidural block. Another difference is that epidural block allows production of segmental anesthesia. Thus, if a thoracic injection is made and an appropriate amount of local anesthetic is injected, a band of anesthesia that does not block the lower extremities can be produced.

Patient Selection. Epidural block is appropriate for virtually the same patients who are candidates for spinal anesthesia, except that epidural anesthesia can be used in the cervical and thoracic areas as well—levels at which spinal anesthesia is not advised. As with spinal anesthesia, if epidural block is to be used for intra-abdominal procedures involving the upper abdomen, it is advisable to combine this technique with a light general anesthetic because diaphragmatic irritation can make the patient, surgeon, and anesthesiologist uncomfortable. Other candidates for epidural anesthesia are patients in whom a continuous technique has increasingly been found to be helpful in providing epidural local anesthesia or opioid analgesia after major surgical procedures. This clinical application likely explains the increased interest in epidural block over the last 20 years.

Pharmacologic Choice. To use epidural local anesthetics effectively, one must combine an understanding of the potency and duration of local anesthetics with estimates of the length of the operation and the postoperative analgesia requirements. Drugs available for epidural use can be categorized as short-acting, intermediate-acting, and long-acting agents; with the addition of epinephrine to these agents, surgical anesthesia ranging from 45 to 240 minutes after a single injection is possible.

Chloroprocaine, an amino ester local anesthetic, is a short-acting agent that allows efficient matching of the length of the surgical procedure and the duration of epidural analgesia, even in outpatients. 2-Chloroprocaine is available in 2% and 3% concentrations; the latter is prefer-

able for surgical anesthesia and the former for techniques not requiring muscle relaxation.

Lidocaine is the prototypical amino amide local anesthetic and is used in 1.5% and 2% concentrations epidurally. Concentrations of mepivacaine necessary for epidural anesthesia are similar to those of lidocaine; however, mepivacaine lasts from 15 to 30 minutes longer at equivalent dosages. Epinephrine significantly prolongs (i.e., by approximately 50%) the duration of surgical anesthesia with 2-chloroprocaine and either lidocaine and mepivacaine. Plain lidocaine produces surgical anesthesia that lasts from 60 to 100 minutes.

Bupivacaine, an amino amide, is a widely used long-acting local anesthetic for epidural anesthesia. It is used in 0.5% and 0.75% concentrations, but analgesic techniques can be performed with concentrations ranging from 0.125% to 0.25%. Its duration of action is not prolonged as consistently by the addition of epinephrine, although up to 240 minutes of surgical anesthesia can be obtained when epinephrine is added.

Ropivacaine, another long-acting amino amide, is also used for regional and epidural anesthesia. For surgical anesthesia it is used in 0.5%, 0.75%, and 1% concentrations. Analgesia can be obtained with concentrations of 0.2%. Its duration of action is slightly less than that of bupivacaine in the epidural technique, and it appears to produce slightly less motor blockade than a comparable concentration of bupivacaine.

In addition to the use of epinephrine as an epidural additive, some anesthesiologists recommend modifying epidural local anesthetic solutions to increase both the speed of onset and the quality of the block produced. One recommendation is to alkalinize the local anesthetic solution by adding bicarbonate to it to achieve both these purposes. Nevertheless, the clinical advisability of routinely adding bicarbonate to local anesthetic solutions should be determined by local practice protocols.

PLACEMENT

Anatomy. As with spinal anesthesia, the key to carrying out successful epidural anesthesia is understanding the three-dimensional midline neuraxial anatomy that underlies the palpating fingers (Fig. 41-1). When a lumbar approach to the epidural space is used in adults, the depth from the skin to the ligamentum flavum is commonly near 4 cm; in 80% of patients the epidural space is cannulated at a distance of 3.5 to 6 cm from the skin. In a small number of patients the lumbar epidural space is as near as 2 cm from the skin. In the lumbar region, the ligamentum

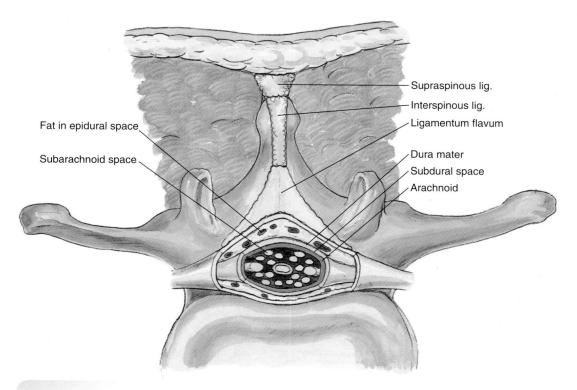

Fat in epidural space

Subarachnoid space

Supraspinous lig.

Interspinous lig.

Ligamentum flavum

Dura mater

Subdural space

Arachnoid

Figure 41-1. Epidural block: cross-sectional anatomy.

flavum is 5 to 6 mm thick in the midline, whereas in the thoracic region it is 3 to 5 mm thick. In the thoracic region, the depth from the skin to the epidural space depends on the degree of cephalad angulation used for the paramedian approach as well as the body habitus of the patient (Fig. 41-2). In the cervical region the depth to the ligamentum flavum is approximately the same as that in the lumbar region, 4 to 6 cm.

The ligamentum flavum will be perceived as a thicker ligament if the needle is kept in the midline than if the needle is inserted off the midline and enters the lateral extension of the ligamentum flavum. Figure 41-3 illustrates how important it is to maintain the midline position of the epidural needle (*needle A*) during lumbar epidural techniques. If an oblique approach is taken, a "false release" can be produced (*needle C*) or the perception of a thin ligament can be reinforced (*needle B*).

Position. Patient positioning for epidural anesthesia is similar to that for spinal anesthesia, with lateral decubitus, sitting, and prone jackknife positions all applicable. The lateral decubitus position is applicable for both lumbar and thoracic epidural techniques, and the sitting position allows the administration of lumbar, thoracic, and cervical epidural anesthetics. The prone jackknife position allows access to the caudal epidural space.

Needle Puncture: Lumbar Epidural. A technique similar to that used for spinal anesthesia should be carried out to identify the midline structures, and the bony landmarks should be used to determine the vertebral level appropriate for needle insertion (Fig. 41-4). When choosing a needle for epidural anesthesia, one must decide whether a continuous or single-shot technique is desired. This is the principal

determinant of needle selection. If a single-shot epidural technique is chosen, a Crawford needle is appropriate; if a continuous catheter technique is indicated, a Tuohy or other needle with a lateral-facing opening is chosen.

The midline approach is most often indicated for a lumbar epidural procedure. The needle is inserted into the midline in the same way as for spinal anesthesia. In the epidural technique, the needle is slowly advanced until the change in tissue resistance is noted as the needle abuts the ligamentum flavum. At this point, a 3- to 5-mL glass syringe is filled with 2 mL of saline solution, and a small (0.25 mL) air bubble is added. The syringe is attached to the needle, and if the needle tip is in the substance of the ligamentum flavum, the air bubble will be compressible (Fig. 41-5A). If the ligamentum flavum has not yet been reached, pressure on the syringe plunger will not compress the air bubble (Fig. 41-5B). Once compression of the air bubble has been achieved, the needle is grasped with the nondominant hand and pulled toward the epidural space, while the dominant hand (thumb) applies constant steady pressure on the syringe plunger, thus compressing the air bubble. When the epidural space is entered, the pressure applied to the syringe plunger will allow the solution to flow without resistance into the epidural space. An alternative technique, although one that I believe has a less precise end point, is the hanging-drop technique for identifying entry into the epidural space. In this technique, when the needle is placed in the ligamentum flavum a drop of solution is introduced into the hub of the needle (Fig. 41-6A). No syringe is attached, and when the needle is advanced into the epidural space, the solution should be "sucked into" the space (Fig. 41-6B).

No matter what method is chosen for needle insertion, when the epidural space is cannulated with a catheter,

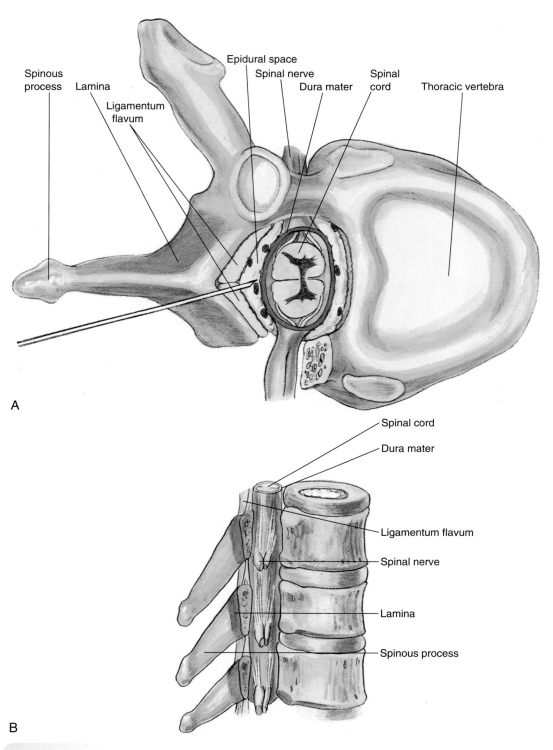

Spinous
process   Lamina

Ligamentum
flavum

Epidural space
          Spinal nerve
              Dura mater

Spinal
cord

Thoracic vertebra

A

Spinal cord

Dura mater

Ligamentum flavum

Spinal nerve

Lamina

Spinous process

B

Figure 41-2. Thoracic epidural block anatomy: overlapping of mid-thoracic spinous processes requires a paramedian technique. **A,** Cross-section, superior view. **B,** Lateral view, paramedian section.

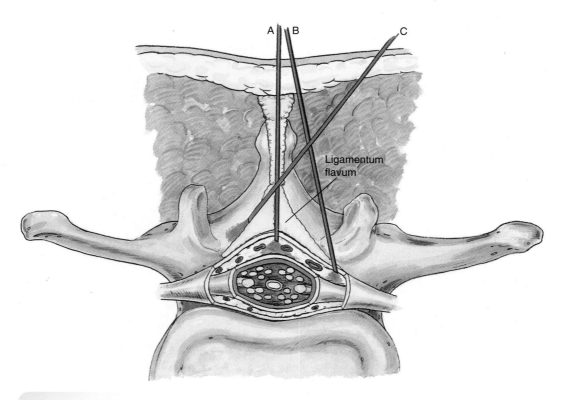

Figure 41-3. Epidural block: functional anatomy of ligamentum flavum.

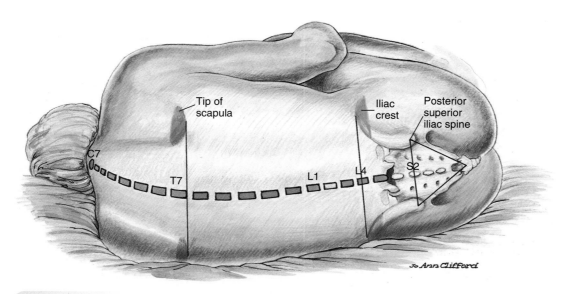

Figure 41-4. Neuraxial anatomy: surface relationships.

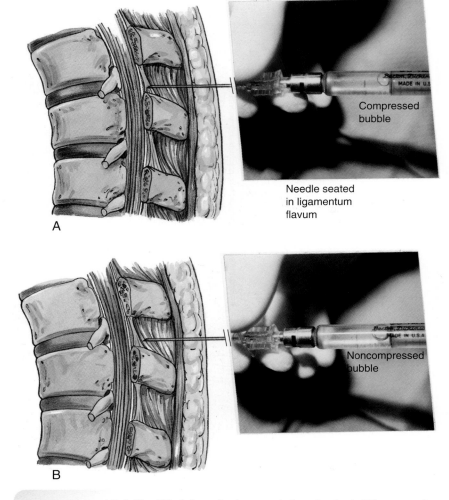

Figure 41-5. A and **B,** Epidural block: loss-of-resistance technique showing bubble compression (**A**) and noncompression (**B**).

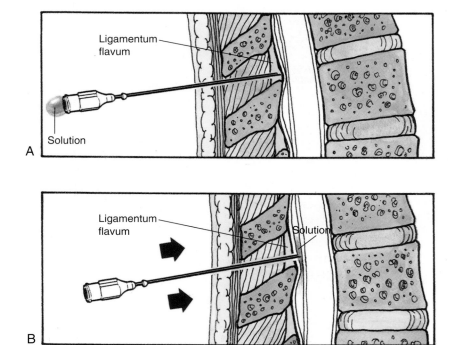

Figure 41-6. Epidural block: hanging-drop technique.

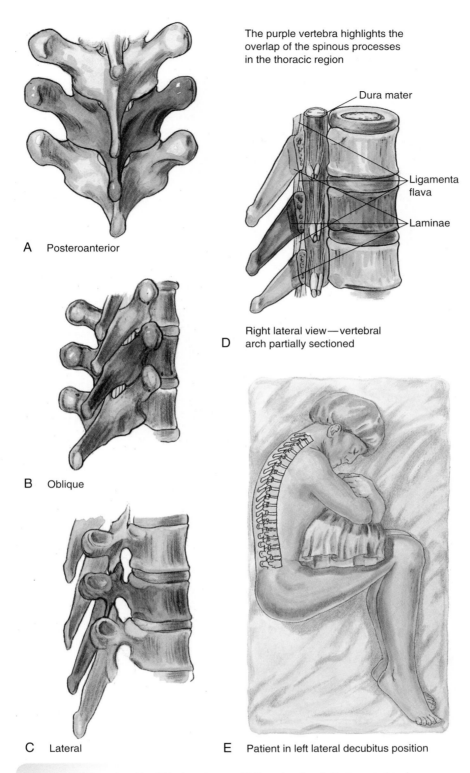

The purple vertebra highlights the overlap of the spinous processes in the thoracic region

A   Posteroanterior

B   Oblique

C   Lateral

Dura mater

Ligamenta flava

Laminae

D   Right lateral view—vertebral arch partially sectioned

E   Patient in left lateral decubitus position

Figure 41-7. Thoracic epidural block anatomy: mid-thoracic spine. **A,** Posteroanterior view. **B,** Oblique view. **C,** Lateral view. **D,** Lateral view after removal of right vertebral arch. **E,** Patient in left lateral decubitus position for thoracic epidural anesthesia.

success may be increased by advancing the needle 1 to 2 mm farther once the space has been identified. In addition, the incidence of unintentional intravenous cannulation with an epidural catheter may be decreased by injecting 5 to 10 mL of solution before threading the catheter. If a catheter is inserted, it should be inserted only 2 to 3 cm into the epidural space because threading it farther may increase the likelihood of catheter malposition. Obstetric patients require catheters to be inserted to 3 to 5 cm into the epidural space to minimize dislodgement during labor analgesia.

Needle Puncture: Thoracic Epidural. As with lumbar epidural anesthesia, patients are usually placed into a lateral decubitus position for needle insertion into the thoracic epidural space (Fig. 41-7). In this technique,

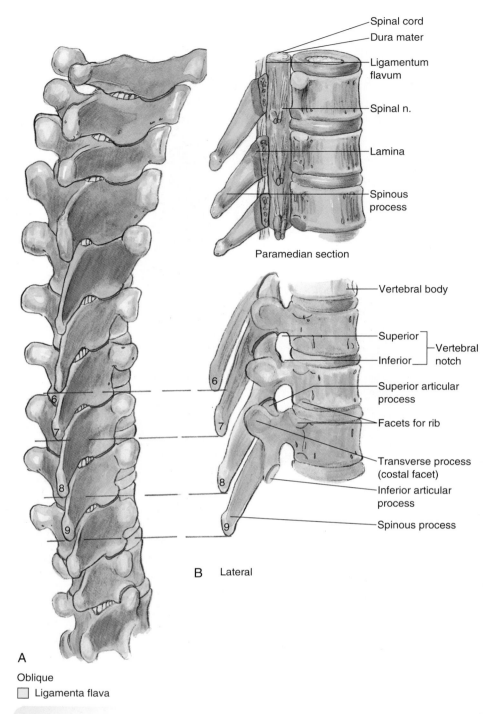

Spinal cord
Dura mater
Ligamentum flavum
Spinal n.
Lamina
Spinous process

Paramedian section

Vertebral body

Superior
Inferior
Vertebral notch

Superior articular process

Facets for rib

Transverse process (costal facet)

Inferior articular process

Spinous process

B   Lateral

A

Oblique

☐ Ligamenta flava

Figure 41-8. Thoracic vertebral anatomy: degree of spinous process overlap changes from high thoracic to mid-thoracic to low thoracic. **A,** Oblique view. **B,** Lateral view and paramedian section.

the paramedian approach is preferred because it allows easier access to the epidural space. This is because the spinous processes in the mid-thoracic region overlap each other from cephalad to caudad (Fig. 41-8). The paramedian approach is carried out in a manner similar to that used for the lumbar epidural space, although in almost every instance the initial needle insertion will result in contact with the thoracic vertebral lamina by the epidural needle (Fig. 41-9). When this occurs, the needle is withdrawn slightly and the tip redirected cephalad in small, incremental steps until the needle is firmly seated in the ligamentum flavum. At this point, the loss-of-

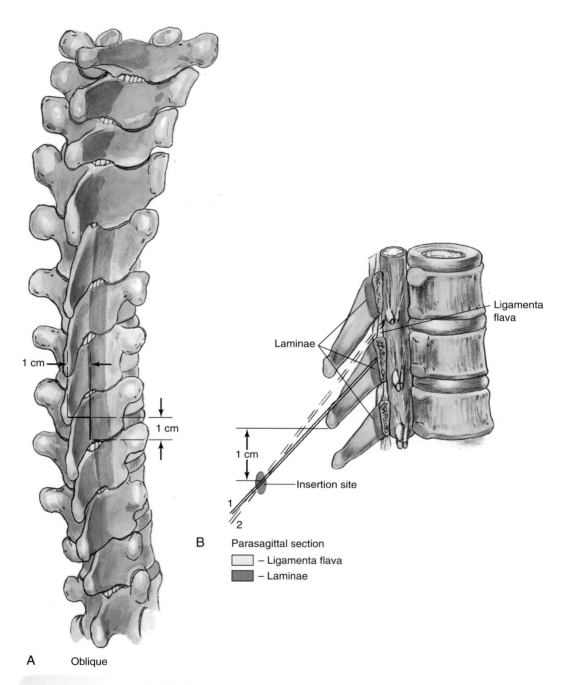

A   Oblique

1 cm

1 cm

1 cm

Ligamenta
flava

Laminae

Insertion site

1

2

B   Parasagittal section

☐ – Ligamenta flava

■ – Laminae

Figure 41-9. Thoracic epidural block technique. **A,** Using the paramedian approach, needle insertion site is 1 cm caudad and 1 cm lateral to the tip of the more cephalad spinous process, similar to the needle insertion used in the lumbar paramedian technique. **B,** Parasagittal view of needle insertion and initial contact with lamina *(blue shading)*.

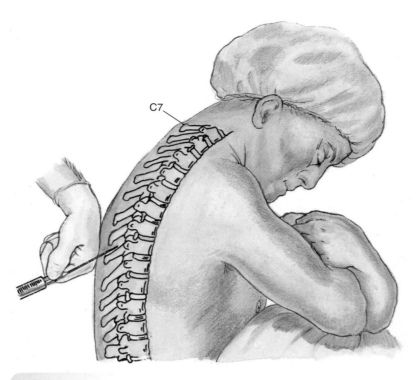

C7

Figure 41-10. Thoracic epidural block technique: Bromage grip for loss-of-resistance technique in thoracic block.

resistance technique and insertion of the catheter are carried out in a manner identical to that used for lumbar epidural block. Again, the hanging-drop technique is an alternative method of identifying the thoracic epidural space, although the classic Bromage needle–syringe grip is my first choice for the thoracic epidural block (Fig. 41-10).

Needle Puncture: Cervical Epidural. In the cervical epidural technique, the patient is typically in a sitting position with the head bent forward and supported on a table (Fig. 41-11). A comparison of the cervical epidural block with the lumbar epidural block reveals many similarities. The spinous processes of the cervical vertebrae are nearly perpendicular to the long axis of the vertebral column;

thus, a midline technique is applicable for the cervical epidural block. The most prominent vertebral spinous processes, those of C7 and T1, are identified with the neck flexed (Fig. 41-12). The second (index) and third fingers of the palpating hand straddle the space between C7 and T1, and the epidural needle is slowly inserted in a plane approximately parallel to the floor (or parallel to the long axis of the cervical vertebral spinous processes). Abutment of the needle onto the ligamentum flavum will be appreciated at a depth similar to that seen in the lumbar epidural block (i.e., 3.5 to 5.5 cm), and needle placement is then performed using the loss-of-resistance technique as in the other epidural methods. The hanging-drop method is also an option for identification of the cervical epidural space.

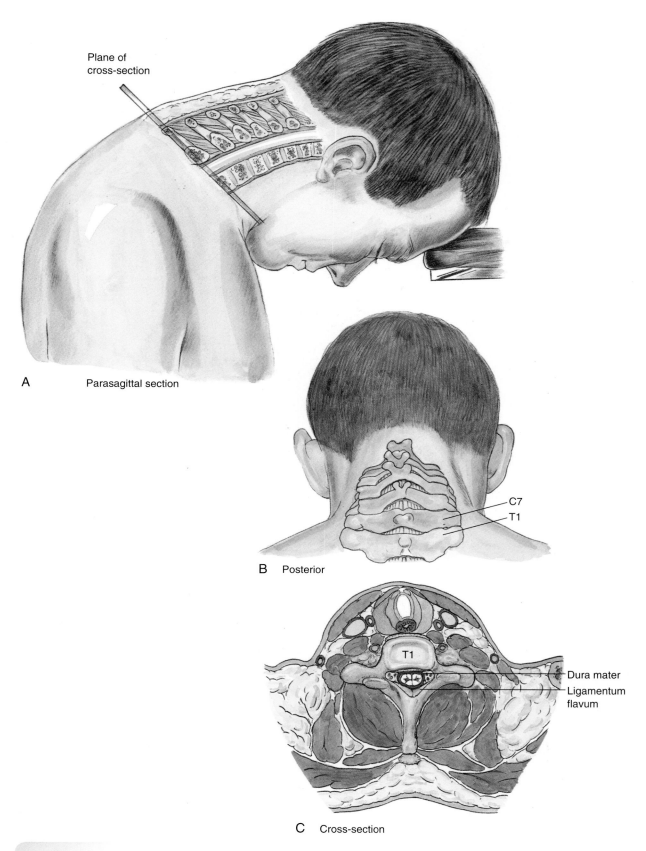

Plane of cross-section

A   Parasagittal section

B   Posterior

C7

T1

T1

Dura mater

Ligamentum flavum

C   Cross-section

Figure 41-11. Cervical epidural anatomy. **A,** Patient sitting with head supported by table, and plane of vertebral cross-section. **B,** Posterior view. **C,** Vertebral cross-section at C7-T1.

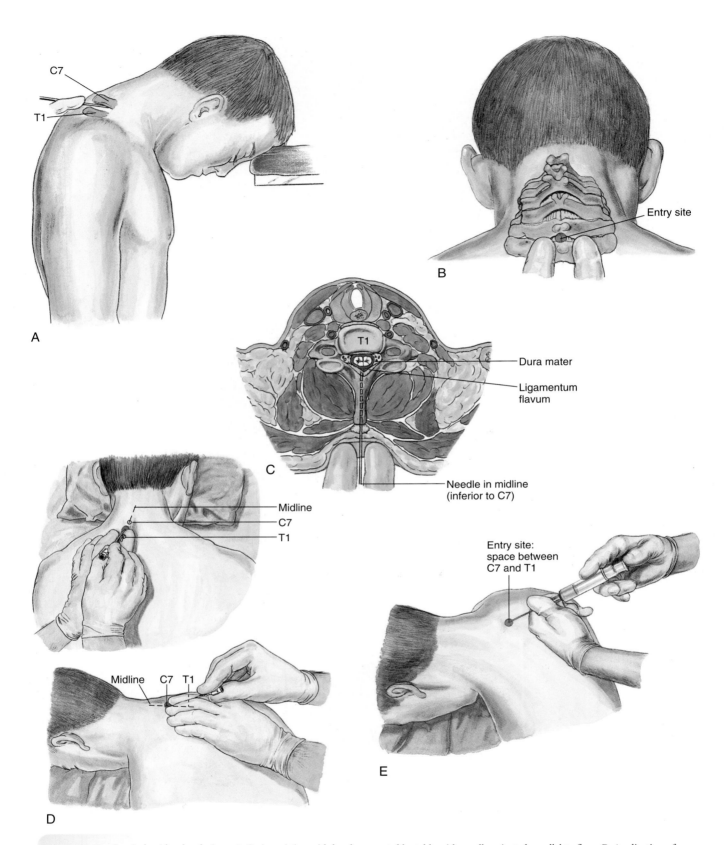

Figure 41-12. Cervical epidural technique. **A,** Patient sitting with head supported by table with needle oriented parallel to floor. **B,** Application of fingers to posterior neck to facilitate cervical epidural block. **C,** Insertion of needle into ligamentum flavum. **D,** Insertion of needle during palpation. **E,** Bromage grip during needle advancement.

POTENTIAL PROBLEMS

One of the most feared complications of epidural anesthesia is systemic toxicity resulting from intravenous injection of the intended epidural anesthetic (Fig. 41-13). This can occur with either catheter or needle injection. One way to minimize intravenous injection of the pharmacologic doses of local anesthetic needed for epidural anesthesia is to verify needle or catheter placement by administering a test dose before the definitive epidural anesthetic injection. The current recommendation for the test dose is 3 mL of local anesthetic solution containing 1:200,000 epinephrine (15 µg of epinephrine). Even if the test dose is negative, the anesthesiologist should inject the epidural solution incrementally, be vigilant for unintentional intravascular injection, and have all necessary equipment and drugs available to treat local anesthetic–induced systemic toxicity.

Another problem that can occur with epidural anesthesia is the unintentional administration of an epidural dose into the spinal fluid. In this event, as when any neuraxial block reaches high sensory levels, blood pressure and heart rate should be supported pharmacologically and ventilation should be assisted as indicated. Usually atropine and ephedrine will suffice to manage this situation, or at least will provide time to administer more potent catecholamines. If the entire dose (20 to 25 mL) of local anesthetic is administered into the cerebrospinal fluid, tracheal intubation and mechanical ventilation are indicated because it will be approximately 1 to 2 hours before the patient can

consistently maintain adequate spontaneous ventilation. When epidural anesthesia is performed and a higher-than-expected block develops after a delay of only 15 to 30 minutes, subdural placement of the local anesthetic must be considered. Treatment is symptomatic, with the most difficult part involving recognition that a subdural injection is possible.

As with spinal anesthesia, if neurologic injury occurs after epidural anesthesia, a systematic approach to the problem is necessary. No particular local anesthetic, use of needle versus catheter technique, addition or omission of epinephrine, or location of epidural puncture seems to be associated with an increased incidence of neurologic injury. Despite this observation, the performance of cervical or thoracic epidural techniques demands special care with hand and needle control because the spinal cord is immediately deep to the site of both these epidural blocks.

An additional problem with epidural anesthesia is the fear of creating an epidural hematoma with the needles or catheters. This probably happens less frequently than severe neurologic injury after general anesthesia. Concern about epidural hematoma formation is greater in patients who have been taking antiplatelet drugs such as aspirin or who have been receiving preoperative anticoagulants. The magnitude of an acceptable level of preoperative anticoagulation and the risk–benefit calculation of performing epidural anesthesia in the anticoagulated patient remain indeterminate at this time. The use of epidural techniques in patients receiving subcutaneous heparin therapy is

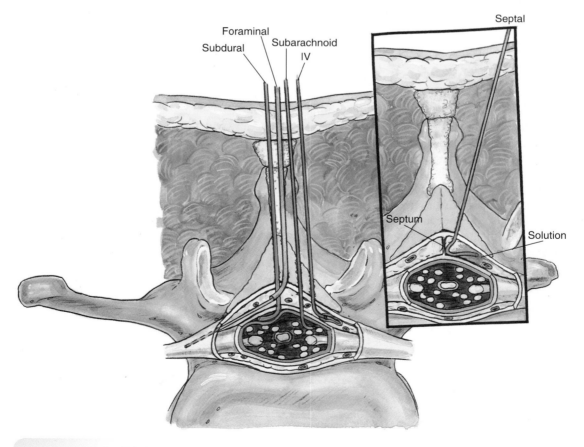

Figure 41-13. Epidural block: cross-sectional anatomy, showing potential incorrect injection sites. IV, intravenous.

probably acceptable if the block can be performed atraumatically, although the risk–benefit ratio of the technique must be weighed for each patient. Perioperative anticoagulant regimens that demand special consideration are the use of low–molecular-weight heparin (LMWH) or potent antiplatelet drugs concurrently with epidural block. LMWH is used for prophylaxis of deep venous thrombosis and produces more profound effects than other intermittently dosed heparin products. It is currently recommended that no procedure, including withdrawal or manipulation of an epidural catheter, should occur within 12 hours after a dose of LMWH, and the next dose of LMWH should be delayed for at least 2 hours after atraumatic epidural needle or catheter insertion or manipulation. The antiplatelet drugs (e.g., ticlopidine, clopidogrel, and platelet glycoprotein IIb/IIIa receptor antagonists) are sometimes combined with aspirin and other anticoagulants. Expert guidelines need to be consulted when using regional blocks in the increasing number of patients on antiplatelet compounds.

As in spinal anesthesia, post–dural puncture headache can result from epidural anesthesia when unintentional subarachnoid puncture accompanies the technique. When using the larger-diameter epidural needles (18 and 19 gauge), it can be expected that at least 50% of patients experiencing unintentional dural puncture will have a postoperative headache.

PEARLS

Avoiding catheters during epidural anesthesia—that is, by selecting an appropriate local anesthetic—can avoid a potential source of difficulty with the technique. Epidural catheters can be malpositioned in a number of ways. If a catheter is inserted too far into the epidural space, it can be routed out of foramina, resulting in patchy epidural block. The catheter can also be inserted into the subdural or subarachnoid space or into an epidural vein. Similarly, the use of epidural catheters may be complicated by a prominent dorsomedian connective tissue band (epidural septum or fat pad), which is found in some patients.

Another means of facilitating the success of epidural anesthesia is to allow the block enough "soak time" before beginning the surgical procedure. This is most effectively accomplished if the block is carried out in an induction room separate from the operating room. There appears to be a plateau effect in the doses of epidural local anesthetics; that is, once a certain quantity of local anesthetic has been injected, more of the same agent does not significantly increase the block height but rather may make the block denser, perhaps improving quality.

One observation about epidural anesthesia through a catheter that needs to be emphasized is the often faulty clinical logic that, by giving incremental doses through a catheter, the level of sensory anesthesia can be slowly developed, thereby allowing frail and physiologically compromised patients to undergo epidural anesthesia. However, when this approach is taken, anesthesiologists usually do not allow enough time between injections because of the reality of time pressures in the normal operating room. They inject small doses through the catheter but then do not allow sufficient time to pass before performing the next incremental injection. Often the clinical result is high block levels in just those patients in whom lower levels were the goal. Furthermore, this approach to epidural anesthesia unnecessarily delays preparing the patient for the operation and makes surgical and nursing colleagues less accepting of the technique.

Epidural catheters are indicated in many situations, especially when the technique is used for postoperative analgesia. To place a known length of catheter into the epidural space, either the catheter and needle must have distance markers, or a way must be found to maintain the catheter position once the needle has been withdrawn over the catheter. Because some epidural needles do not have distance markers, a method of maintaining catheter position while the needle is withdrawn over the catheter is required. One technique of positioning the catheter is illustrated in Figure 41-14. An object of known length, such as a syringe or the anesthesiologist's finger, is selected, and that object is placed next to the needle–catheter assembly after the catheter has been inserted 3 cm (or other known distance) into the epidural space. Because the catheter is marked, a known point on the catheter can be related to a known point on either the finger or the syringe. As shown in Figure 41-14A, the 15-cm mark is opposite the plunger on the syringe or the anesthesiologist's knuckle. Once this relationship has been noted, the needle is removed while the catheter position is maintained. The measurement object is then placed next to the catheter, as illustrated in Figure 41-14B, and the catheter is withdrawn to the point at which the distance marker on the catheter relates to the previously identified point. In this example, the 15-cm mark on the catheter is placed opposite the plunger of the syringe or the anesthesiologist's knuckle. By using this technique, the epidural catheter can be accurately placed without the need for either a marked needle or a ruler.

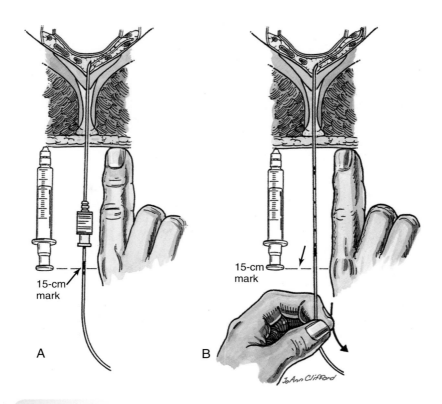

Figure 41-14. **A** and **B,** Epidural block: catheter measurement technique.

Caudal Block

42

PERSPECTIVE

With advances in lumbar epidural anesthesia, caudal anesthesia has become an infrequently used and taught technique. Nevertheless, caudal anesthesia can be effectively used for anorectal and perineal procedures, as well as some lower extremity operations.

Patient Selection. Patient selection for caudal anesthesia should be determined by examining the anatomy of the sacral hiatus. In approximately 5% of adult patients, the sacral hiatus is nearly impossible to cannulate with needle or catheter; thus, in 1 of 20 patients the technique is clinically unusable. Likewise, there are patients in whom the tissue mass overlying the sacrum makes the technique difficult, and if another technique is applicable, caudal anesthesia should be avoided. Probably more so than for any other block, experience and confidence on the anesthesiologist's part are necessary to carry out the technique effectively.

Pharmacologic Choice. When choosing local anesthetics for caudal anesthesia, the same considerations as those applied to epidural anesthesia are needed. Volumes of local anesthetic in the 25- to 35-mL range are necessary to predictably provide a sensory level of T12 to T10 with caudal injection for adults.

PLACEMENT

Anatomy. Anatomy pertinent to caudal anesthesia centers on the sacral hiatus (Fig. 42-1). This can be most effectively localized by finding the posterior superior iliac spines bilaterally, drawing a line to join them, and then completing an equilateral triangle caudad. The tip of the equilateral triangle will overlie the sacral hiatus (Fig. 42-2). The caudal tip of the triangle will rest near the sacral cornua, which are unfused remnants of the spinous processes of the fifth sacral vertebra. Overlying the sacral hiatus is a fibroelastic membrane, which is the functional counterpart of the

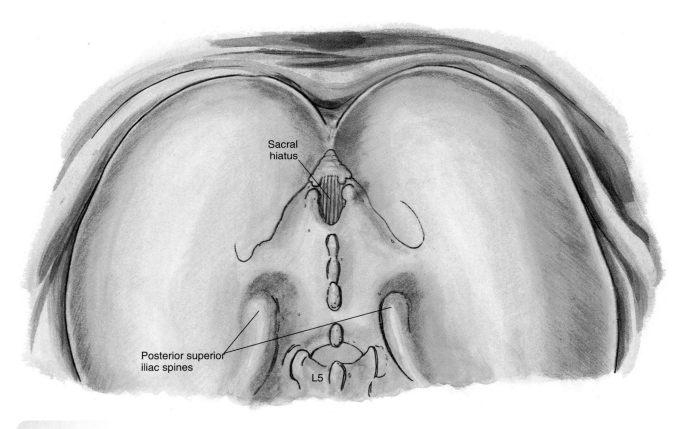

Figure 42-1. Caudal block: surface anatomy.

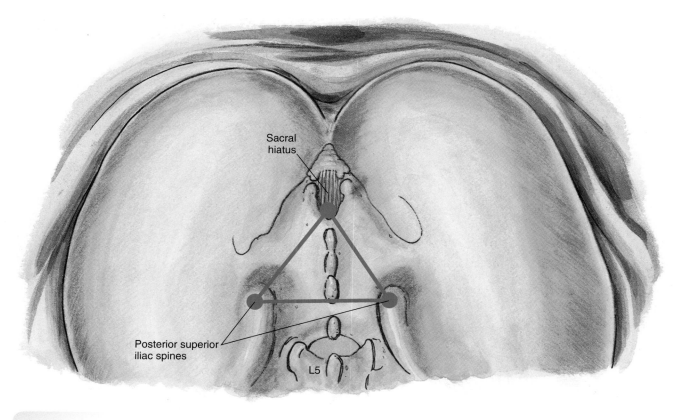

Figure 42-2. Caudal block: surface anatomy showing sacral hiatus localization.

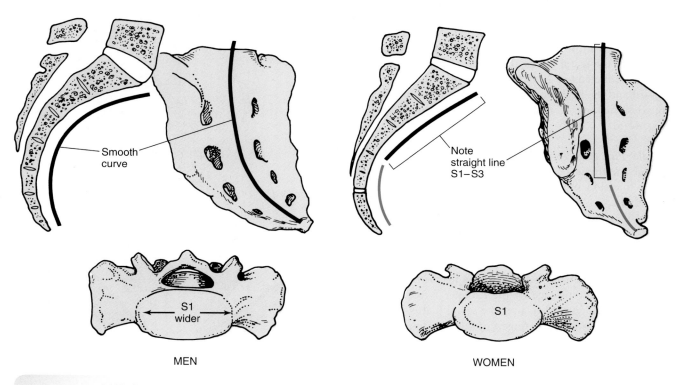

Figure 42-3. Caudal block: relationship of sacral anatomy to sex.

ligamentum flavum. Perhaps more than with any other sex difference found in regional anesthesia, the sacrum is distinctly different in men and women. In men, the cavity of the sacrum has a smooth curve from S1 to S5. Conversely, in women the sacrum is quite flat from S1 to S3, with a more pronounced curve in the S4 to S5 region (Fig. 42-3).

Position. Caudal block can be carried out in a lateral decubitus position or a prone position. In adults, I find the prone position with a pillow placed beneath the lower abdomen most effective. In this position, patients can be sufficiently sedated to make the block comfortable, and it makes the midline more easily identifiable than in the

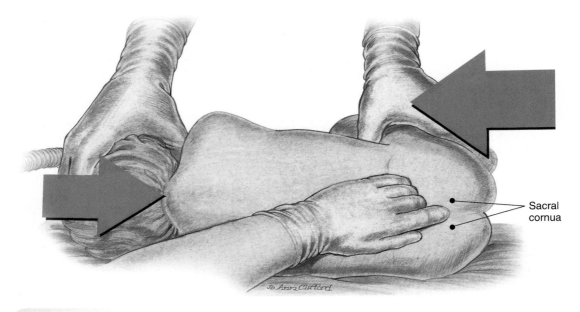

Figure 42-4. Caudal block: pediatric position.

lateral position. As illustrated in Figure 42-4, pediatric caudal anesthesia is commonly carried out with the child in the lateral decubitus position. Because most pediatric caudal blocks are performed after induction with general anesthesia, the lateral position is almost mandatory. Identification of the midline and performance of the block are less complicated in the pediatric patient, thus making the lateral position clinically practical. To optimize identification of the sacral hiatus, the prone patient should have the legs abducted to a 20-degree angle with the toes rotated inward and the heels outward. This helps relax the gluteal muscles, making it easier to identify the sacral hiatus (Fig. 42-5).

Needle Puncture. As with lumbar epidural anesthesia, caudal anesthesia requires a decision about the use of a single-injection or a catheter technique. If a single-shot caudal block is to be performed, almost any needle of sufficient length to reach the caudal canal is acceptable. In adults, a needle of at least 22 gauge is recommended because it is large enough to allow sufficiently rapid injection of solution to help detect misplaced local anesthetic injections. If a catheter is to be used, a needle that is large enough to allow passage of the catheter is required. As illustrated in Figure 42-6, after the sacral hiatus is identified, the index and middle fingers of the palpating hand are each placed on the sacral cornua, and the caudal needle is inserted at an angle of approximately 45 degrees to the sacrum. As the anesthesiologist advances the needle, he or she will become aware of a decrease in resistance as the needle enters the caudal canal (*needle position 1*). The needle is then advanced until it contacts bone; this should be the dorsal aspect of the ventral plate of the sacrum. The needle is then withdrawn slightly and redirected so that the angle of insertion relative to the skin surface is decreased. In male patients, this angle will be almost parallel with the tabletop, whereas in female patients a slightly steeper angle will be necessary (*needle position 2*).

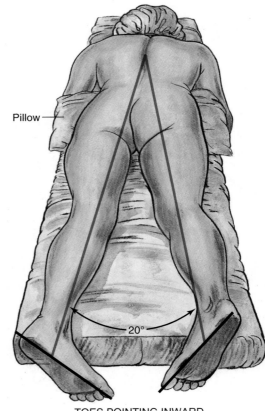

Figure 42-5. Caudal block: prone position.

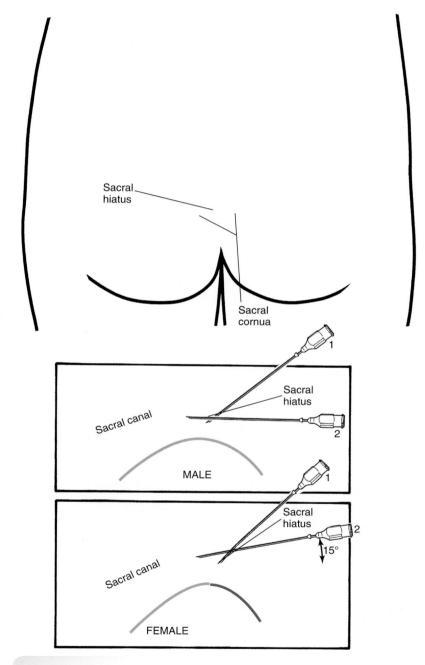

Figure 42-6. Caudal block: technique.

During the redirection of the needle and after noting loss of resistance, the needle should be advanced approximately 1 to 1.5 cm into the caudal canal. Further advance is not advised because dural puncture and unintentional intravascular cannulation become more likely. Before the injection of the therapeutic dose of local anesthetic, aspiration should be performed and a test dose administered because a vein or the subarachnoid space can be entered unintentionally, as is the case in lumbar epidural anesthesia.

POTENTIAL PROBLEMS

Caudal anesthesia entails most of the same complications that can accompany lumbar epidural anesthesia, although there are some differences. The frequency of local anesthetic toxicity after caudal anesthesia appears to be higher than it is with lumbar epidural block. Another distinct difference is that the incidence of subarachnoid puncture is exceedingly low with the caudal technique. The dural sac ends at approximately the level of S2; thus, unless a needle is inserted deeply within the caudal canal, subarachnoid puncture is unlikely. In children the dural sac is more distally placed in the caudal canal, and this should be considered when carrying out pediatric caudal anesthesia.

Perhaps the most frequent problem with caudal anesthesia is ineffective blockade, which results from the considerable variation in the anatomy of the sacral hiatus. If anesthesiologists are unfamiliar with caudal technique and the needle passes anterior to the ventral plate of the sacrum, puncture of the rectum or, in obstetric anesthesia, of fetal parts is possible. As illustrated in Figure 42-7, the area surrounding the sacral hiatus can be imagined as a potential "circle of errors." The practitioner may be faced with a slitlike hiatus that does not allow easy needle insertion; the hiatus may be located more cephalad than anticipated or in fact may be closed. Likewise, loss of resistance may be encountered as the needle is inserted into one of the sacral foramina rather than the hiatus. In the lateral view, it is obvious that needles may be misdirected into subcutaneous or periosteal locations as well as into the marrow of sacral bones.

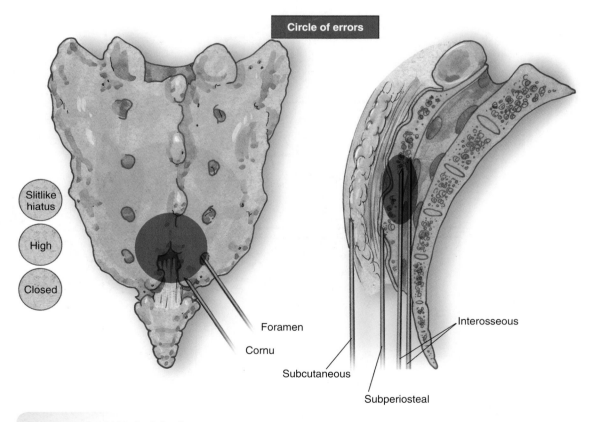

Figure 42-7. Caudal block: circle of errors.

PEARLS

To produce effective caudal anesthesia, anesthesiologists should be selective about the patients in whom it is attempted. It makes no sense to use the technique in a patient whose anatomy is unfavorable. Because of the anatomic variations in the area around the sacral hiatus, this block seems to require more operator experience and a longer time to attain proficiency than many other regional blocks. As a result, anesthesiologists should develop their technique in patients whose anatomy is favorable.

One helpful hint that will confirm needle location when carrying out caudal anesthesia is illustrated in Figure 42-8. Once the needle has entered what is thought to be the caudal canal, the anesthesiologist should place a palpating hand across the sacral region dorsally. Then, 5 mL of saline solution should be rapidly injected through the caudal needle. By placing the hand as shown, the anesthesiologist should be immediately aware of the subcutaneous needle position overlying the sacrum. If the needle is mispositioned subcutaneously, a bulge during injection will develop in the midline. If the needle is correctly positioned in the caudal canal, no midline bulge should be palpable. In thin individuals, accurate needle placement in the caudal canal and rapid injection of solution may allow the anesthesiologist to feel small pressure waves more laterally overlying the sacral foramina. These smaller pressure waves should not be confused with those associated with a misplaced subcutaneous needle.

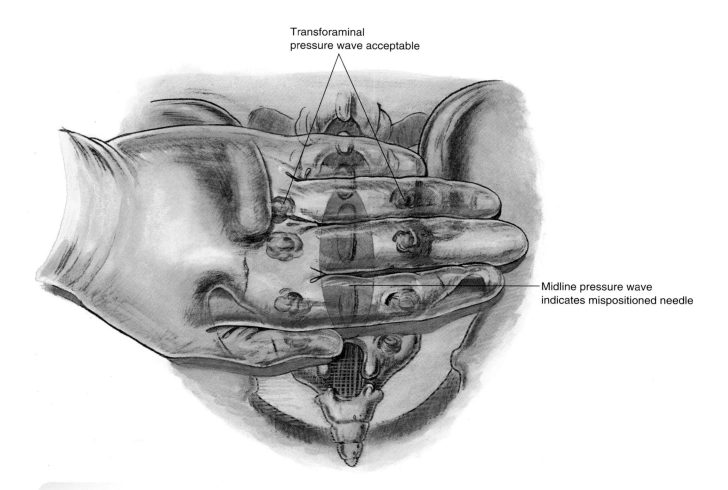

Transforaminal
pressure wave acceptable

Midline pressure wave
indicates mispositioned needle

Figure 42-8. Caudal block: palpation technique.

SECTION VIII:
Chronic Pain Blocks

Chronic and Cancer Pain Care: An Introduction and Perspective

43

Chronic pain and cancer pain invokes many images to physicians, patients, and families. For too long, chronic pain and cancer pain have been an undertreated and neglected part of our society's medical care delivery system. Those of us involved in pain medicine, as physicians and patients, know that these pain states are very real and often poorly managed by colleagues and patients.

Many have considered short-term approaches to pain care as the ideal, using nerve blocks to the exclusion of other therapies. Other colleagues have vigorously and actively avoided any use of regional analgesia techniques in the patient with chronic pain or cancer pain. As a physician with a practice of pain medicine spanning nearly three decades, I believe that the polar ends of this conceptual continuum (Fig. 43-1) represent incomplete and inappropriate approaches to pain medicine. Over the long years of my practice treating a wide selection of patients, increas-

ingly fewer of my patients receive recommendations for an exclusive regional analgesic/anesthetic approach to their pain control or rehabilitation regimen. In fact, many of my patients receive oral analgesia options with a physical rehabilitation and activity regimen, without any regional techniques as part of their therapy. These practices do not suggest that regional analgesic/anesthetic/neuromodulation regimens are not indicated in our patients. In fact, they are indicated in many patients, but they should be used with a clear indication for how they help in diagnosis or in the pain control and rehabilitation regimen in the patient with chronic pain. Their use should be incorporated into a chronic rehabilitation and cancer pain control regimen that focuses on return of function, always keeping in mind our charge as physicians to balance risk and benefit for each individual patient.

I ask that each of us use the techniques described in the following chapters on chronic pain medicine without

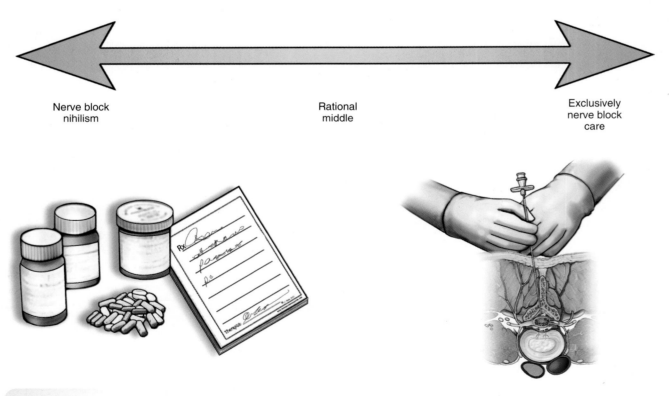

Nerve block
nihilism

Rational
middle

Exclusively
nerve block
care

Figure 43-1. The continuum of pain medicine for patient care.

seeking to establish positions at either polar end of the regional anesthesia technique continuum, represented by *nerve block nihilism* and *exclusively nerve block care*. Our patients will be best cared for by a mature and logical application of the rehabilitation and palliation options so well outlined in the following chapters. I particularly thank Dr. James Rathmell for providing his sound insights in the new chapters found in this section of the fourth edition of the *Atlas*.

The techniques outlined represent a select group of techniques in pain medicine practice. The list is not exhaustive, but rather a group of techniques that my contributors and I have found helpful in our own pain medicine practices. Most important in the use of any of these techniques is to approach each patient as an individual with unique needs, while always thinking first like a physician and holding that age-old tenet of "first do no harm" close to our decision making.

Facet Block

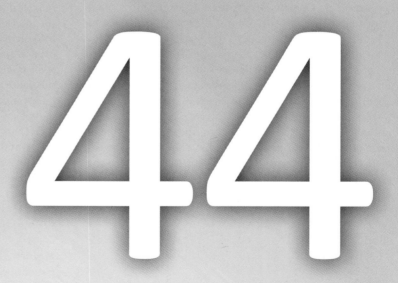

PERSPECTIVE

Facet blocks are used to diagnose and treat subsets of patients with chronic low-back and neck pain. Difficulties may arise in interpreting the results of facet blocks because the innervation of facet joints is diffuse, and radiographic changes in facet joints may or may not be linked to a specific patient's pain. Despite the caveats, the pain relief attained with facet injection seems convincing, although in contrast to many other pain management techniques, extra care must be taken in balancing the patient, the pain syndrome, and the treatment regimen with the individual clinical setting.

Patient Selection. Facet-related pain remains a diagnosis of exclusion, supported by reproduction of the pain during arthrography and relief of pain after diagnostic facet injection. In patients with lumbar pain syndromes, facet-related pain is often located in the low back and is described as a deep, dull ache that is difficult to localize. It may be referred to the buttocks or to the posterior leg, and infrequently it extends more distally into the lower leg. The pain is often made worse by lumbar extension, especially with lateral flexion to the affected side because this maneuver opposes the facet joints more forcefully. In cervical facet pain syndromes, the pain remains deep and aching, and the level of the facet involvement dictates the referral pattern of the pain. There are distinct upper, lower, and pancervical neck facet pain syndromes.

Pharmacologic Choice. Diagnostic blocks are most often performed with 1 to 2 mL of local anesthetic, either 1% to 1.5% lidocaine, 0.25% to 0.5% bupivacaine, or 0.2% to 0.5% ropivacaine. Lidocaine is chosen if immediate interpretation is sought, whereas bupivacaine or ropivacaine is used if diagnostic information is sought over a longer interval. For therapeutic injection, the total volume of solution is kept at 1.5 to 2.0 mL, although 20 mg of methylprednisolone is added to the local anesthetic (most often a longer-acting agent for a therapeutic injection). For either diagnostic or therapeutic injection, the needle position is confirmed with 0.25 to 0.5 mL of a radiocontrast agent, Hypaque-M 60% (Sanofi Winthrop, Irving, Tex).

PLACEMENT

Anatomy. The 33 vertebrae that make up the spinal column are linked by intervertebral disks and longitudinal ligaments anteriorly and through facet joints posteriorly.

The posterior facet joints allow flexion, extension, and rotation of the vertebral column while providing a means for the axial nerves to exit the vertebral column on their way to becoming peripheral nerves. The facet joints are synovial joints formed by the inferior articular processes of one vertebra and the superior articular processes of the adjacent caudad vertebra. These articular processes are projections, two superior and two inferior, from the junction of the pedicles and the laminae. In the cervical and lumbar portions of the vertebral column, the facet joints are posterior to the transverse processes, whereas in the thoracic region the facet joints are anterior to the transverse processes (Fig. 44-1). In the cervical vertebrae, the joint surfaces are midway between a coronal and an axial plane, whereas in the lumbar region, the joints (at least the posterior portion) assume an orientation approximately 30 degrees oblique to the sagittal plane (Fig. 44-2).

The capsule of a facet joint varies by location relative to the joint. A tough fibrous capsule is present on the posterolateral aspect of the joint, whereas on the anteromedial aspect of the joint, the facet synovial membrane is in direct contact with the ligamentum flavum.

The facet joints are innervated through the segmental sensory nerves that overlap the vertebral levels. Each joint has a dual innervation from the segmental nerve at its vertebral level as well as from the nerve at the level caudad to it. In the lumbar region, the posterior and anterior primary rami of a segmental nerve diverge at the intervertebral foramen (Fig. 44-3A). The posterior ramus, also known as the sinuvertebral nerve of Luschka, passes dorsally and caudally to enter the spine through a foramen in the intertransverse ligament. Almost immediately it divides into medial, lateral, and intermediate branches. The medial branch supplies the lower pole of the facet joint at its own level and the upper pole of the facet joint caudad to it. Each medial branch of the lumbar posterior ramus also supplies paraspinous muscles, such as the multifidus and interspinalis, as well as ligaments and the periosteum of the neural arch (Fig. 44-3B). In the cervical region, the medial branch innervates primarily the facet joint and not the paraspinous musculature. Further, in the cervical region, the nerves of Luschka wrap around the waists of their respective articular pillars and are bound to the periosteum by an investing fascia and held against the articular pillars by tendons of the semispinalis capitis muscle (Fig. 44-4).

Position. Lumbar facet blocks are performed with the patient prone on an imaging table with the hips and lower abdomen supported by a pillow. After the level of the facet joint is identified, the fluoroscopy unit is angled approximately 30 degrees off the parasagittal plane to obtain

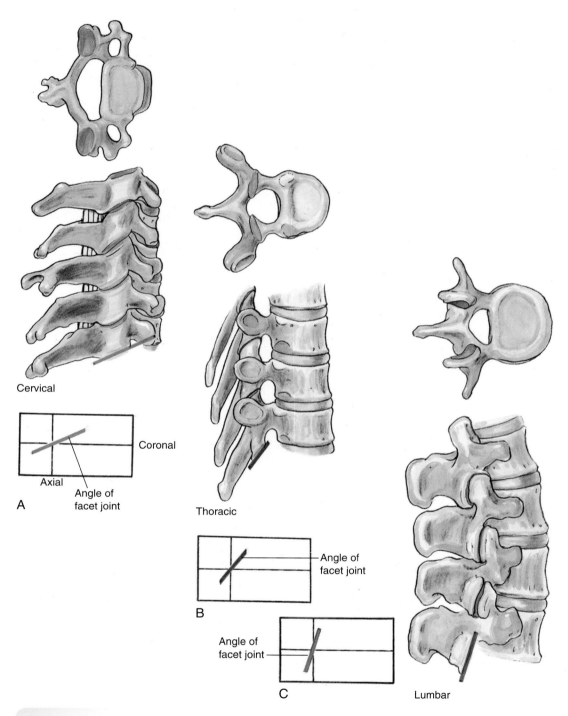

Cervical

Coronal

Axial

Angle of
facet joint

A

Thoracic

Angle of
facet joint

B

Angle of
facet joint

C

Lumbar

Figure 44-1. Superior and lateral views of cervical (**A**), thoracic (**B**), and lumbar (**C**) facet joints. Angle of the facet joints in the sagittal plane is indicated in the *insets*. Transverse processes are highlighted in *purple* in each image.

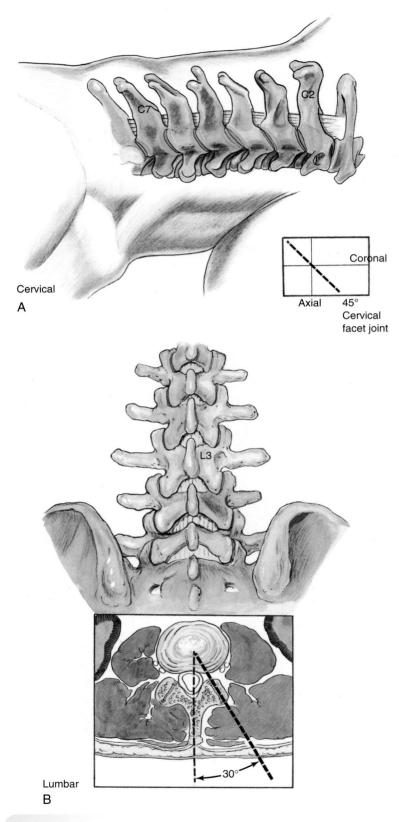

Cervical

A

Coronal

Axial   45°
Cervical
facet joint

Lumbar

B

Figure 44-2. Facet joint orientation. **A,** Cervical facet joint orientation is midway between axial and coronal. **B,** Lumbar facet joint orientation is 30 degrees oblique to the parasagittal plane.

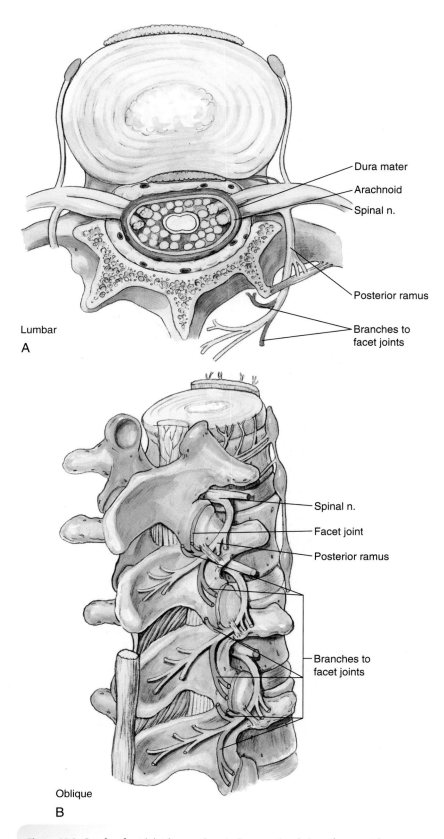

Figure 44-3. Lumbar facet joint innervation. **A,** Cross-sectional view of segmental nerve innervation of facet joint. **B,** Oblique parasagittal view of overlapping segmental innervation of facet joint.

Labels in figure A: Dura mater, Arachnoid, Spinal n., Posterior ramus, Branches to facet joints, Lumbar

Labels in figure B: Spinal n., Facet joint, Posterior ramus, Branches to facet joints, Oblique

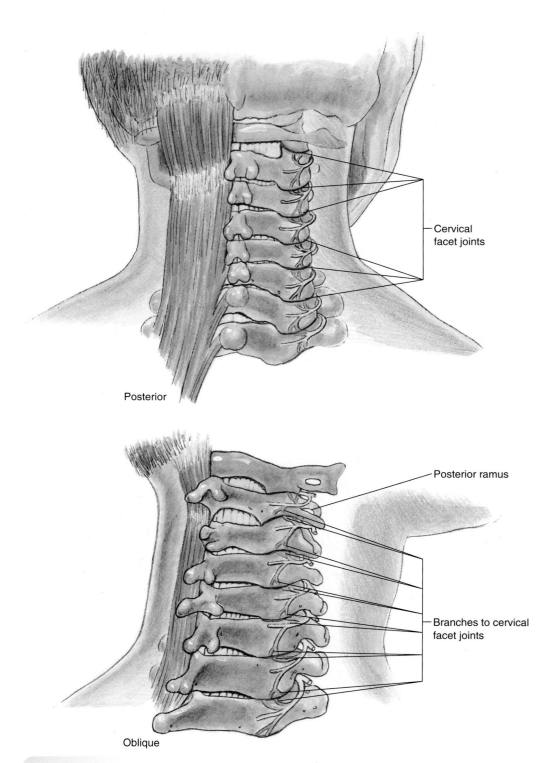

Cervical facet joints

Posterior

Posterior ramus

Branches to cervical facet joints

Oblique

Figure 44-4. Cervical facet joint innervation. Posterior and oblique parasagittal views of overlapping segmental innervation of facet joint.

optimum visualization of the lumbar facet joint (Fig. 44-5). Cervical facet blocks are also performed with the patient prone on an imaging table with the forehead and chest supported by pillows or individual silicone pads (Fig. 44-6A). Again, fluoroscopy is used to identify the facet joint, and after its position has been marked, the fluoroscopy unit is rotated to produce a lateral image of the cervical spine.

Needle Puncture. The facet joint is often located at the cephalocaudad level of the inferior extent of the more cephalad spinous process of the vertebra contributing to the facet joint. For example, the inferior extent of the spinous process of L3 corresponds to the L3-L4 facet joint. After the level of the facet joint has been marked, the fluoroscopy unit is angled approximately 30 degrees off the parasagittal plane, as described previously (see Fig. 44-5). A mark is then made 5 cm lateral to the vertebral midline at the previously identified facet joint level. After aseptic skin preparation, a 22-gauge, 6- to 10-cm needle is inserted at a slightly medial parasagittal angle. Under fluoroscopic guidance, the needle tip is placed in the facet joint (Fig. 44-7). Then a radiocontrast agent is injected to verify the

position of the needle tip (see Fig. 44-6B). Once the needle position is confirmed, the therapeutic or diagnostic injection is performed.

Cervical facet blocks are also performed with the patient prone on an imaging table, as described earlier. Fluoroscopy is used to identify the facet joint to be blocked, and its cephalocaudad vertebral level is marked. After the paravertebral cephalocaudad and mediolateral positions of the facet joint have been marked, the fluoroscopy unit is rotated to produce a lateral image of the cervical spine. This allows optimum visualization of the cervical facet joint during needle placement. A needle entry skin mark is made 3 to 4 cm caudad to the facet joint previously identified and approximately 3 cm lateral to the vertebral midline (Fig. 44-8A). After the skin has been aseptically prepared, a 22-gauge, 6- to 8-cm needle is inserted in a cephaloanterior direction and guided with fluoroscopic assistance into the previously identified cervical facet joint (Fig. 44-8B). Radiocontrast medium is then injected to verify the position of the needle tip (Fig. 44-8C). Once the needle position has been confirmed, the therapeutic or diagnostic injection is performed.

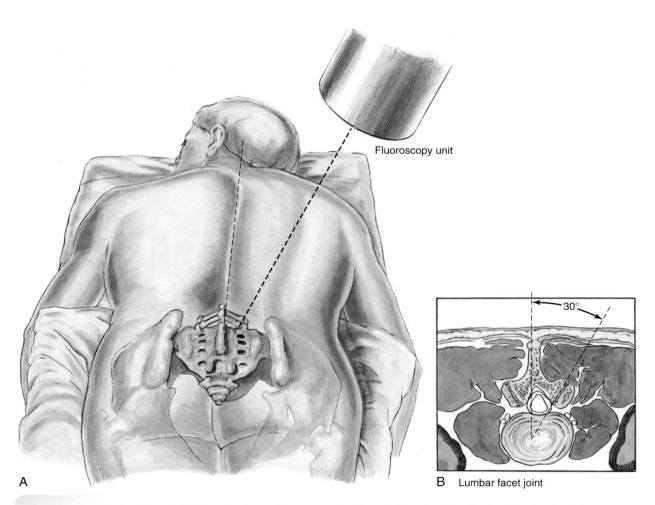

Fluoroscopy unit

30°

A

B   Lumbar facet joint

Figure 44-5. Lumbar facet joint. **A,** Position of patient and fluoroscopic imaging unit for optimal visualization of lumbar facet joint. **B,** Cross-sectional image of lumbar facet joint.

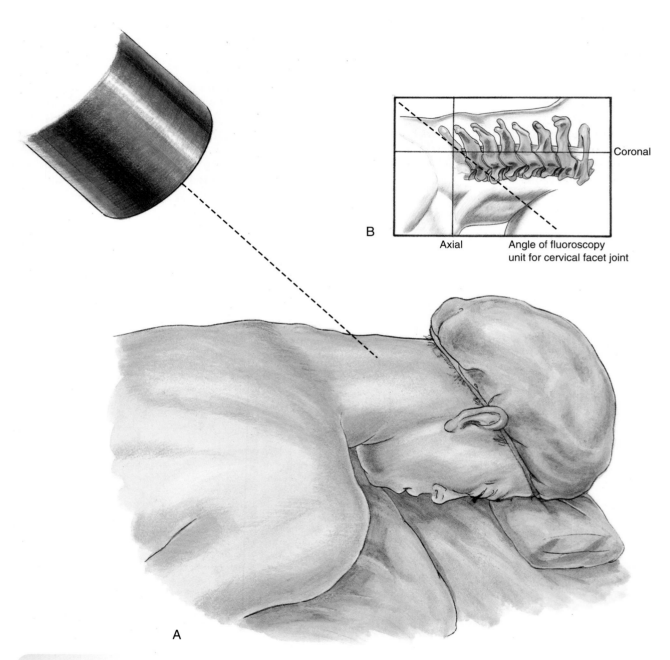

B

Coronal

Axial

Angle of fluoroscopy
unit for cervical facet joint

A

Figure 44-6. Cervical facet joint. **A,** Position of patient and fluoroscopic imaging unit for optimal visualization of cervical facet joint. **B,** Oblique posteroanterior image of cervical facet joints, showing cephalad angulation of fluoroscopic unit.

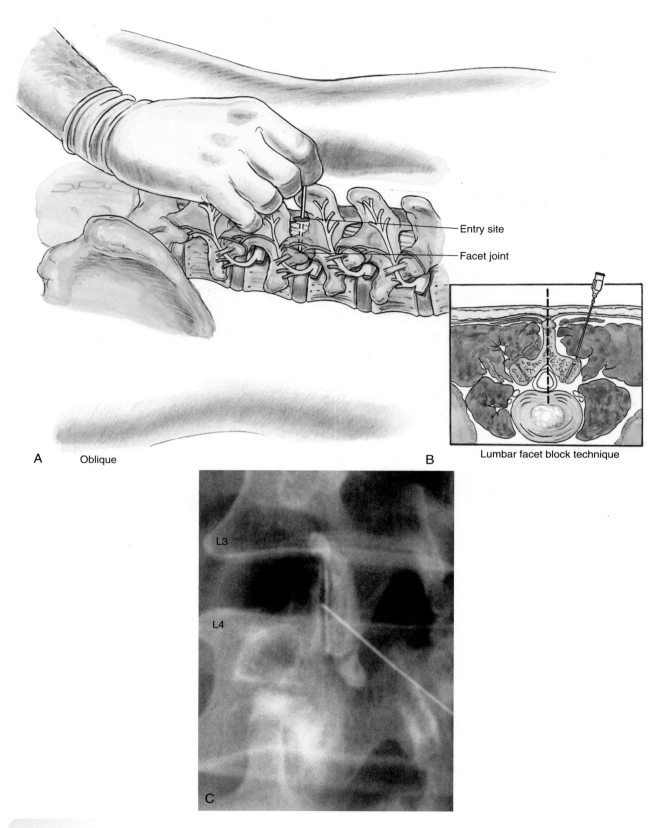

Entry site

Facet joint

A   Oblique

B   Lumbar facet block technique

L3

L4

C

Figure 44-7. Lumbar facet joint injection. Oblique (**A**) and cross-sectional (**B**) views of lumbar facet block technique. **C,** Radiographic image of injection of 1.5 mL of contrast into lumbar facet joint.

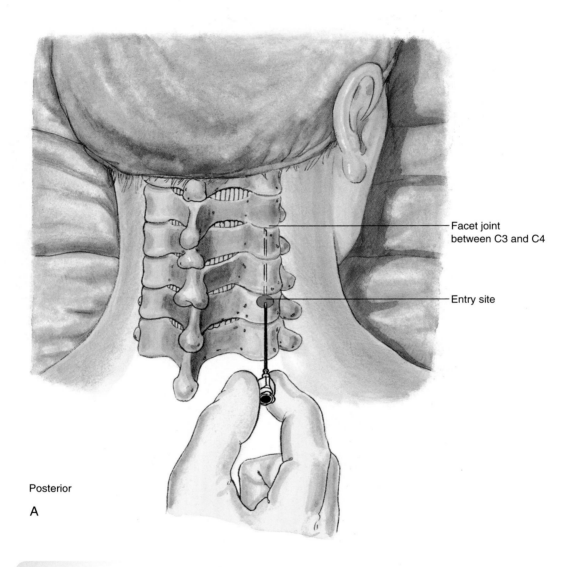

Facet joint
between C3 and C4

Entry site

Posterior

A

Figure 44-8. Cervical facet joint injection. **A,** Posteroanterior view of needle insertion for a cervical facet block.

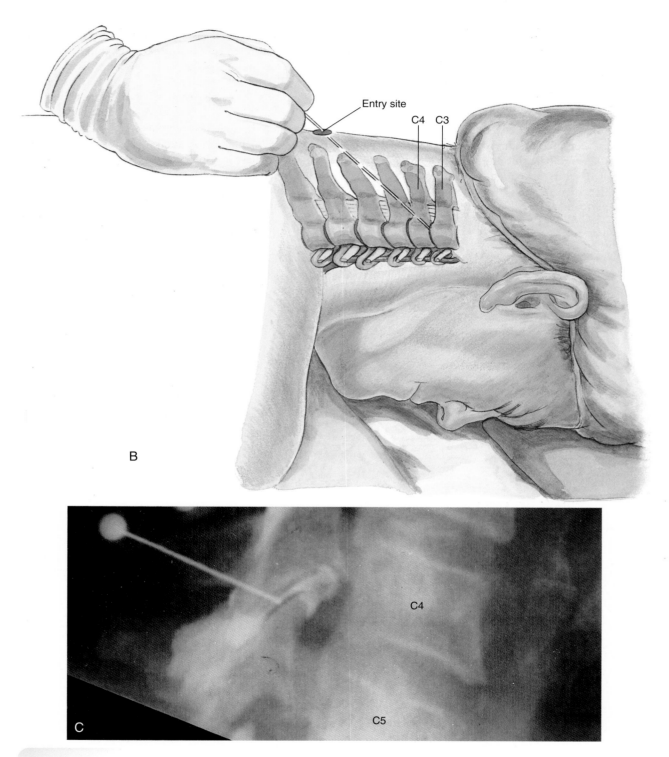

Entry site

C4 C3

B

C4

C5

C

Figure 44-8, cont'd. B, Lateral view of needle insertion for a cervical facet block. **C,** Radiographic image of injection of 1.0 mL of contrast into C4-C5 cervical facet joint.

POTENTIAL PROBLEMS

As in any other regional block, facet injections should be avoided if the patient has a coagulopathy or infection at the site of the injection. Because these injections are administered near the neuraxis, epidural or intrathecal effects are possible, as is injection of the vertebral artery in the cervical region.

PEARLS

The most important word of advice about facet blocks is that they should be used selectively after a thorough history and physical examination directed at the patient's pain complaints. The radiographic and neurodiagnostic studies are integrated with the patient's signs and symptoms. Heeding this advice allows the anesthesiologist to be more precise in performing facet blocks and minimizes frustration over any lack of diagnostic or therapeutic results. Also, to use facet blocks effectively it is important to understand the innervation of both the lumbar and the cervical facet joints. Such an understanding helps to minimize diagnostic confusion.

Another help in minimizing diagnostic confusion is to become comfortable with radiocontrast agents and their use near the neuraxis; Hypaque-M 60% is currently the preferred agent. It is also important to constantly remind oneself and one's colleagues that radiographic changes in the facet joints have never been effectively linked to specific facet pain states. If larger volumes (4 to 5 mL) of therapeutic solutions are injected at the lumbar facet joints, the results may be difficult to interpret because the solution will not be contained within the facet joint but will spread to the segmental nerves and the paraspinous muscles. Finally, I believe it is important to warn patients that neuraxial block effects are possible (although rare) after facet injections; thus, the blocks should be performed only when complete stabilization or resuscitation of unintentional postinjection effects is possible.

Sacroiliac Block

45

PERSPECTIVE

The sacroiliac block is most often used for patients with chronic low-back pain, both diagnostically and therapeutically. Patients with low-back pain treated at chronic pain centers often experience relief of low-back pain after a sacroiliac block. Pain secondary to sacroiliac arthropathy is a cause of low-back pain that is often overlooked by physicians infrequently involved in comprehensive pain programs.

Patient Selection. Patients undergoing evaluation for low-back pain should be evaluated clinically for sacroiliac pain. These patients typically complain of unilateral low-back pain, which often radiates into the ipsilateral buttock, groin, or leg. Often these patients have symptoms similar to those characteristic of facet joint syndromes. During the clinical examination, an increase in pain with pressure over the sacroiliac joint suggests sacroiliac pain. If such pain is present, provocative maneuvers that increase sacroiliac joint motion should be performed, such as Gaenslen's test and the flamingo test (Fig. 45-1).

Pharmacologic Choice. During fluoroscopically guided provocative diagnostic sacroiliac joint injection, 1 to 2 mL of radiocontrast solution (e.g., Isovue-300 [Bracco Diagnostics, Princeton, NJ] mixed with an equal volume of isotonic saline solution) should be used. This injection often provokes pain similar to that experienced by the patient with activity. After sacroiliac joint involvement has been confirmed, a therapeutic injection of 5 to 10 mL of 1% lidocaine mixed with 20 to 40 mg of methylprednisolone can be performed. If fluoroscopy is unavailable and a combined diagnostic–therapeutic injection is performed

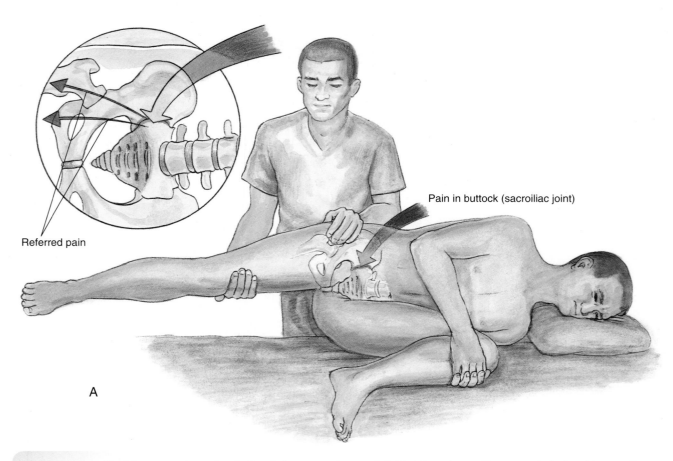

Referred pain

Pain in buttock (sacroiliac joint)

A

Figure 45-1. Sacroiliac joint provocative testing. **A,** Gaenslen's test: examiner stands behind the patient and hyperextends the leg of the sacroiliac joint being tested while stabilizing the pelvis. Pain with this maneuver may indicate sacroiliac joint involvement but may also indicate a hip lesion or lumbar root problem.

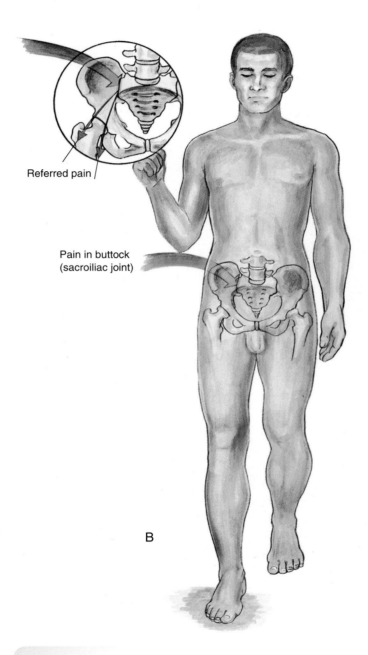

Referred pain

Pain in buttock
(sacroiliac joint)

B

Figure 45-1, cont'd. B, Flamingo test: the patient is asked to stand on the involved leg alone and then hop. Pain in the region of the sacroiliac joint is a positive test result.

empirically, 5 to 10 mL of 1% lidocaine, 0.25% bupivacaine, or 0.2% ropivacaine mixed with 20 to 40 mg of methylprednisolone is used.

PLACEMENT

Anatomy. The sacroiliac joint has a well-developed joint space lined by synovial membrane with typical hyaline articular cartilage on the sacral side of the joint and a thinner layer of fibrocartilage on the iliac side. Anteriorly,

the joint capsule is well developed, forming the thin anterior sacroiliac ligament. There is no joint capsule posteriorly, and the joint space is in continuity with the interosseous sacroiliac ligament. Immediately posterior to the interosseous sacroiliac ligament is the large and strong posterior sacroiliac ligament (Fig. 45-2A). The joint surfaces can rotate 3 to 5 degrees in younger, symptom-free patients, and the joint provides elasticity to the pelvic rim and serves as a buffer between the lumbosacral joint and the hip joint.

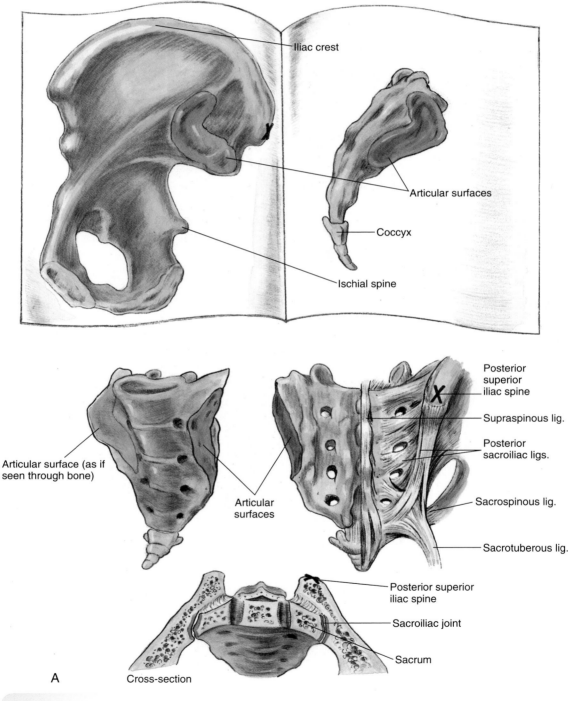

Figure 45-2. **A,** Sacroiliac joint anatomy.

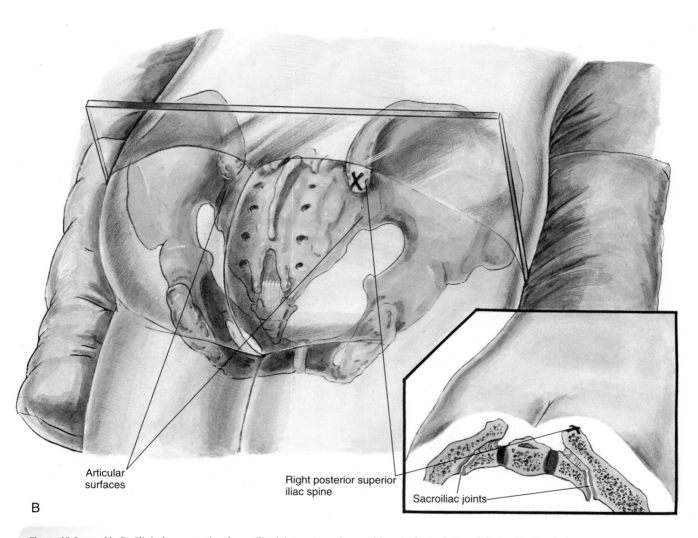

Articular
surfaces

Right posterior superior
iliac spine

Sacroiliac joints

B

Figure 45-2, cont'd. B, Clinical cross-sectional sacroiliac joint anatomy in a position similar to that used during block technique.

Position. Patient position depends on whether fluoroscopy is used to confirm the position of the needle. When fluoroscopy is used, the patient is placed prone with the contralateral hip raised slightly on a pillow (approximately 20 degrees off the horizontal). This position allows the anterior and posterior orifices of the lower third of the joint to be superimposed, maximizing visualization of the joint. If fluoroscopy is not used, a pillow can simply be placed beneath the pelvis and lower abdomen with the patient prone (Fig. 45-2B).

The anesthesiologist can approach the technique in one of two ways. He or she can stand on the side of the sacroiliac joint undergoing injection. This allows palpation of the sacroiliac joint with the fingers of the dominant hand from a lateral position and frees more space medially for joint injection (Fig. 45-3A). Conversely, the anesthesiologist can stand opposite the sacroiliac joint to be blocked, allowing needle insertion with the dominant hand (Fig. 45-3B).

Needle Puncture. When fluoroscopy is used for needle guidance, the patient is placed in the slightly oblique position described in the section on "Patient Position." Fluoroscopy is used to superimpose the lower third of the

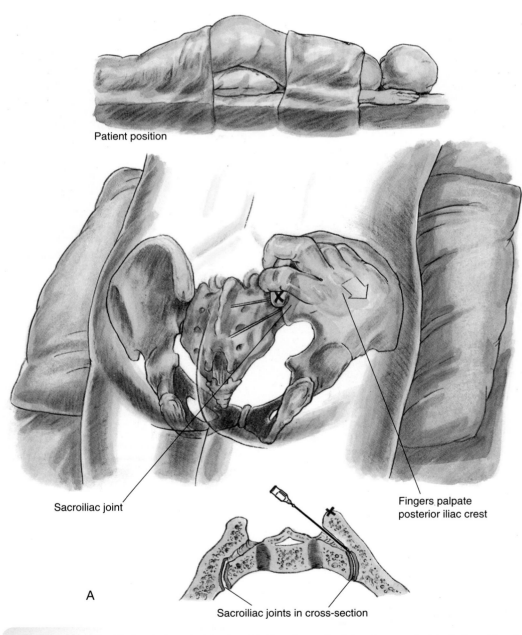

Patient position

Sacroiliac joint

Fingers palpate posterior iliac crest

Sacroiliac joints in cross-section

A

Figure 45-3. Sacroiliac block technique. **A,** Palpation of ipsilateral sacroiliac joint when anesthesiologist is positioned on the side being blocked.

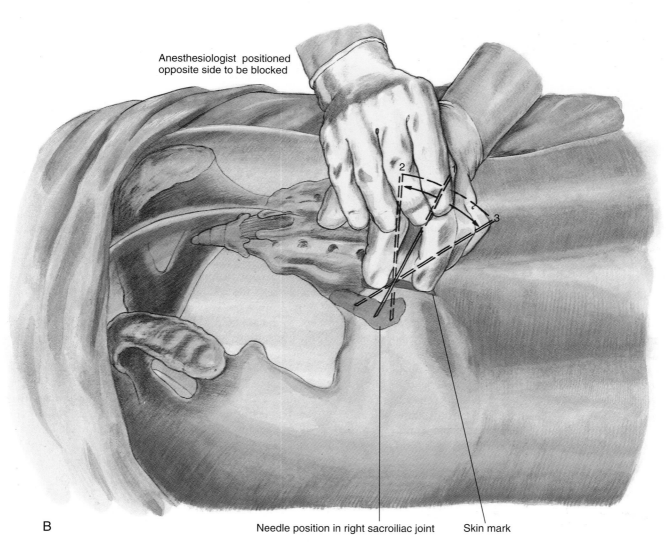

Anesthesiologist positioned
opposite side to be blocked

B

Needle position in right sacroiliac joint   Skin mark

Figure 45-3, cont'd. B, Needle insertion for block when anesthesiologist is positioned opposite the side being blocked.

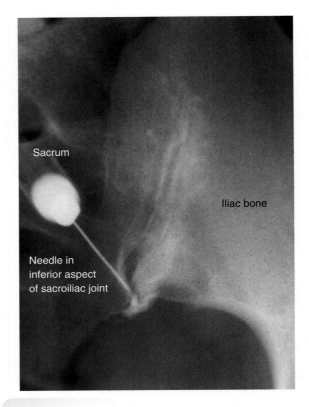

Sacrum

Iliac bone

Needle in
inferior aspect
of sacroiliac joint

Figure 45-4. Sacroiliac joint fluoroscopic anatomy. The needle is in the inferior aspect of the sacroiliac joint; a small amount of contrast material is seen outlining the joint and spilling out inferiorly.

anterior and posterior orifices of the sacroiliac joint, which should appear as a "Y"-shaped image (Fig. 45-4). After aseptic skin preparation and skin infiltration with local anesthetic, a 22-gauge, 7- to 9-cm needle is advanced into the lower third of the joint and its position is confirmed with radiocontrast injection. If inadequate spread of contrast medium is noted, the needle can be repositioned under fluoroscopic guidance and the cycle repeated. If no fluoroscopic needle guidance is planned, after aseptic skin preparation and local anesthetic skin infiltration, a 22-gauge, 7- to 9-cm needle on a 10-mL, three-ring control syringe is inserted in an anterolateral direction into the

region between the posterior superior and the posterior inferior iliac spines. The needle may be repositioned along an arc extending between the posterior superior and the posterior inferior iliac spines, and the solution can be reinjected incrementally (see Fig. 45-3B). Again, it is typical to use approximately 5 to 10 mL of solution during these injections. In the nonfluoroscopic needle insertion, the local anesthetic–steroid solution is directed primarily at and deep to the posterior sacroiliac ligament and some of the solution may find its way into the joint. Verification of joint injection is possible only through fluoroscopy.

POTENTIAL PROBLEMS

Like any block performed near the sacrum, sciatic or sacral root block is a possible outcome, especially if larger volumes of local anesthetic are used. Misdiagnosis is also possible when fluoroscopy is not used to guide needle placement and the patient reports no pain relief. In this situation, it may simply be that the drug did not reach the sacroiliac joint.

PEARLS

Sacroiliac block appears to be an underused diagnostic and therapeutic pain control technique. One of the first requirements in using this block effectively is to consider the possibility that sacroiliac joint pain is a source of the patient's low-back pain. In addition, a logical, prospectively planned sequence of fluoroscopically guided sacroiliac block injections should be developed. Although radiographic guidance validates correct injection, it is not used in all cases. An underappreciated symptom of sacroiliac joint pain is referral of pain to the ipsilateral groin. Relief of groin pain after sacroiliac block seems to be linked to the sacroiliac joint as a real source of low-back pain. Finally, before performing a sacroiliac block it is helpful to warn the patient that a small percentage of patients will experience a temporarily numb ipsilateral leg. Advance comment about this phenomenon seems to smooth clinical care even if the procedure results in a lower extremity block.

Lumbar Sympathetic Block

46

PERSPECTIVE

Lumbar sympathetic blocks are typically carried out to improve blood flow to the lower extremities or provide pain relief to the lower extremities.

Patient Selection. Patients requiring lumbar sympathetic block can be divided into two primary groups: (1) those requiring sympathetic block because of ischemic vascular disease to the lower extremities (these patients are often older); and (2) patients requiring the block for diagnosis or treatment of complex regional pain syndromes of the lower extremities (these patients have a much wider age range).

Pharmacologic Choice. Block of the sympathetic nervous system can be performed with lower concentrations of local anesthetics than almost any other regional block. For example, 0.5% lidocaine, 0.125% or 0.25% bupivacaine, or 0.1% or 0.2% ropivacaine are appropriate choices.

PLACEMENT

Anatomy. The lumbar sympathetic chain, with its accompanying ganglia, is located in the fascial plane immediately anterolateral to the lumbar vertebral bodies (Fig. 46-1). The sympathetic chain is separated from the somatic nerves by the psoas muscle and fascia. The lumbar regions L1, L2, and sometimes L3 provide white rami communicantes to the sympathetic chain, and all five lumbar vertebrae are associated with gray rami communicantes. These rami are longer in the lumbar region than in the thoracic region. This is anatomically important because it allows needle placement nearer the anterolateral border of the vertebral body in the lumbar region. Conceptually, the anatomy important to anesthesiologists performing lumbar sympathetic nerve block is also the anatomy important for celiac plexus nerve block.

Position. My experience suggests that lumbar sympathetic nerve block is most effectively carried out in a manner similar to that used for celiac plexus block (see Chapter 47, Celiac Plexus Block). The patient should be prone with a pillow under the mid-abdomen to help reduce lumbar lordosis. (Despite this recommendation, many clinicians continue to use the lateral position successfully.)

Needle Puncture. Most experienced anesthesiologists now carry out this block through a single needle. This is possible because placing the needle tip at the anterolateral border of the second or third lumbar vertebral body allows the local anesthetic solution to spread along the fascial plane enveloping the sympathetic chain. As an example, the second lumbar vertebral spine is identified, and a mark is made lateral to it in the horizontal plane, 7 to 9 cm from the midline, as illustrated in Figure 46-2. A skin wheal is raised, and a 15-cm, 20- or 22-gauge needle is directed in the horizontal plane at an angle of 30 to 45 degrees from a

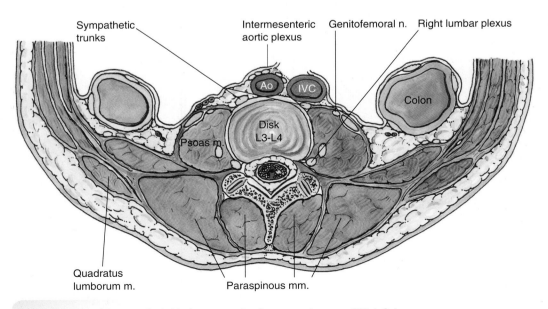

Figure 46-1. Lumbar sympathetic block: cross-sectional anatomy. Ao, aorta; IVC, inferior vena cava.

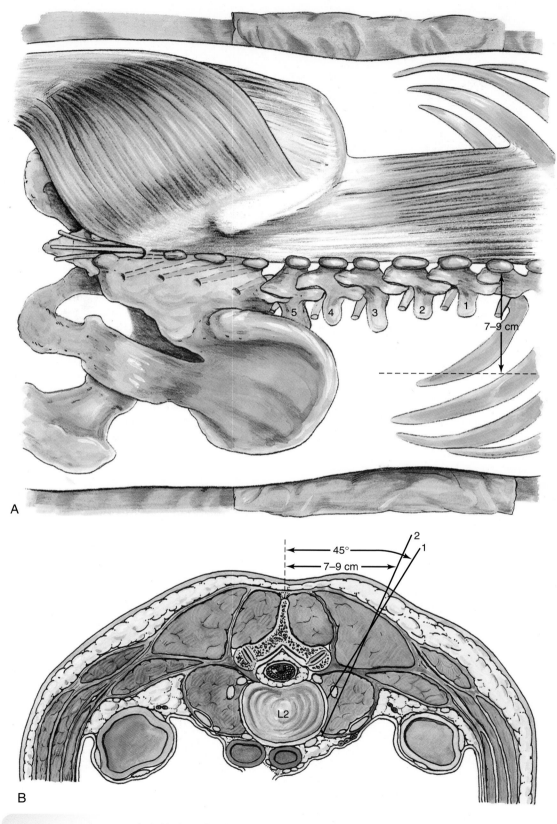

Figure 46-2. Lumbar sympathetic block: surface (**A**) and cross-sectional (**B**) technique.

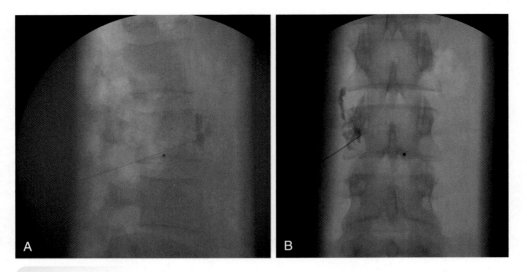

Figure 46-3. Lumbar sympathetic block: fluoroscopic spread of contrast in typical lumbar sympathetic block. Needle placement anterolateral to L3 and spread of 1.5 mL of contrast. **A,** Posteroanterior view. **B,** Lateral view.

vertical plane through the patient's midline. It is inserted until it contacts the lateral aspect of the L2 vertebral body. If it comes into contact with the vertebral transverse process at a more superficial level (at only 3 to 5 cm), the needle can simply be redirected cephalad or caudad to avoid the transverse process. The vertebral body is usually located at a depth of 7 to 12 cm.

Once the needle's position on the lateral aspect of the vertebral body is certain, the needle is withdrawn and redirected at a steeper angle until it slides off the anterolateral surface of L2. This needle insertion and redirection process is almost identical to that described for the celiac plexus block. For the lumbar sympathetic block, once the needle is in position, approximately 15 to 20 mL of local anesthetic solution is injected. With proper needle tip position, this volume will allow spread along the axis of the sympathetic chain (Fig. 46-3).

POTENTIAL PROBLEMS

As illustrated in Figure 46-4, a potential problem with the lumbar sympathetic block is puncture of the aorta. Most

often this results in no sequelae. Nevertheless, anesthesiologists should be aware that the position of the aorta relative to the vertebral body ranges from an anterolateral position to a midline position. Because the needle is directed toward the neuraxial structures, both epidural and spinal block can result from an errantly placed needle. Thus, development of a postural headache after a lumbar sympathetic block should lead the anesthesiologist to think of unrecognized dural puncture. Also, when using neurolytic agents, one should be aware that spillover onto lumbar roots is a possibility, although it happens rarely.

PEARLS

Few regional blocks are as similar as the lumbar sympathetic block and celiac plexus block. Thus, it is easy to translate the anatomic understanding of one technique into successful performance of the other. Adequate sedation for placing the needle against the lateral portion of the second lumbar vertebra is also essential for patient—and thus anesthesiologist—satisfaction.

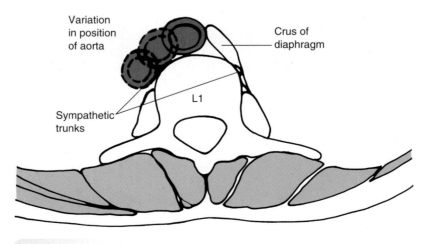

Figure 46-4. Lumbar sympathetic block: variable aortic position.

Celiac Plexus Block

47

PERSPECTIVE

Celiac plexus block can be used for many types of intra-abdominal visceral pain syndromes. Its most frequent application is to relieve pain associated with intra-abdominal cancer, using a neurolytic solution. Visceral analgesia can also be provided for patients undergoing upper abdominal surgery; combining celiac plexus block with intercostal nerve block provides an unrivaled quality of immediate postoperative analgesia.

Patient Selection. Most celiac plexus blocks are carried out for cancer pain therapy, and the majority of blocks used for cancer pain are related to gastric or pancreatic malignancies. The celiac plexus provides innervation to most of the gut from the lower esophagus to the level of the splenic flexure of the colon. Therefore, celiac plexus block may be applicable to a wide variety of patients with intra-abdominal malignancy.

Pharmacologic Choice. The celiac plexus is primarily a sympathetic ganglion; thus, low concentrations of local anesthetics are successful in blocking the celiac plexus. For example, 0.5% lidocaine, 0.125% or 0.25% bupivacaine, or 0.1% or 0.2% ropivacaine is adequate. If celiac plexus neurolysis is sought, my choice is 50% alcohol, which is formulated by combining equal volumes of 100% alcohol with 0.25% bupivacaine or 0.2% ropivacaine, to a total of 50 mL.

PLACEMENT

Anatomy. The celiac plexus has also been called the *solar plexus*, the *celiac ganglion*, and the *splanchnic plexus* (Fig. 47-1). It is the largest of the three great plexuses of the sympathetic nervous system in the chest and abdomen: the cardiac plexus innervates the thoracic structures, the celiac plexus innervates the abdominal organs, and the hypogastric plexus supplies the pelvic organs. All three of these plexuses contain visceral afferent and efferent fibers. In addition, they contain some parasympathetic fibers that pass through after originating in cranial or sacral areas of the parasympathetic nervous system.

The celiac plexus innervates most of the abdominal viscera, including the stomach, liver, biliary tract, pancreas, spleen, kidneys, adrenals, omentum, small bowel, and large bowel to the level of the splenic flexure. The celiac plexus receives its primary innervation from the greater, lesser, and least splanchnic nerves, which arise from T5 through T12. The splanchnic nerves innervate the celiac plexus after traversing the posterior mediastinum and entering the abdomen through the crura of the diaphragm, a variable distance above L1 (Figs. 47-2 and 47-3). The splanchnic nerves are preganglionic, and after they synapse in the celiac ganglion proper (or associated ganglia), their postganglionic fibers radiate to the abdominal viscera (Fig. 47-4). Autopsy examination has shown that the number of ganglia making up the celiac plexus ranges from one to five, with the size of ganglia ranging from 0.5 to 4.5 cm in diameter.

The celiac plexus is found anterolateral to the celiac artery. In addition, the vena cava is often anterolateral on the right, the aorta is posterior to the plexus in the midline, the kidneys are lateral, and the pancreas lies anteriorly (Figs. 47-5 and 47-6).

One point of anatomic clarification that is essential for understanding the celiac plexus block is that there are two basic methods of carrying out the block. In the longest-used method, the needles are inserted to perform a deep splanchnic block. This results in spread of the solution (*blue*, as illustrated in Fig. 47-7) cephalad and posterior to the diaphragmatic crura. The second method involves placing the needle through one crus of the diaphragm from a posterior approach, or through the anterior abdominal wall, to end up with the needle placed anterior to the aorta in the region of the celiac plexus. As illustrated in Figure 47-7, this results in spread of solution (*pink*) in the vicinity of the celiac artery, anterior to the diaphragmatic crura.

Position. The patient should be positioned for the celiac plexus block in the prone position, with a pillow placed beneath the abdomen to reduce lumbar lordosis.

Needle Puncture: Method. The lumbar vertebral spinous processes, as well as the 12th thoracic vertebral spinous process, should be identified and marked. Parallel lines should then be drawn 7 to 8 cm off the midline, as shown in Figure 47-8. The 12th rib should be palpated and a mark placed where the paramedian lines cross the 12th rib bilaterally. Another mark should be placed in the midline between the 12th thoracic and 1st lumbar vertebral spinous processes. By drawing lines between the three marks, a flat isosceles triangle is created. The equal sides of this triangle (*A and B*) serve as directional guides for the bilaterally placed needles.

Skin wheals should then be raised on the marks immediately below the 12th rib, and a 12- to 15-cm, 20- or 22-gauge needle is inserted without the syringe attached, as shown in Figure 47-9. The needle is inserted 45 degrees off the plane of the tabletop, directed at the space between the T12 and the L1 vertebral spinous processes. This place-

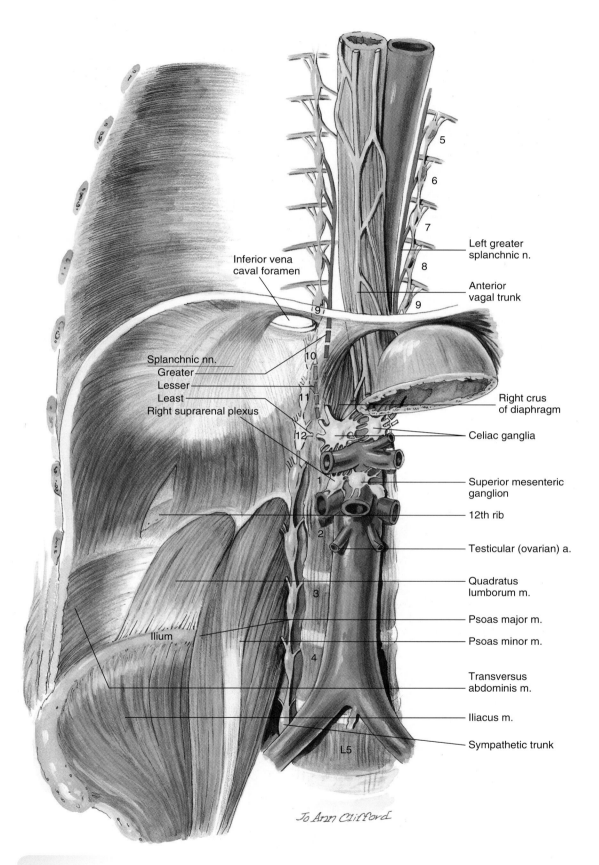

Inferior vena
caval foramen

Left greater
splanchnic n.

Anterior
vagal trunk

Splanchnic nn.
Greater
Lesser
Least
Right suprarenal plexus

Right crus
of diaphragm

Celiac ganglia

Superior mesenteric
ganglion

12th rib

Testicular (ovarian) a.

Quadratus
lumborum m.

Psoas major m.

Psoas minor m.

Transversus
abdominis m.

Iliacus m.

Sympathetic trunk

Ilium

5

6

7

8

9

9

10

11

12

1

2

3

4

L5

Jo Ann Clifford

Figure 47-1. Celiac plexus block: anatomy.

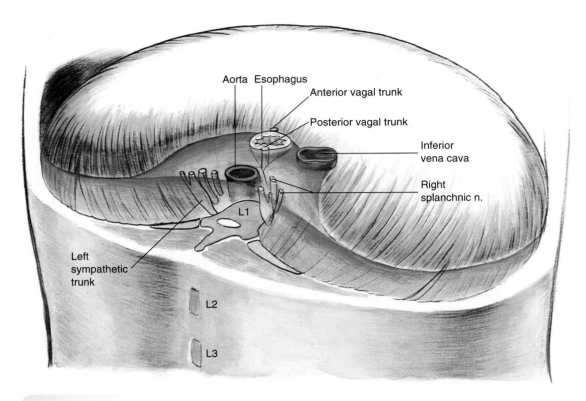

Figure 47-2. Celiac plexus block: cross-sectional anatomy.

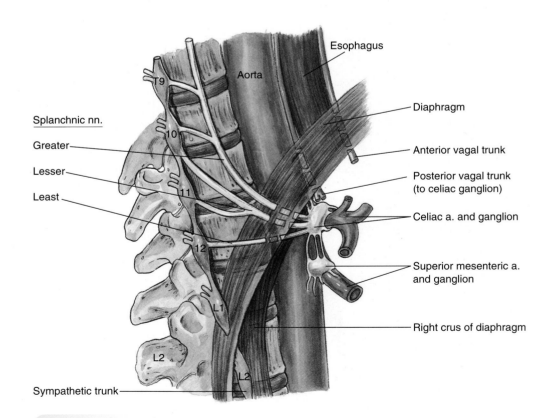

Figure 47-3. Celiac plexus block: parasagittal anatomy.

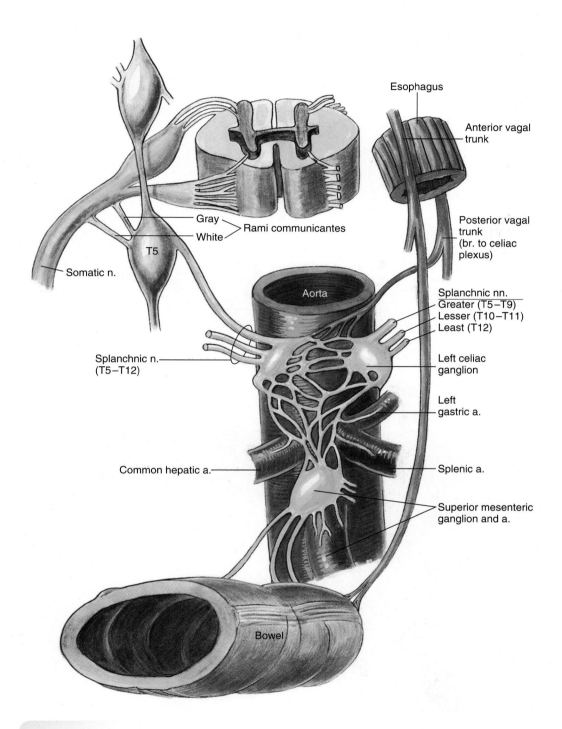

Esophagus

Anterior vagal trunk

Gray
White
Rami communicantes

T5

Somatic n.

Posterior vagal trunk (br. to celiac plexus)

Aorta

Splanchnic nn.
Greater (T5–T9)
Lesser (T10–T11)
Least (T12)

Splanchnic n. (T5–T12)

Left celiac ganglion

Left gastric a.

Common hepatic a.

Splenic a.

Superior mesenteric ganglion and a.

Bowel

Figure 47-4. Celiac plexus block: functional anatomy.

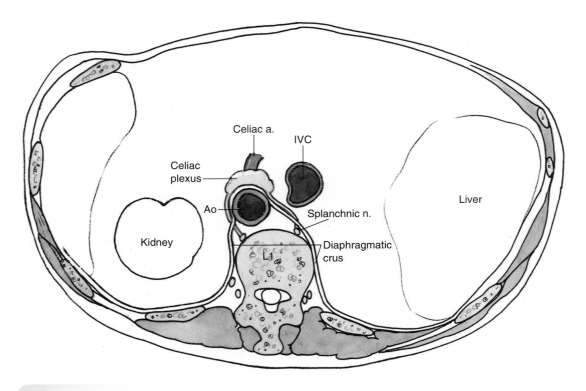

Figure 47-5. Celiac plexus block: interpretation of cross-sectional magnetic resonance imaging anatomy. Ao, aorta; IVC, inferior vena cava.

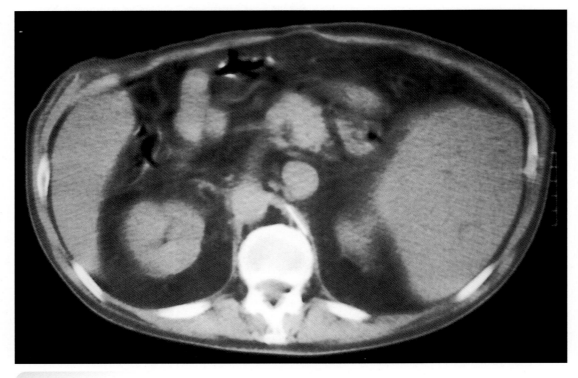

Figure 47-6. Celiac plexus block: anatomy on cross-sectional magnetic resonance imaging scan.

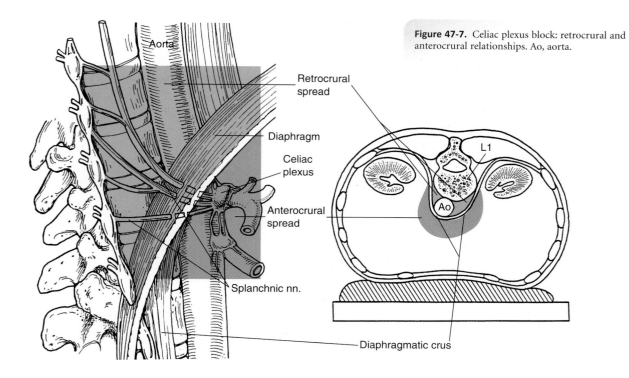

Figure 47-7. Celiac plexus block: retrocrural and anterocrural relationships. Ao, aorta.

Aorta

Retrocrural spread

Diaphragm

Celiac plexus

Anterocrural spread

Splanchnic nn.

L1

Ao

Diaphragmatic crus

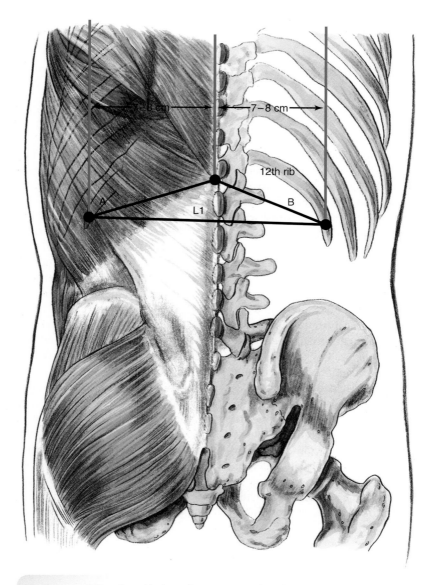

7–8 cm

7–8 cm

12th rib

A

B

L1

Figure 47-8. Celiac plexus block: surface anatomy and markings.

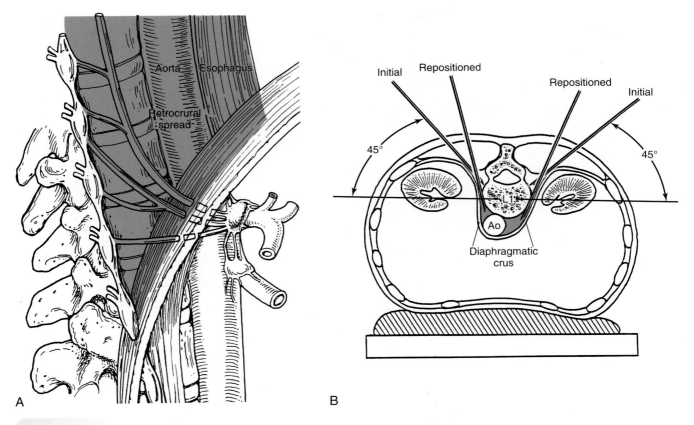

Figure 47-9. Celiac plexus block: retrocrural (deep splanchnic) technique. Ao, aorta.

ment will allow contact with the L1 vertebral body at a depth of 7 to 9 cm. If bony contact is made at a more superficial level, it is likely that a vertebral transverse process has been contacted. In today's practice of pain care, most patients will have their celiac block performed with fluoroscopic guidance, simplifying needle insertion.

When the vertebral body is confidently identified, the needle is withdrawn to a subcutaneous level and the angle is increased to allow the tip to pass the lateral border of the vertebral body. On the left side (the side of the aorta), once the needle passes off the vertebral body, it should be inserted an additional 1.5 to 2 cm or until the aortic wall is identified by pulsations transmitted through the length of the needle. On the right side, the needle can be inserted 2 to 3 cm after it "walks off" the vertebral body. It is helpful in inserting the needles to the proper depth to insert the left needle first because it can be advanced slowly until the operator's sensitive fingertips (Fig. 47-10) appreciate the aortic pulsations transmitted up the needle shaft. When this aortic depth is identified, the right needle can then be inserted and readily advanced to a slightly deeper level.

Before local anesthetic or neurolytic agent is injected, the needle should be carefully examined for leakage of blood, urine, or cerebrospinal fluid. If the needle is misplaced, leakage of these fluids should be spontaneous. Injection of local anesthetic solution through the needle should be

similar to when an epidural needle is properly placed. There should be very little resistance to injection if a 20- or 22-gauge needle is correctly placed in the retrocrural area.

Needle Puncture: Anterocrural Method. The second basic method of celiac plexus block is the anterocrural approach, which results in the needle tip's being placed anterior to the crus of the diaphragm on the right side, as illustrated in Figure 47-11. To carry out this block, all the foregoing steps are the same, except that the paramedian line on the right is drawn 5 to 6 cm off the midline, rather than 7 to 8 cm as in the classic retrocrural approach. The needle is inserted to strike the vertebral body. Often an angle larger than 45 degrees is necessary to contact the vertebral body initially. When the vertebral body is contacted, the needle is withdrawn and redirected until it "walks off" the antero-lateral edge of the vertebral body. To place an anterocrural needle properly, radiographic assistance is necessary. Commonly, the needle must be inserted 10 to 13 cm to place its tip anterior to the crus of the diaphragm. It is helpful to use a supplementary imaging technique for the transcrural approach because passage of the needle tip through the crus of the diaphragm is difficult to appreciate by palpation unless a transaortic method similar to the method of Ischia is used. Once the needle tip is in position anterior to the crus of the diaphragm, local anesthetic solution is injected through the single right-sided needle.

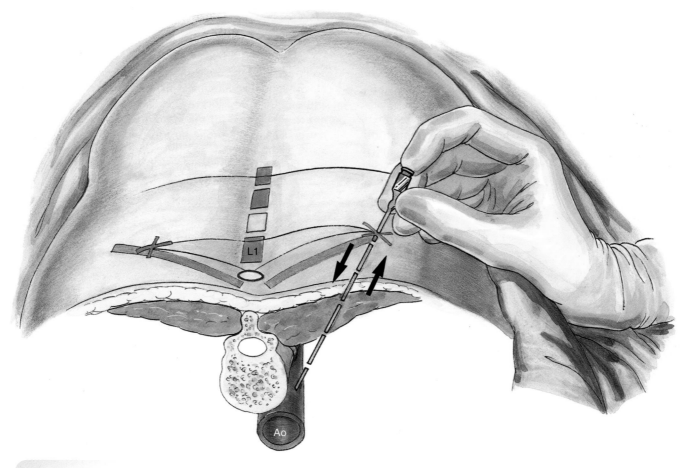

Figure 47-10. Celiac plexus block: technique of using finger as "pressure transducer." Ao, aorta.

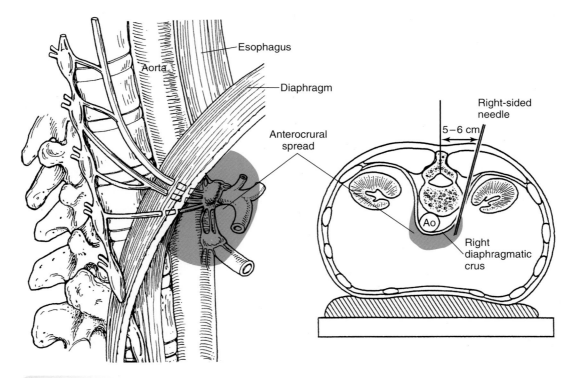

Esophagus

Aorta

Diaphragm

Anterocrural
spread

Right-sided
needle

5–6 cm

Ao

Right
diaphragmatic
crus

Figure 47-11. Celiac plexus block: anterocrural technique. Ao, aorta.

POTENTIAL PROBLEMS

Because of the location of the celiac plexus near the neuraxis, epidural or spinal anesthesia may develop with this technique. In addition, because of the close relationship of the celiac plexus to the aorta, aortic puncture occurs in approximately one third of patients. Nevertheless, this rarely results in serious problems. As in lumbar sympathetic block, the placement of the needle tip for a celiac block may allow tracking of local anesthetic or neurolytic solution in the region of the lumbar roots, although this also appears to happen infrequently. An even less frequent neurologic injury after neurolytic celiac block, paraplegia, may result from drug-induced spasm of a major lumbar feeding artery (artery of Adamkiewicz). This most likely hypothesis awaits clinical proof.

PEARLS

To understand the celiac plexus block fully, the anesthesiologist should be familiar with the concepts of retrocrural and anterocrural block, which help to develop a three-dimensional "feel" for the location of the needle tip. With the patient in the prone position, adequate sedation can also be administered, and this will go a long way toward making the anesthesiologist and the patient comfortable during the celiac plexus block.

Superior Hypogastric Plexus Block

48

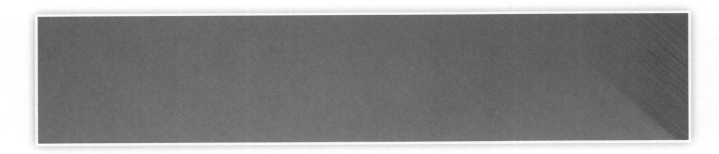

PERSPECTIVE

The superior hypogastric plexus block is conceptually patterned after the use of neurolysis of paravertebral neural plexuses to provide intra-abdominal or lower extremity pain relief. Gynecologic surgeons have performed presacral neurectomy for many years to treat a variety of pelvic pain syndromes, and this surgical procedure is designed to interrupt the superior hypogastric plexus. The superior hypogastric plexus block is used for both diagnostic and therapeutic purposes in patients with both benign and cancer pain syndromes. Nevertheless, much of the focus remains on neurolysis to provide pain relief for patients with pelvic cancer pain syndromes who are otherwise difficult to treat.

Patient Selection. When superior hypogastric plexus block is used diagnostically in patients with chronic benign pelvic pain syndromes, it is designed to help define the source of the pain. It is used less frequently for this purpose than for neurolysis of the plexus to produce long-lasting pain relief in patients with pelvic cancers. Cancer pain syndromes that may be amenable to relief with a superior hypogastric plexus block include cervical, proximal vaginal, uterine, ovarian, testicular, prostatic, and rectal cancers. The technique has also been used to relieve pain in patients with distal colonic or rectal inflammatory bowel disease.

Pharmacologic Choice. During diagnostic blocks, the choice of local anesthetic should be determined by the desired duration of the block. Often, 0.25% bupivacaine or 0.2% ropivacaine with 1:200,000 epinephrine is used through bilaterally placed needles to a total dose of 20 to 30 mL. Shorter-acting local anesthetics such as 1% lidocaine, again often with 1:200,000 epinephrine, are also used effectively. When neurolysis is the goal, a radiocontrast agent, 2 to 4 mL through each needle, is used to ensure correct needle position; 8 to 10 mL of 10% aqueous phenol or 50% alcohol can be used as the neurolytic agent.

PLACEMENT

Anatomy. The superior hypogastric plexus is continuous with the intermesenteric plexus and is located retroperito-

neally, caudad to the origin of the inferior mesenteric artery. It lies anterior to the lower part of the abdominal aorta, its bifurcation, and the middle sacral vessels; more specifically, it is anterior to the fourth and fifth lumbar vertebrae and the first sacral vertebra. The plexus is composed of a flattened band of intercommunicating nerve bundles that descend over the aortic bifurcation (Figs. 48-1 and 48-2). Broadening below, it divides into the right and left hypogastric nerves. In addition to its continuity with the intermesenteric plexus, the superior hypogastric plexus receives input from the lower two lumbar splanchnic nerves (Fig. 48-3). Figure 48-3 identifies with a *red triangle* a key concept in the superior hypogastric plexus nerve block. The red triangle highlights the anatomic window between the iliac crest, the L5 transverse process, and the L5-S1 vertebral bodies, which allows successful needle insertion.

In addition to sympathetic fibers, the superior hypogastric plexus usually also contains parasympathetic fibers that originate in the ventral roots of S2-S4 and travel as slender nervi erigentes (pelvic splanchnic nerves) through the inferior hypogastric plexus.

The left and right hypogastric nerves descend lateral to the sigmoid colon and rectosigmoid junction to reach the two inferior hypogastric plexuses. The inferior hypogastric plexus is a bilateral structure situated on each side of the rectum, the lower portion of the bladder, and the prostate and seminal vesicles (in the male) or the uterine cervix and vaginal fornices (in the female). Because of its location and configuration, the inferior hypogastric plexus does not lend itself to neurolysis.

Position. Patients undergoing superior hypogastric plexus block are placed prone on a radiographic imaging table with a pillow beneath the lower abdomen to reduce lumbar lordosis (see Fig. 48-2A). Ideally, biplane fluoroscopy is available to assess needle placement, for which oblique posteroanterior and lateral images are needed.

Needle Puncture. The L4-L5 interspace is identified fluoroscopically and skin marks are placed 5 to 7 cm lateral to the midline at the level of the L4-L5 interspace (Fig. 48-4). This preparation is needed for the insertion of the needles through the area of bony access (shown by the *red triangle* in Figs. 48-3 through 48-5) to the superior hypogastric plexus. After aseptic skin preparation, skin infiltration with

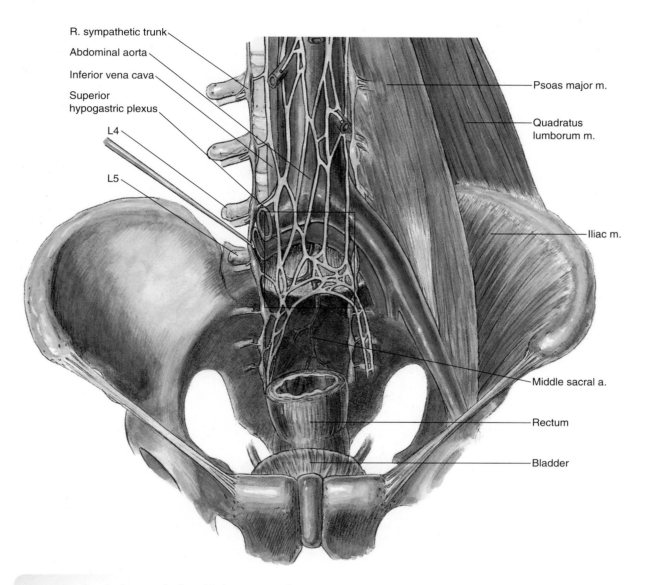

R. sympathetic trunk

Abdominal aorta

Inferior vena cava

Superior
hypogastric plexus

L4

L5

Psoas major m.

Quadratus
lumborum m.

Iliac m.

Middle sacral a.

Rectum

Bladder

Figure 48-1. Superior hypogastric plexus block: anteroposterior anatomy.

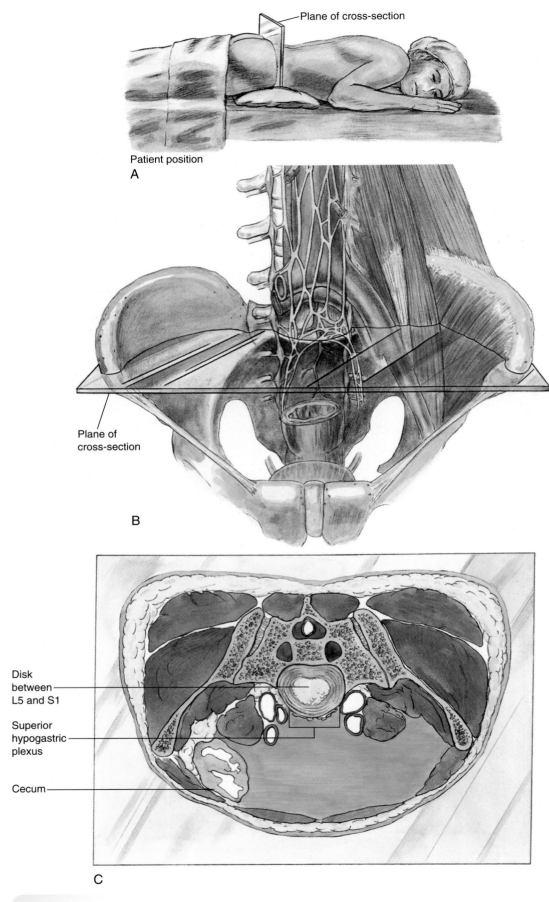

Plane of cross-section

Patient position

A

Plane of
cross-section

B

Disk
between
L5 and S1

Superior
hypogastric
plexus

Cecum

C

Figure 48-2. Superior hypogastric plexus block: cross-sectional anatomy.

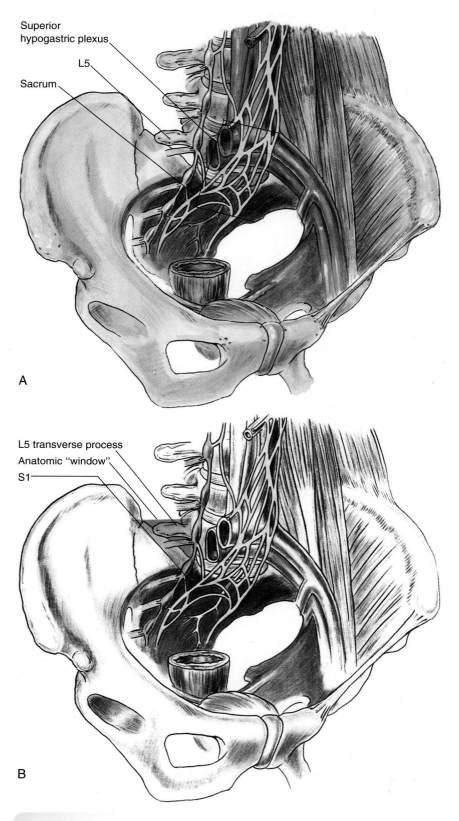

Superior
hypogastric plexus

L5

Sacrum

A

L5 transverse process
Anatomic "window"
S1

B

Figure 48-3. Oblique anatomy of the superior hypogastric plexus. **A,** Anatomy. **B,** Concept of the red triangle for access to the superior hypogastric plexus.

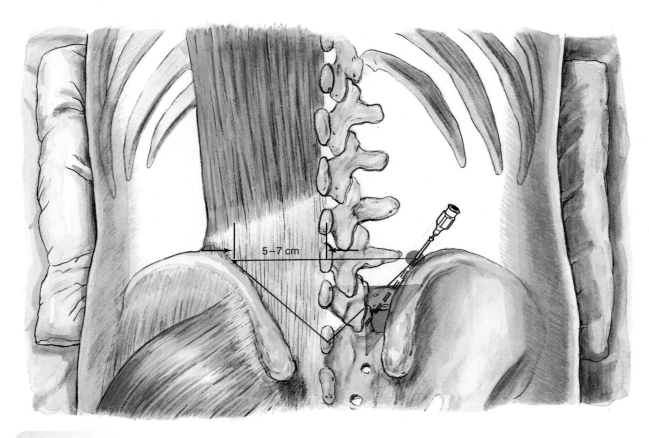

Figure 48-4. Surface anatomy and skin markings important for superior hypogastric plexus block: posteroanterior view.

local anesthetic is performed with a 30-gauge, 2-cm needle at the previously marked bilateral sites (Fig. 48-5). Local anesthetic infiltration is continued subcutaneously with a 22-gauge, 5- to 9-cm needle along the eventual caudo-medial oblique needle path. The fluoroscopic beam is directed along the projected needle path to simplify needle insertion. The needle is then directed under fluoroscopic guidance to reach a point immediately anterior to the L5-S1 vertebral junction; the fluoroscopic beam is directed to minimize the needle hub's radiographic size. If the fluoroscopic beam is directed properly, this approach should guide the needle tip to the correct position. The iliac crest and the L5 transverse process may obstruct passage of the needle; if this is the case, the needle is withdrawn and redirected in a cephalad or caudad angle to bypass the obstruction. As in the approach taken with either the celiac

or lumbar sympathetic block, if the needle tip contacts the body of the vertebra (in this case, L5), the needle is simply redirected to "walk off" the body to its desired position immediately anterior to the L5-S1 junction (the sacral prominence).

Once the needle tip is positioned adequately and the position has been confirmed with biplanar fluoroscopy, the contralateral needle is inserted in a similar manner. Once both needles are positioned, radiocontrast medium (2 to 4 mL of Hypaque-M 60 [Sanofi Winthrop, Irving, Tex]) is injected to verify adequate placement. The radiocontrast agent should spread in a band immediately anterior to the sacral promontory; its smooth posterior margin should identify needle tip placement anterior to the psoas fascia. The contrast should spread toward the midline from the bilaterally placed paramedian sites.

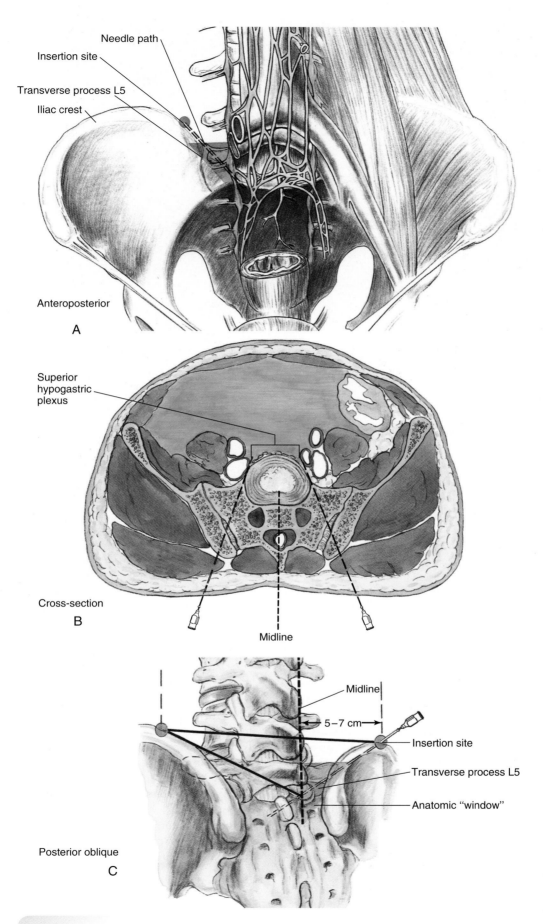

Needle path

Insertion site

Transverse process L5

Iliac crest

Anteroposterior

A

Superior
hypogastric
plexus

Cross-section

B

Midline

Midline

5–7 cm

Insertion site

Transverse process L5

Anatomic "window"

Posterior oblique

C

Figure 48-5. Technique for superior hypogastric plexus block using the red triangle to identify route of needle insertion and access to the superior hypogastric plexus. **A,** Anteroposterior view. **B,** Cross-section. **C,** Posterior oblique view.

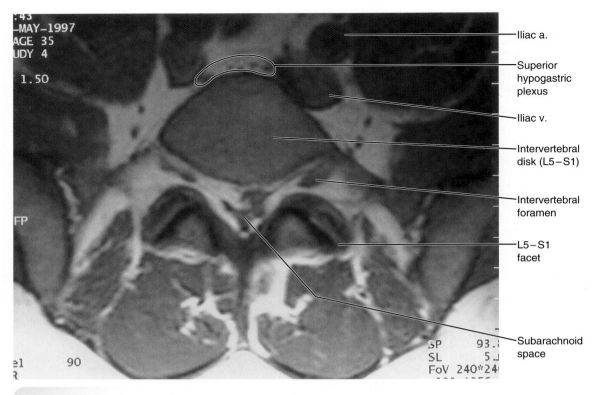

Iliac a.

Superior
hypogastric
plexus

Iliac v.

Intervertebral
disk (L5–S1)

Intervertebral
foramen

L5–S1
facet

Subarachnoid
space

Figure 48-6. Anatomy on magnetic resonance imaging scan of the superior hypogastric plexus.

POTENTIAL PROBLEMS

Owing to the proximity of the iliac vessels (arteries and veins) to the needle paths, care should be taken to minimize the potential for intravascular injection (Fig. 48-6). This anatomic relationship also makes hematoma formation possible. If the position of the needle tip is not accurately verified, both intramuscular and intraperitoneal injection are possible. Even when the needle is inserted correctly, paraspinous muscle spasm may result from needle-induced paraspinous muscle irritation. This usually lasts only a few days. Less frequent problems are lumbar or sacral somatic nerve injury and renal or ureteral puncture. It is advisable to caution the patient about the potential for bowel or bladder habit changes as well as decreases in sexual function after the neurolytic superior hypogastric plexus block, despite the rarity of these side effects.

PEARLS

When this block is used diagnostically for patients with pelvic pain syndromes, the anesthesiologist should emphasize that the block is being performed for diagnostic purposes, and no neurolytic block is planned. To use a superior hypogastric plexus block most effectively, the anesthesiologist must become comfortable with the anatomy, both bony and neurovascular. This block is not possible in my hands without fluoroscopy; thus, another strong recommendation is to develop facility with fluoroscopic needle placement for this block. Lining up the needle path with the fluoroscopic beam is a radiographic guidance technique that simplifies placement of the needle.

Some subsets of patients with cancer who may be candidates for neurolysis have previously undergone extensive pelvic surgery, perhaps combined with radiation therapy of the pelvis. In these patients extra time should be spent to ensure that the pattern of radiocontrast spread appears typical. This recommendation stems from experience with patients in whom extensive prior surgery and radiation therapy has altered the typical neurovascular anatomy. As with celiac neurolysis, complete pain relief after this block is not frequent, but the block often increases patient comfort and minimizes the need for opioid therapy, which can improve the patient's quality of life during the remaining months of life.

Selective Nerve Root Block

James P. Rathmell

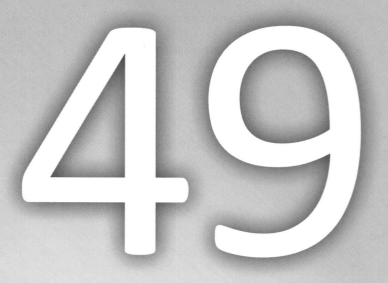

The term *transforaminal injection* is often used interchangeably with the term *selective nerve root injection*. The spinal nerves enter and exit the bony spinal canal through the intervertebral foramina. Just lateral to the foramen, a small volume of injectate can be placed directly adjacent to a single nerve. Blocking of a single spinal nerve with local anesthetic can be used diagnostically to clarify which nerve root is contributing to clinical symptoms in patients with pathology at multiple levels and a confusing pattern of symptoms. In this way, selective nerve root injection can be used to assist the surgeon's decision making when pondering the proper operative approach. The results must be interpreted cautiously because the potential space surrounding the spinal nerves in the paravertebral region is contiguous with the epidural space. Indeed, as the volume of injectate is increased, the material spreads laterally along the spinal nerve and proximally through the intervertebral foramen to the epidural space directly surrounding the spinal nerve within the dural cuff. Although some physicians conduct selective nerve root injection just outside the intervertebral foramen and transforaminal injection by advancing the needle tip a few millimeters farther to enter the foramen, this distinction likely carries little practical meaning. Even a small volume of material injected at either location often enters the epidural space by contiguous spread.

The most common application of transforaminal injection is to inject steroids. The rationale for injecting steroids is that they suppress inflammation of the nerve, which in many instances is believed to be the basis for radicular pain. A transforaminal route of injection rather than an interlaminar route is used so that the injectate is delivered directly onto the target nerve, which ensures that the medication reaches the site of the suspected lesion in maximum concentration.

Cervical Transforaminal Injection

Anatomy. At typical cervical levels, the ventral and dorsal roots of the spinal nerves traverse laterally and caudally in the vertebral canal to form the spinal nerve in the intervertebral foramen. The foramen is oriented obliquely anteriorly and laterally. Its roof and floor are formed by the pedicles of consecutive vertebrae. Its posterolateral wall is formed largely by the superior articular process of the lower vertebra and in part by the inferior articular process of the upper vertebra and the capsule of the zygapophyseal joint formed between the two articular processes. The anteromedial wall is formed by the caudad portion of the upper vertebral body, the uncinate process of the lower vertebra, and the posterolateral corner of the intervertebral disk. Immediately lateral to the external opening of the foramen, the vertebral artery rises closely anterior to the articular pillars of the zygapophyseal joint.

The spinal nerve, in its dural sleeve, lies in the caudad half of the foramen. The cephalad half is occupied by epiradicular veins. The ventral ramus of the spinal nerve arises just lateral to the intervertebral foramen and passes anteriorly and laterally onto the transverse process. Radicular and spinal medullary arteries arise from the vertebral artery and the ascending cervical artery; radicular arteries supply the spinal nerve itself, whereas spinal medullary arteries continue medially to join the anterior and or posterior spinal arteries, which provide critical perfusion to the spinal cord itself.

Position. The procedure can be performed with the patient lying in a supine, oblique, or lateral decubitus position, depending on the operator's preference and the patient's comfort. The position must allow adequate visualization of the cervical intervertebral foramina in the anteroposterior (AP), lateral, and oblique planes (Fig. 49-1A). The important first step is to obtain a correct oblique view of the target foramen (Fig. 49-1B). In this view the foramen is maximally wide transversely, and the anterior wall of the superior articular process projects onto the silhouette of the lamina. If these criteria are not satisfied, the inclination of the fluoroscope must be adjusted until they are. The correct oblique view is essential because in less oblique views, which may nevertheless show a foramen, the vertebral artery lies along the course of the needle. Older C-arm fluoroscopy units often restrict the degree of rotation of the side opposite the unit to less than 45 degrees, which can prevent adequate visualization of the cervical intervertebral foramina on the patient's right side when the C-arm is positioned from the patient's left. The 60 degrees of anterior oblique angulation often needed for good visualization can be achieved simply by placing a foam cushion under the patient's right side, thereby tilting him or her to the left, or by tilting the surface of the table to the patient's left.

Needle Puncture. A 25-gauge, 2.5- to 3.5-inch needle is passed into the neck through a skin puncture at a point overlying the posterior half of the target foramen. Some

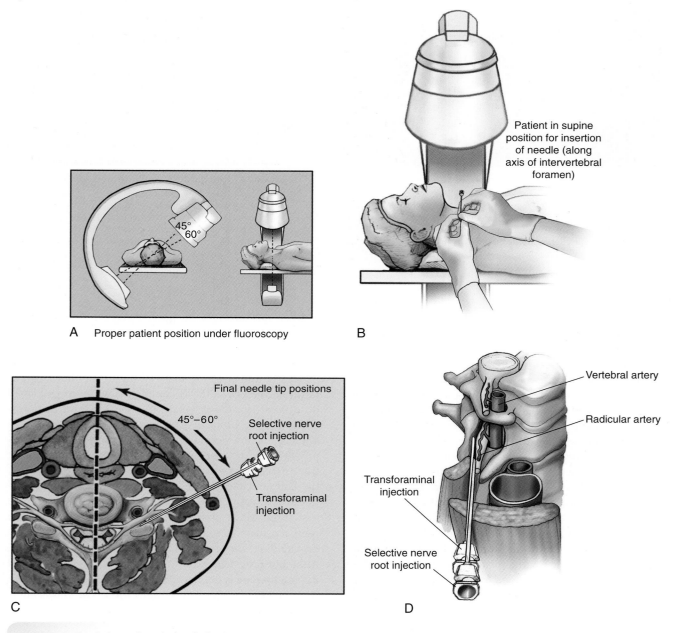

A Proper patient position under fluoroscopy

Patient in supine position for insertion of needle (along axis of intervertebral foramen)

B

Final needle tip positions

45°–60°

Selective nerve root injection

Transforaminal injection

C

Vertebral artery

Radicular artery

Transforaminal injection

Selective nerve root injection

D

Figure 49-1. Cervical transforaminal and selective nerve root injection. **A,** Proper patient positioning and fluoroscopic C-arm angulation. **B,** Needle placement along axis of intervertebral foramen under fluoroscopic guidance. **C,** Axial view of final needle positions for transforaminal and selective nerve root injection, demonstrating the angle of the foramen and adjacent structures. **D,** Final needle positions for transforaminal injection within intervertebral foramen and selective nerve root injection just lateral to the foramen.

Continued

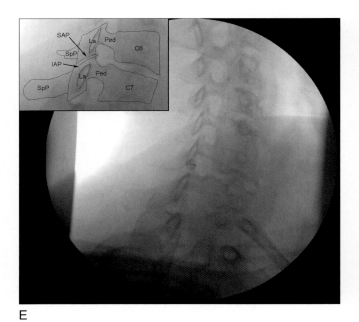

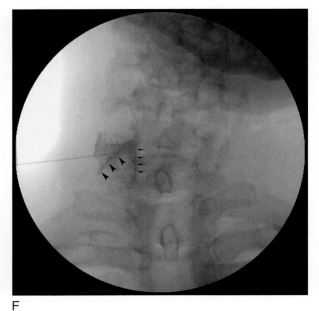

E

F

Figure 49-1, cont'd. E, Right anterior oblique radiograph demonstrating a needle in position along the posterior aspect of the right C6-C7 intervertebral foramen. *Inset:* Mid-portion of image with bony structures labeled: C6, C6 vertebral body; C7, C7 vertebral body; Ped, pedicle; La, lamina; SpP, spinous process; SAP, superior articular process; IAP, inferior articular process. **F,** Final anteroposterior radiograph after cervical transforaminal injection, with the needle in its final position and radiographic contrast outlining the spinal nerve *(arrowheads)* and extending into the lateral epidural space *(arrows).*

experts advocate the use of a blunt-tipped needle to reduce the likelihood of penetration into an arterial structure. The needle tip should always lie over the anterior half of the superior articular process lest it be inserted prematurely and too far into the foramen. Once the needle has reached the superior articular process, its depth is noted. Subsequent insertion should not be more than a few millimeters beyond this depth. The needle is then repositioned to enter the foramen tangential to its posterior wall, opposite the equator of the foramen (Fig. 49-1C through E). Cephalad to this level, the needle may encounter veins; caudad to this level, the needle may encounter the spinal nerve and its arteries. The needle must stay in contact with the posterior wall lest it encounter the vertebral artery.

Under an AP fluoroscopic view, the tip of the needle is finally adjusted so that it lies opposite the midline of the articular pillars in the sagittal plane. Insertion beyond this depth increases the likelihood of puncturing the dural sleeve or thecal sac. The final needle position is checked and radiographically recorded on an oblique view, which documents needle placement against the posterior wall of the foramen, and on an AP view (Fig. 49-1F), which documents the depth of needle insertion.

To ensure that the final needle position does not change with attempts to connect and disconnect syringes directly to the needle, a short length of sterile connecting tubing is attached to the needle and further injections carried out through the distal end of this tubing. Under direct, real-time fluoroscopy, a small volume of nonionic contrast medium (≤1.0 mL) is injected. The solution should outline the proximal end of the spinal nerve and spread centrally toward the epidural space (see Fig. 49-1F).

Once the target nerve has been correctly outlined, a small volume of a short-acting local anesthetic (1% lidocaine, 0.5 to 1.5 mL) is injected to block the target nerve and render the subsequent injection of corticosteroid less painful. While ensuring that the needle has not changed position, the procedure is completed by injecting a small dose of corticosteroid (betamethasone 3 to 6 mg or triamcinolone 20 to 40 mg). Although the size of the particles in available depot steroid solutions varies widely (methylprednisolone > triamcinolone > betamethasone), all of these preparations have particles of sufficient size to block the end-arterioles supplying the brain or spinal cord, if injected directly into an artery supplying one of these structures. Much attention has been given to use of the nonparticulate steroid dexamethasone, with experts recommending use of 4 mg (1 mL of a 4 mg/mL solution). Although early evidence from animal models suggests that dexamethasone is not harmful when injected into the cerebral circulation, the safety and efficacy of this soluble steroid have not been carefully examined in humans.

POTENTIAL PROBLEMS

Real-time fluoroscopy is essential to verify that there is no unintentional intra-arterial injection, which may occur even if the needle is correctly placed using radiographic landmarks. Intra-arterial injection manifests by extremely rapid clearance of the injected contrast material. In a vertebral artery, the contrast material streaks cephalad. In a radicular artery, it blushes briefly in a transverse fashion medially toward the spinal cord. In either instance, the needle is withdrawn and no further injections are attempted. The procedure is then rescheduled after a period long enough for the puncture wound to have healed.

Sometimes the contrast medium fills epiradicular veins. This situation is recognized by slow clearance of the contrast medium, which is characteristic of venous flow. In that event, the needle is adjusted either by slightly withdrawing it or redirecting it to a position slightly more caudad on the posterior wall or the foramen.

Only a small volume of contrast medium (≤1.0 mL) is required to outline the dural sleeve of the spinal nerve. As it spreads onto the thecal sac, the contrast medium assumes a linear configuration. Rapid dilution of the contrast medium implies subarachnoid spread, which may occur if the needle punctures the thecal sac when there is lateral dilation of the dural root sleeve into the intervertebral foramen. In that event, the procedure is abandoned and rescheduled lest subsequently injected material penetrate the puncture made through the dura.

Lumbar Transforaminal Injection

PLACEMENT

Anatomy. At lumbar levels, the ventral and dorsal roots of the spinal nerves traverse laterally and caudally in the vertebral canal to form the spinal nerve in their respective intervertebral foramina. The foramina are oriented laterally. The foraminal roof and floor are formed by the pedicles of consecutive vertebrae. The posterolateral wall is formed largely by the superior articular process of the lower vertebra and in part by the inferior articular process of the upper vertebra and the capsule of the zygapophyseal joint formed between the two articular processes. The anteromedial wall is formed by the caudad end of the upper vertebral body and the posterolateral corner of the intervertebral disk.

The spinal nerve, in its dural sleeve, traverses obliquely through the foramen. In the cephalad half of the foramen, the dorsal root ganglion lies just deep to the pedicle of the cephalad vertebra; this region is also occupied by epiradicular veins. As the root traverses inferolaterally through the foramen, it divides into a ventral ramus and a dorsal ramus. The ventral ramus of the spinal nerve passes anteriorly and laterally adjacent to the transverse process of the caudad vertebra bounding the foramen. Radicular arteries arise from the abdominal aorta and its branches and accompany the spinal nerve and its roots to the spinal cord. As in the cervical region, the location and size of the radicular arteries are variable, and the importance of recognizing their presence for carrying out this block safely and effectively must be emphasized.

Position. The procedure is typically performed with the patient in the prone position, with a pillow under the abdomen above the iliac crests and the pelvis tilted anteriorly (Fig. 49-2A). The first step is to obtain a 10- to 20-degree oblique view of the target foramen that allows the needle to pass into the lateral aspect of the intervertebral foramen. This is most difficult for the LS-Sl level, where the iliac crest blocks entry to the foramen when the oblique angle is too extreme.

Needle Puncture. Through a skin puncture point overlying the superior portion of the target foramen, just caudad to the pars interarticularis (the junction of the transverse process with the lamina or just caudad to the most proximal portion of the transverse process), a 25-gauge, 2.5- to 3.5-inch needle is passed into the back (Fig. 49-2B). Some experts advocate the use of blunt-tipped needles to reduce the likelihood of penetration into an arterial structure. The needle tip should always lie over the posterior aspect of the intervertebral foramen (Fig. 49-2C). Once the needle has reached the pars interarticularis, its depth should be noted; the radiographic image orientation is then switched to the lateral projection (Fig. 49-2D). Subsequent insertion is carried out using the lateral projection, observing the needle as it enters the foramen. The needle is advanced slowly; further insertion is halted if the patient reports a paresthesia or the needle reaches the mid-portion of the foramen in the AP dimension.

The final needle position is checked and recorded on an AP view, which documents the medial extent of the needle's advancement. To ensure that the final needle position does not change with attempts to connect and disconnect syringes directly to the needle, a short length of sterile connecting tubing is attached to the needle and further injections carried out through the distal end of this tubing. Under direct, real-time fluoroscopy in the AP view, a small volume of nonionic contrast medium (≤1.0 mL) is injected. The solution should outline the proximal end of the exiting nerve root and spread centrally underneath the pedicle toward the epidural space (Fig. 49-2E).

Once the target nerve has been correctly outlined, a small volume of a short-acting local anesthetic (1% lidocaine, 0.5 to 1.5 mL) is injected to anesthetize the target nerve and render the subsequent injection of corticosteroid painless. While ensuring that the needle has not changed position, the procedure is completed by injecting a small dose of corticosteroid (betamethasone 3 to 6 mg or triamcinolone 20 to 40 mg). Although the size of the particles in available depot steroid solutions varies widely (methylprednisolone > triamcinolone > betamethasone), all of these preparations have particles of sufficient size to block the end-arterioles supplying the spinal cord, if injected directly into an artery supplying this structure. Although much attention has been given to use of the nonparticulate steroid dexamethasone for cervical transforaminal injection, with experts recommending use of 4 mg (1 mL of a 4 mg/mL solution), the incidence of intra-arterial injection is much lower in the lumbar region than at cervical levels, and thus less emphasis has been placed on use on nonparticulate steroids at lumbar levels. Although early evidence from animal models suggests that dexamethasone is not harmful when injected into the cerebral circulation, the safety and efficacy of soluble steroid have not been carefully examined in humans.

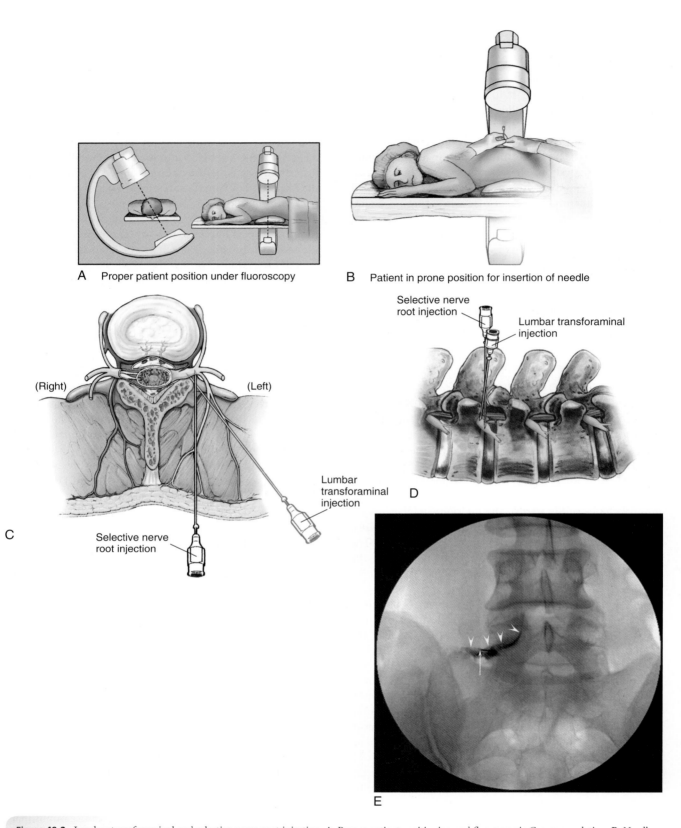

A   Proper patient position under fluoroscopy

B   Patient in prone position for insertion of needle

(Right)   (Left)

Lumbar transforaminal injection

Selective nerve root injection

C

Selective nerve root injection

Lumbar transforaminal injection

D

E

Figure 49-2. Lumbar transforaminal and selective nerve root injection. **A,** Proper patient positioning and fluoroscopic C-arm angulation. **B,** Needle placement under fluoroscopic guidance. **C,** Axial view of final needle positions for transforaminal and selective nerve root injection. **D,** Lateral view of final needle positions for transforaminal and selective nerve root injection. **E,** Final anteroposterior radiograph after contrast injection and selective nerve root injection (left L5), with the needle tip along the superior surface of the nerve root *(arrow)* and contrast outlining the spinal nerve and extending into the lateral epidural space *(arrowheads)*.

POTENTIAL PROBLEMS

As with cervical transforaminal injection, real-time fluoroscopy is essential to check for unintentional intra-arterial injection, which may occur even if the needle is correctly placed using radiographic landmarks. Intra-arterial injection manifests by extremely rapid clearance of the injected contrast material. In a radicular artery, the contrast blushes briefly in a transverse fashion medially toward the spinal canal. In this instance, the needle is withdrawn and no further injections are attempted. The procedure is then rescheduled after a period long enough for the puncture wound to have healed.

Contrast medium may also fill epiradicular veins, which is recognized as slow clearance of the contrast medium (characteristic of venous flow). In this setting, the needle is adjusted by slightly withdrawing it or redirecting it to a position slightly more caudad within the foramen.

Only a small volume of contrast medium (≤1.0 mL) is required to outline the dural sleeve of the spinal nerve. As it spreads onto the thecal sac, the contrast medium assumes a linear configuration (see Fig. 49-2E). Rapid dilution of the contrast medium implies subarachnoid spread, which may occur if the needle has punctured the thecal sac when there is lateral dilation of the dural root sleeve into the intervertebral foramen. In that case, the procedure should be abandoned and rescheduled lest subsequently injected material penetrate the puncture made through the dura.

CERVICAL AND LUMBAR TRANSFORAMINAL PEARLS

A coaxial technique should be used for both cervical and lumbar transforaminal injections. By aligning the x-ray beam so that it shares a common axis with the advancing needle, the needle can be advanced with a high degree of precision in one pass without the need for redirection. This improves the success rate of the block as well as patient comfort. Maintaining the needle in a coaxial plane at the cervical level can be difficult. The needle tends to flop to one side or the other when it is in the superficial tissues. By using a small clamp (e.g., a surgical clamp such as a Kelly clamp), the operator can hold the needle in a coaxial orientation until it is firmly seated. Once the needle is in final position, the operator should inject a small volume of radiographic contrast material using real-time fluoroscopic imaging to identify needle penetration of an artery.

Intrathecal Catheter Implantation

James P. Rathmell

50

PERSPECTIVE

After thousands of years of empiric use of opioids for treating pain, in the early 1970s a class of highly specific opioid receptors was identified. Soon thereafter, opioid receptors were localized in the brain and spinal cord. Investigators developed a model of chronic catheterization of the spinal subarachnoid space in experimental animals, and evidence that direct application of morphine at the spinal cord level produces selective spinal analgesia soon followed. Based on this limited experimental evidence, intrathecal morphine was administered to patients with severe pain associated with advanced cancer, and it produced profound and long-lasting pain reduction.

Since these first bold clinical experiments, we have witnessed a rapid transition from the laboratory to clinical practice. Intrathecal morphine and other opioids are now widely used as adjuncts in the treatment of acute and chronic pain, and a number of agents show promise as analgesic agents with spinal selectivity. Continuous delivery of analgesic agents at the spinal level can be carried out using percutaneous epidural or intrathecal catheters, but vulnerability to infection and the cost of external systems typically limits them to short-term use, in most cases less than 6 weeks. Reliable implanted drug delivery systems that make long-term delivery of medications to the intrathecal space feasible are available. These systems consist of a drug reservoir/pump implanted in the subcutaneous tissue of the abdominal wall that is refilled periodically through an access port. The pump may be a fixed-rate, constant-flow device or a variable-rate pump that can be programmed using a wireless radiofrequency transmitter, similar to the programming possible with implanted cardiac pacemakers.

Patient selection for spinal pain therapy is empiric and remains the subject of some debate. In general, intrathecal drug delivery is reserved for patients with severe pain that does not respond to conservative treatment. Most patients with cancer-related pain have ongoing pain despite appropriate oral opioid therapy, or they may have developed intolerable side effects related to these medications. Randomized controlled trials comparing maximal medical therapy with intrathecal drug delivery for cancer-related pain have demonstrated improved pain control and reduced opioid-related side effects with intrathecal pain therapy. Intrathecal drug delivery has also been widely used for noncancer pain, particularly for the treatment of chronic low-back pain. Use of this therapy for noncancer pain, however, has not been subject to controlled trials and remains controversial.

Once a patient is selected for intrathecal therapy, a trial is carried out. Most physicians now conduct trials by placing a temporary percutaneous intrathecal catheter and infusing the analgesic agent over several days to judge the effectiveness of this therapy before a permanent system is implanted. Some carry out the trial of intrathecal therapy using a single dose or a continuous epidural infusion. The most common analgesic agent used for spinal delivery is morphine, which remains the only opioid approved for intrathecal use by the U.S. Food and Drug Administration.

PLACEMENT

Anatomy. The intrathecal catheter is placed directly in the cerebrospinal fluid (CSF) of the lumbar cistern by advancing a needle between the vertebral laminae at the L2-L3 level or below. Direct delivery of the opioid at the spinal level corresponding to the dermatome(s) in which the patient is experiencing pain may improve analgesia, particularly when local anesthetics or lipophilic opioids (e.g., fentanyl or sufentanil) are used. Thus, some practitioners have advocated threading the catheter cephalad to the appropriate dermatome. In recent years, there have been some reports of granuloma formation surrounding the tip of some chronic indwelling intrathecal catheters. These inflammatory masses often present with sudden neurologic deterioration caused by spinal cord compression. Many physicians now recommend that implanted intrathecal catheters be placed only within the lumbar cistern below the conus medullaris (at about L2), where the appearance of an inflammatory mass is less likely to impinge directly on the spinal cord.

Position. Before the procedure, discuss with the patient the location of the pocket for the intrathecal pump. Most devices are large, and the only region suitable for placement is the left or right lower quadrant of the abdomen. Once the site is determined, the proposed skin incision is marked with a permanent marker while the patient is in the sitting position. The position of the pocket on the abdominal wall is deceptively difficult to determine once the patient is lying on his or her side. If the location is not marked, the pocket is often placed too far laterally in the abdominal wall.

Implantation of an intrathecal drug delivery system is a minor surgical procedure that is carried out in the operating room using aseptic precautions, including skin preparation, sterile draping, and full surgical attire (Fig. 50-1A). The procedure can be conducted under regional anesthesia or general anesthesia using dedicated anesthesia personnel. Performing the initial spinal catheter placement under general anesthesia is controversial, and concerns about neural injury are similar to those when performing any neuraxial technique under general anesthesia.

The patient is positioned on a radiolucent table in the lateral decubitus position with the patient's side for the pump pocket nondependent (see Fig. 50-1A). The arms are extended at the shoulders and secured so that they are well away from the surgical field. The skin is prepared and sterile drapes are applied. The fluoroscopic C-arm is positioned across the lumbar region to provide a cross-table anteroposterior view of the lumbar spine. Care must be taken to ensure that the radiographic view is not rotated by observing that the spinous processes are in the midline, halfway between the vertebral pedicles (see Fig. 50-1E).

Procedure for Intrathecal Catheter Placement. The L3-L4 interspace is identified using fluoroscopy The spinal needle supplied by the intrathecal device manufacturer must be used to ensure that the catheter can advance through the needle without damage. The needle is advanced using a paramedian approach starting 1 to 1.5 cm lateral to the spinous processes. The needle is directed to enter the spinal space in the midline; the stylet is removed to ensure adequate flow of CSF (Fig. 50-1B). The spinal catheter is then advanced through the needle until the tip is well into the spinal space but below L2 in the lumbar cistern (Fig. 50-1C). The position of the catheter tip is verified using fluoroscopy in the anteroposterior and lateral planes (Fig. 50-1D and E). The needle is then withdrawn slightly (about 1 to 2 cm) but left in place around the catheter in the subcutaneous tissues to protect the catheter during the subsequent incision and dissection (Fig. 50-1F). The catheter is secured to the surgical field using a small clamp to ensure that it does not fall from the sterile field (see Fig. 50-1F).

A 5- to 8-cm incision parallel to the axis of the spine is extended from just cephalad to just caudad to the needle, extending directly through the needle's entry point on the skin (Fig. 50-1G). The subcutaneous tissues are divided using blunt dissection until the lumbar paraspinous fascia is visible surrounding the needle shaft (Fig. 50-1H). A pursestring suture is created in the fascia surrounding the needle shaft site (Fig. 50-1I). This suture is used to tighten the fascia around the catheter and prevent backflow of CSF, which may lead to a chronic subcutaneous CSF collection. The needle and stylet are then removed simultaneously, using care not to dislodge the spinal catheter (Fig. 50-1J). Free flow of CSF from the catheter should be evident; if there is no CSF flowing from the catheter, a blunt needle can be inserted in the end of the catheter and gentle aspiration used to ensure that the catheter remains in the thecal sac. If CSF cannot be aspirated from the catheter, the catheter is removed and replaced. The catheter is then secured to the paraspinous fascia using a specific anchoring device supplied by the manufacturer (Fig. 50-1K).

Attention is now turned to creating the pocket in the patient's abdominal wall. A 10- to 12-cm transverse incision is made along the previously marked line, and a subcutaneous pocket is created using blunt dissection (Fig. 50-1L). The pocket should always be created caudad to the incision; if the pocket is placed cephalad to the incision, the weight of the pump on the suture line is likely to cause wound dehiscence. In many patients, the blunt dissection can be accomplished using gentle but firm pressure with the fingers. It is simpler and less traumatic to use a small surgical scissors to perform the blunt dissection, using repeated opening motions rather than closing or cutting motions that are likely to cut vascular structures and provoke marked bleeding. An alternative to blunt dissection is the use of a monopolar electrocautery device in the "cut" mode, an effective means to carry out the necessary dissection without excessive tissue trauma or blood loss. After the pocket has been created, the pump is placed in the pocket to ensure that the pocket is large enough. The pump should fit completely within the pocket without any part of the device extending into the incision. With the device in place, the wound margins should fall into close apposition. There should be no tension on the sutures during closure of the incision, or the wound is more likely to undergo dehiscence.

After the pocket has been created, a tunneling device is extended within the subcutaneous tissues between the paraspinous incision and the pocket (Fig. 50-1M). The catheter is then advanced through the tunnel, leaving a small tension-relief loop of catheter in the subcutaneous area of the paraspinous dissection (commonly used tunneling devices place a hollow plastic sleeve through which the catheter can be advanced from the patient's back to the pump pocket). The catheter is then trimmed to a length that allows a small loop of catheter to remain deep to the pump and attached to it. The pump is placed in the pocket with a loop of catheter deep to the device (Fig. 50-1N). This loop and the small loop of catheter in the paraspinous region allow patient movement without placing tension on the distal catheter, causing it to be pulled from the thecal sac. Two or more sutures are then placed through the suture loops or mesh enclosure surrounding the pump and are used to secure the pump to the abdominal fascia. These simple retaining sutures prevent the pump from rotating or flipping within the pocket. The skin incisions are then closed in two layers: a series of interrupted subcutaneous sutures to close the fascia securely overlying the pump and the catheter, followed by skin closure using suture or staples.

Procedure for Permanent Epidural Catheter Placement. Patient positioning and use of fluoroscopy when placing a permanent epidural catheter are similar to those described for intrathecal catheter placement. The interspace of entry varies with the dermatomes to be covered, particularly if local anesthetic solution is to be used. A typical loss-of-resistance technique is used to identify the epidural space, and a Silastic catheter is threaded into the epidural space. A paraspinous incision is created and the catheter is secured to the paraspinous fascia as described previously for intrathecal catheter placement.

Two permanent epidural systems are available: (1) a totally implanted system using a subcutaneous port that is accessed by a needle placed into the port through the skin, and (2) a percutaneous catheter that is tunneled subcutaneously but exits the skin to be connected directly to an external infusion device.

To place a permanent epidural system with a subcutaneous port, a 6- to 8-cm transverse incision is made overlying the costal margin halfway between the xiphoid process and the anterior axillary line. A pocket is created overlying the

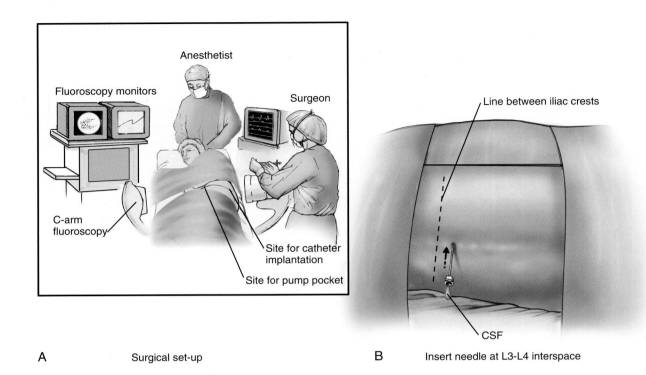

Anesthetist

Fluoroscopy monitors

Surgeon

C-arm
fluoroscopy

Site for catheter
implantation

Site for pump pocket

A   Surgical set-up

Line between iliac crests

CSF

B   Insert needle at L3-L4 interspace

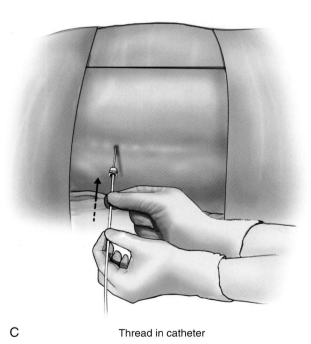

C   Thread in catheter

Figure 50-1. Intrathecal drug delivery system implantation. **A,** View of a typical operating room arrangement during intrathecal implantation. The patient is placed in the lateral position with the fluoroscopic C-arm in place for a cross-table anteroposterior view of the lumbar spine. **B,** Initial spinal needle placement at the L3-L4 interspace using a paramedian approach. Free flow of cerebrospinal fluid (CSF) indicates an intrathecal location. **C,** Intrathecal catheter placement through the spinal needle under fluoroscopic guidance.

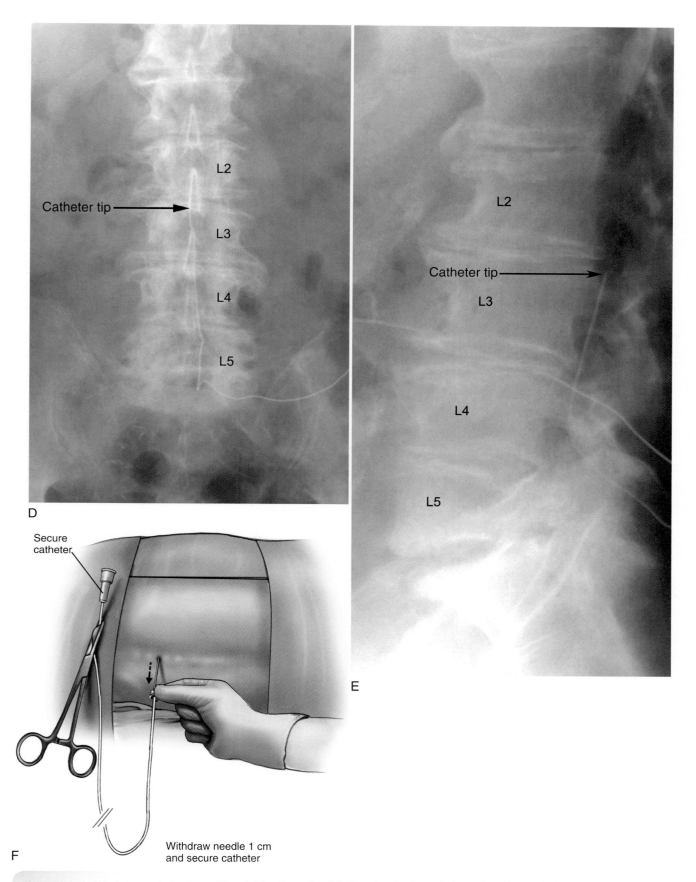

Labels in figure D (anteroposterior radiograph):
Catheter tip →
L2
L3
L4
L5

Labels in figure E (lateral radiograph):
L2
Catheter tip —
L3
L4
L5

Labels in figure F:
Secure catheter
Withdraw needle 1 cm and secure catheter

Figure 50-1, cont'd. Anteroposterior (**D**) and lateral (**E**) radiographs of the intrathecal catheter tip in good position, with the tip adjacent to the L2-L3 intervertebral disk. **F,** After confirming the final position of the catheter tip, the proximal portion of the catheter is fastened to the surgical field and the spinal needle is withdrawn about 1 cm to lie in the subcutaneous tissue. Leaving the needle in place protects the catheter during subsequent dissection.

Continued

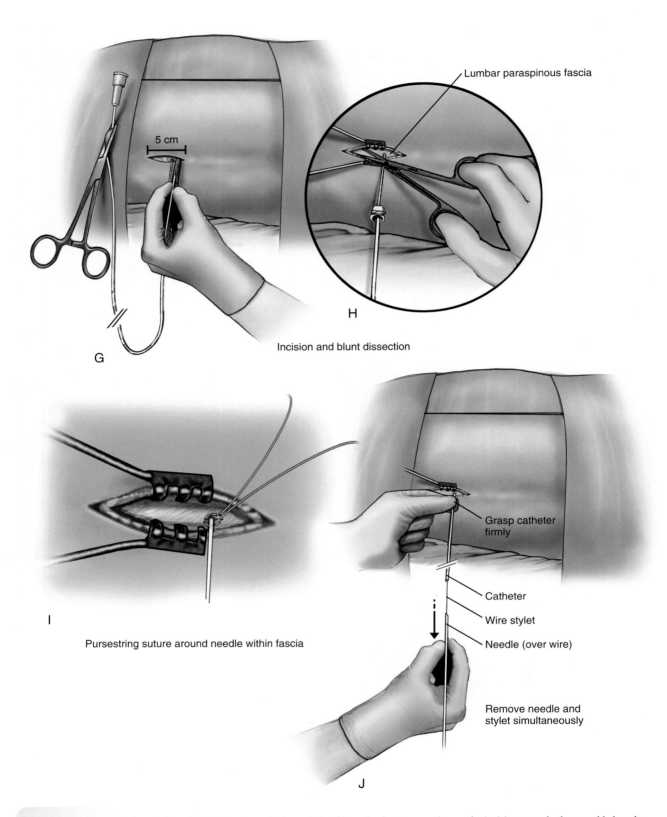

5 cm

Lumbar paraspinous fascia

H

Incision and blunt dissection

G

I

Pursestring suture around needle within fascia

Grasp catheter firmly

Catheter

Wire stylet

Needle (over wire)

Remove needle and stylet simultaneously

J

Figure 50-1, cont'd. G, A cephalocaudad incision is made through the skin and subcutaneous tissues; the incision extends above and below the needle entry point. **H,** Using blunt dissection, the skin and subcutaneous tissues are further divided until the lumbar paravertebral fascia is exposed. **I,** A pursestring suture is placed around the base of the needle in the paravertebral fascia; this suture reduces the likelihood that CSF will track back along the catheter and result in a subcutaneous CSF collection. **J,** The needle and catheter stylet are removed together while the catheter is held firmly in position.

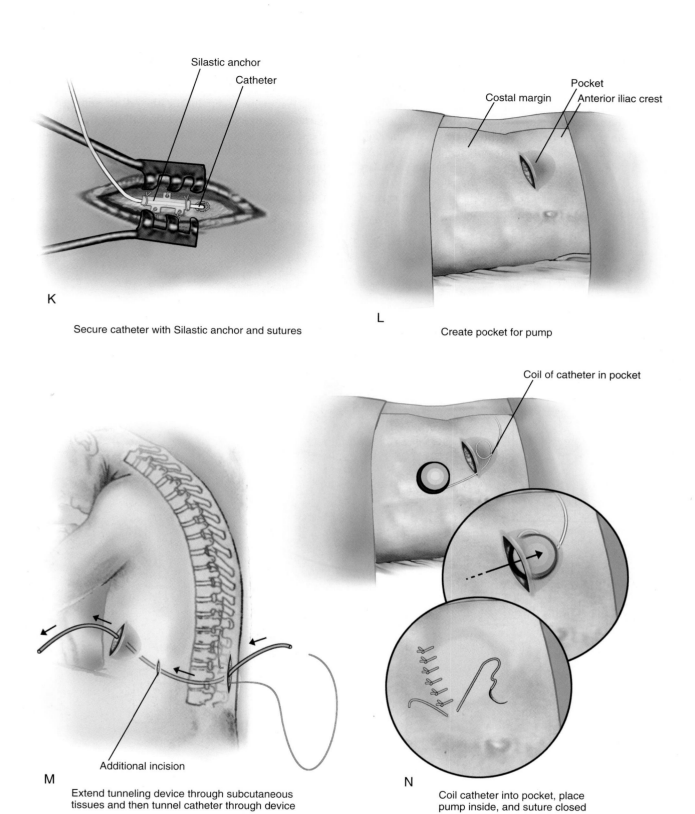

Silastic anchor

Catheter

K

Secure catheter with Silastic anchor and sutures

Costal margin

Pocket

Anterior iliac crest

L

Create pocket for pump

Coil of catheter in pocket

Additional incision

M

Extend tunneling device through subcutaneous tissues and then tunnel catheter through device

N

Coil catheter into pocket, place pump inside, and suture closed

Figure 50-1, cont'd. K, The catheter is secured to the paravertebral fascia using an anchoring device provided by the manufacturer. **L,** A transverse incision is created in the abdominal wall midway between the umbilicus and the anterior axillary line, and a pocket of sufficient size to accommodate the pump is created using blunt dissection. The blunt dissection can be accomplished using the fingertips or surgical scissors and a repeated spreading (rather than cutting) motion. **M,** A tunneling device provided by the manufacturer is used to position the catheter in the subcutaneous tissue between the paravertebral incision and the abdominal pump pocket. **N,** Once good hemostasis has been achieved, the pump is placed in the pocket. The abdominal and paravertebral incisions are then closed in two layers: a layer of interrupted, absorbable sutures in the subcutaneous tissue overlying the pump and a separate layer within the skin.

rib cage using blunt dissection (Fig. 50-2A). The catheter is then tunneled from the paraspinous region to the pocket, as described previously for intrathecal catheter placement, and secured to the port. The port must then be sutured securely to the fascia over the rib cage. Care must be taken to ensure that the port is secured firmly in a region that overlies the rib cage; if the port migrates inferiorly to lie over the abdomen, it becomes difficult to access. The rigid support of the rib cage holds the port firmly from behind, allowing easier access to the port. The skin incisions are then closed in two layers: a series of interrupted subcutaneous sutures to close securely the fascia overlying the catheter, followed by skin closure using sutures or staples.

To place a permanent epidural system without a subcutaneous port, a tunneling device is extended from the paraspinous incision to the right upper abdominal quadrant just inferior to the costal margin. A small incision (about 0.5 cm) is made to allow the tunneling device to exit the skin. Percutaneous epidural catheters are supplied in two parts: the proximal portion of the catheter that is placed in the epidural space and the distal portion of the catheter that enters the abdominal wall and connects with the proximal portion of the catheter. The distal portion of the catheter is now secured to the tunneling device and pulled through the incision in the abdominal wall subcutaneously to emerge from the paraspinous incision (Fig. 50-2B).

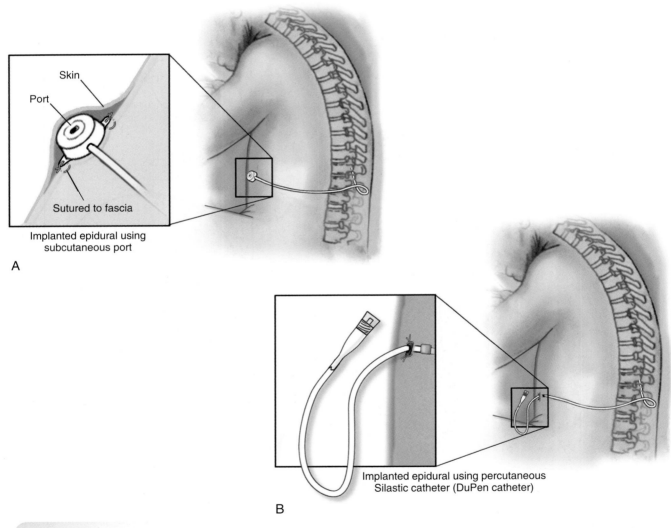

Figure 50-2. Permanent epidural catheter placement. Placement of the epidural catheter is accomplished using a loss-of-resistance technique, and fluoroscopy is used to direct the catheter to the dermatome of the pain to be treated. Creation of a paravertebral incision and securing the catheter to the lumbar paravertebral fascia are carried out as described for intrathecal catheter placement. **A,** Placement of a subcutaneous port. The epidural catheter is placed and tunneled to a pocket over the costal margin, leaving a small tension-relief loop of catheter in the subcutaneous paraspinous pocket. The port is connected to the epidural catheter and sutured to the fascia overlying the inferior rib cage. The port must lie firmly in place over the ribs rather than the abdominal wall; without the support of the firm rib cage behind the port, it would be difficult to access. **B,** Placement of a percutaneous tunneled catheter. This type of catheter typically is supplied in two pieces: a distal, epidural portion and a proximal catheter length with a subcutaneous antibiotic-impregnated cuff and external access port. After placement of the epidural catheter and dissection through a paravertebral incision, the proximal catheter is tunneled from the costal margin to the paravertebral incision and the catheter is pulled into the subcutaneous tissues until the antibiotic-impregnated cuff lies 1 to 2 cm from the chest wall incision in the subcutaneous tissue. The catheter segments are then trimmed, joined together using a connector supplied by the manufacturer, and secured to the paravertebral fascia, leaving a small tension-relief loop of catheter in the subcutaneous paraspinous pocket. The skin entry site on the chest wall is secured around the exiting catheter using interrupted sutures.

Many catheters are supplied with an antibiotic-impregnated cuff that is designed to arrest entry of bacteria along the track of the catheter. This cuff should be placed about 1 cm from the catheter's exit site along the subcutaneous catheter track. The proximal and distal portions of the catheter are then trimmed, leaving enough catheter length to ensure that there is no traction on the catheter with movement. The two ends of the catheter are connected using a stainless steel union supplied by the manufacturer and sutured securely. The paraspinous skin incision is then closed in two layers: a series of interrupted subcutaneous sutures to securely close the fascia overlying the catheter, followed by skin closure using suture or staples. The skin incision at the epidural catheter's exit site in the right upper quadrant is closed around the base of the catheter using one or two simple interrupted sutures.

POTENTIAL PROBLEMS

Bleeding and infection are risks inherent to all open surgical procedures. Bleeding in the pump pocket can lead to a hematoma surrounding the pump and may require surgical drainage. Bleeding along the subcutaneous tunneling track often causes significant bruising in the region but rarely requires treatment. As with other neuraxial techniques, bleeding in the epidural space can lead to significant neural compression. Signs of infection in the pump pocket typically appear between 10 and 14 days after implantation but may occur at any time. Some practitioners have reported successful treatment of superficial infections of the incision overlying the pocket with oral antibiotics aimed at the offending organism and close observation alone. However, infections within the pocket or along the catheter's subcutaneous course almost always require removal of all implanted hardware and treatment with parenteral antibiotics to eradicate infection. Catheter and deep tissue infections can extend to involve the neuraxis and result in epidural abscess formation, meningitis, or both. Permanent epidural catheters without subcutaneous ports have a higher infection rate than those with ports during the first weeks after placement, but both systems have a similar high rate of infection when left in place for more than 6 to 8 weeks.

Spinal cord injury during initial catheter placement has been reported. Most practitioners recommend placing the catheter only in awake patients so that the patients can report paresthesias during needle placement. However, this is a topic of some debate, and placing the intrathecal catheter under general anesthesia using radiographic guidance below the level of the conus medullaris (at about L2) is considered appropriate by some physicians. The catheter can be placed incorrectly in the subdural compartment or the epidural space. In both cases, free flow of CSF does not occur, indicating improper location of the catheter tip.

Wound dehiscence and pump migration are infrequent problems. Ensuring that the size of the pocket is sufficient to prevent tension on the suture line at the time of wound closure is essential to minimize the risk of dehiscence. Pump migration usually occurs because retaining sutures were omitted at the time of pump placement. Placing two or more sutures through the suture loops or mesh on the pump and securely fastening them to the abdominal fascia minimizes the risk of pump migration. Subcutaneous collection of fluid surrounding the pump (seroma formation) can be problematic and typically follows pump replacement. Percutaneous drainage of the sterile fluid collection is often successful in resolving the problem. A subcutaneous collection of CSF, particularly in the paraspinous region, can also develop, even many months after pump placement. This complication can be managed with observation alone unless the fluid collection is large or painful; in these instances, neurosurgical exposure of the spinal catheter as it enters the dura and placement of a pursestring suture around the catheter to eliminate the CSF leak may be needed.

PEARLS

Routine administration of prophylactic antibiotics is warranted before any intrathecal implantation based on the significance of potential infection. Appropriate agents include cefazolin 1 to 2 g intravenously (IV) 30 minutes before incision, clindamycin 900 mg IV 30 minutes before incision, or vancomycin 1 g IV over 60 minutes before incision. It is important to discuss the location of the pump with the patient before surgery and mark the site using a skin marker with the patient in the sitting position. The operator should make sure that CSF flows freely from the intrathecal catheter at each step during the implantation to ensure early detection of incorrect placement or dislodgement. Great care is needed when attempting to pull the catheter back through the needle, as the Silastic catheter used for this purpose is very prone to shearing. If any resistance to withdrawal of the catheter is met, the needle and catheter must be removed as a unit, then the catheter must be removed from the needle and inspected for damage. Then, implantation should be repeated. The operator must ensure that the size of the pocket created for the pump is adequate to prevent tension on the suture line after wound closure. Caution is needed when placing the fascial closure sutures: the operator must know where the catheter lies at all times to avoid damaging the catheter with the suture needle.

Spinal Cord Stimulation

James P. Rathmell

51

PERSPECTIVE

The idea that direct stimulation of the ascending sensory tracts of the spinal cord might interfere with the perception of chronic pain is founded on everyday observations. We are all familiar with the fact that rubbing an area that has just been injured seemingly reduces the amount of pain coming from that injured region. The advent of transcutaneous electrical nerve stimulation (TENS), wherein a light, pleasant electrical current is passed through surface electrodes in the region of ongoing pain, reinforced the observation that stimulation of sensory pathways reduces pain perception in chronic pain states. In 1965, Patrick Wall, a neurophysiologist exploring the basic physiologic mechanisms of pain transmission, and Ronald Melzack, a psychologist working with patients who had chronic pain, together proposed the gate control theory to explain how non-noxious stimulation can reduce pain perception. With their theory, they proposed that second-order neurons at the level of the spinal cord dorsal horn act as a "gate" through which noxious stimuli must pass to reach higher centers in the brain and be perceived as pain. If these same neurons receive input from other sensory fibers entering through the same set of neurons in the spinal cord, the non-noxious input can effectively close the gate, preventing simultaneous transmission of noxious input. Thus, the light touch of rubbing an injured region or the pleasant electrical stimulation of TENS closes the gate to the noxious input of chronic pain. Based on this theory, investigators developed the concept of direct activation of the ascending fibers in the dorsal columns that transmit nonpainful cutaneous stimuli (e.g., light touch) as a means of treating chronic pain. We have learned much about the anatomy and physiology of pain perception since the gate control theory was first proposed. It is unlikely that the simplistic notion of a gate in the dorsal horn is responsible for our observations, but the theory served as a useful concept in the development of spinal cord stimulation. Both the peripheral nerve fibers and second-order neurons in the dorsal horn that transmit pain signals become sensitized after injury, and anatomic changes, cell death, and altered gene expression are all likely to have a role in the development of chronic pain. Direct electrical stimulation of the dorsal columns, referred to as *spinal cord stimulation (SCS)* or *dorsal column stimulation*, has proven effective, particularly in the treatment of chronic radicular pain. The mechanism remains unclear, but direct electrical stimulation in the dorsal columns may produce retrograde changes in the ascending sensory fibers that modulate the intensity of incoming noxious stimuli.

Patient selection for SCS is empiric and remains a subject of some debate. In general, SCS is reserved for patients with severe pain that does not respond to conservative treatment. The pain responds best when it is relatively well localized because the success of SCS depends on the ability to cover the entire painful region with electrical stimulation. Attaining adequate coverage is more difficult when pain is bilateral, often requiring two leads, one on each side of the midline. When the pain is diffuse, it may be impossible to obtain effective coverage with stimulation using SCS. Among the best-established indications for SCS is chronic radicular pain with or without radiculopathy in either the upper or lower extremities. Use of SCS to treat chronic, axial low-back pain has been less satisfactory, but recent results seem more promising with the advent of dual-lead systems and electrode arrays that allow for a broad area of stimulation. Randomized controlled trials comparing SCS with repeat surgery for patients with failed back surgery syndrome have demonstrated greater success in attaining satisfactory pain relief in those treated with SCS. Recent small randomized controlled trials also suggest significantly improved pain relief and physical function in patients with complex regional pain syndrome who are treated with SCS in conjunction with physical therapy compared with physical therapy alone. Prospective observational studies indicate an overall success rate of about 50% (defined as at least 50% pain reduction and ongoing use of SCS 5 years after implantation) in mixed groups of patients with ongoing low-back or extremity pain (or both) after lumbar surgery. The usefulness of psychological screening before SCS remains controversial; some investigators have suggested that screening for patients with personality disorders, somatoform disorder, or hypochondriasis may improve the success rate of SCS.

Once a patient is selected for therapy with SCS, a trial is carried out. Most physicians now conduct trials by placing a temporary percutaneous epidural lead and conducting the screening using an external device as an outpatient procedure to judge the effectiveness of this therapy before a permanent system is implanted. Some carry out the SCS trial using a surgically implanted lead that is tunneled using a lead extension that exits percutaneously. The strictly percutaneous trial lead is simpler to place and does not require a full operating room setup, but the lead must be removed and replaced surgically after a successful trial. The surgically implanted trial lead requires placement in the operating room, with surgical removal if the trial is unsuccessful. If the trial is successful, the implanted trial lead can remain, and the second procedure to place the impulse generator is brief, not requiring placement of a new epidural lead. In either case, after successful trial stimulation, a permanent system is placed and the lead is positioned to produce the same pattern of stimulation that afforded pain relief during the trial stimulation.

PLACEMENT

Anatomy. The epidural SCS lead is placed directly into the dorsal epidural space just to one side of the midline using a paramedian, interlaminar approach. Entry into the epidural space is performed several levels below the final intended level of lead placement. Typically, leads for stimulation of the low back and lower extremities are placed through the L1-L2 interspace, and those for upper extremity stimulation are placed through the C7-T1 interspace. Investigators have mapped the patterns of electrical stimulation of the dorsal columns and the corresponding patterns of coverage reported by patients with leads in various locations. In general, the epidural lead must be positioned just 2 to 3 mm to the left or right of the midline on the same side as the painful region to be covered. For lower extremity stimulation, successful coverage is usually achieved by placing the lead between the T8 and T10 vertebral levels, whereas upper extremity stimulation usually requires lead placement between the occiput and C3 vertebral levels. If the lead ventures too far from the midline, uncomfortable stimulation of the spinal nerves may result. If the lead is placed too low, overlying the conus medullaris (at or below L1-L2), unpredictable patterns of stimulation may result. In the region of the conus, the fibers of the dorsal columns do not lie parallel to the midline; rather, they arc from the corresponding nerve entering the spinal cord toward their eventual paramedian location several levels cephalad.

Position. A percutaneous trial spinal cord stimulator lead can be placed in any location that is suitable for epidural catheter placement. This procedure may be done in the operating room but can easily and safely be carried out in any location that allows adequate sterile preparation of the skin and draping of the operative field and that has fluoroscopy available to guide anatomic placement. In a strictly percutaneous trial, the trial lead is placed in the same fashion as that used for permanent lead placement, but the lead is secured to the skin without any incision for the trial period.

Before permanent spinal cord stimulator implantation, one must discuss with the patient the location of the pocket for the impulse generator. The most suitable regions are the lower quadrant of the abdomen and the lateral aspect of the buttock. Once the site is determined, the proposed skin incision is marked with a permanent marker while the patient is in the sitting position. The position of the pocket is deceptively difficult to determine once a patient is lying on his or her side. If the location is not marked, the pocket is often placed too far laterally in the abdominal wall or buttock. Placing the impulse generator in the buttock allows the entire procedure to be carried out with the patient in the prone position and simplifies the operation by obviating the need to turn from the prone to the lateral position halfway through implantation.

Implantation of a spinal cord stimulator lead and impulse generator is a minor surgical procedure that is carried out in the operating room using aseptic precautions, including skin preparation, sterile draping, and full surgical attire (Fig. 51-1A). The procedure must be conducted using local anesthesia and sedation light enough that the patient can report feeling the electrical stimulation during lead placement. The patient is positioned on a radiolucent table in the prone position (see Fig. 51-1A). Initial lead placement can be carried out with the patient in a lateral decubitus position, but even small degrees of rotation along the spinal axis can make positioning the lead difficult. The arms are extended upward so that they are in a position of comfort well away from the surgical field. The skin is prepared, and sterile drapes are applied. For stimulation in the low back and lower extremities, the fluoroscopic C-arm is positioned directly over the thoracolumbar junction to provide an anteroposterior view of the spine. Care must be taken to ensure that the radiographic view is not rotated by observing that the spinous processes are in the midline, halfway between the vertebral pedicles (Fig. 51-1B).

Procedure. The L1-L2 interspace is identified using fluoroscopy. The epidural needle supplied by the device manufacturer must be used to ensure that the lead can advance through the needle without damage. The needle is advanced using a paramedian approach starting 1 to 1.5 cm lateral to the spinous processes and somewhat caudad to the interspace to be entered. The needle is directed to enter the spinal space in the midline with an angle of entry no greater than 45 degrees from the plane of the epidural space (Fig. 51-1C). If the angle of attack of the needle during the initial entry into the epidural space is too great, the epidural lead is difficult to thread as it negotiates the steep angle between the needle and the plane of the epidural space. The epidural space is identified using a loss-of-resistance technique. The electrode is then advanced through the needle and directed to remain just to one side of midline as it is threaded cephalad under fluoroscopic guidance. The electrode contains a wire stylet with a slight angulation at the tip; gentle rotation of the electrode as it is advanced allows the operator to direct the electrode's path in the epidural space (Fig. 51-1D). For stimulation in the low back and lower extremities, the electrode is initially positioned 2 to 3 mm from the midline on the same side as the patient's pain between the T8 and T10 vertebral levels (see Fig. 51-1B). Final electrode position is attained by connecting the electrode to an external impulse generator and asking the patient where the stimulation is felt. In general, cephalad advancement results in stimulation higher in the extremity, and caudad movement leads to stimulation lower in the extremity. However, if the lead is angled even slightly from medial to lateral, the pattern of stimulation may change less predictably with movement of the electrode; for example, craniad advancement can lead to stimulation lower in the extremity under these circumstances. The final electrode position should be recorded using radiography so that a permanent lead can be placed in the same position (see Fig. 51-1B). For trial stimulation, the needle is removed, the electrode secured to the back, and a sterile occlusive dressing applied (Fig. 51-1E). The patient is

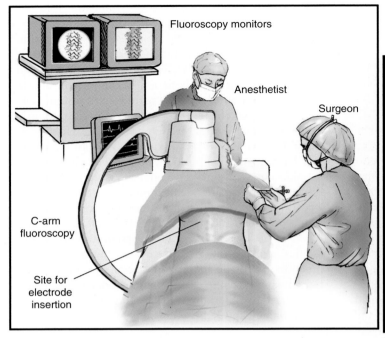

A   Surgical setup

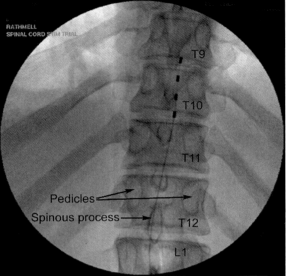

B

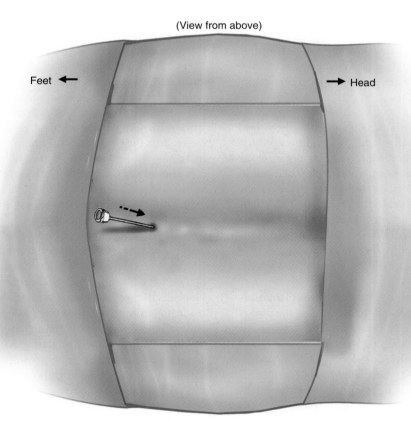

C   Insert needle

Figure 51-1. Spinal cord stimulator trial and permanent implantation. **A,** View of a typical operating room arrangement during spinal cord stimulator implantation; the patient is placed in the prone position with the fluoroscopic C-arm in place for an anteroposterior (AP) view of the thoracolumbar spine. **B,** Posteroanterior radiograph of a spinal cord stimulator lead in position for stimulation of the right lower extremity. The lead lies to the right of midline, with the tip over the inferior endplate of the T9 vertebral body. During initial patient positioning, care must be taken to ensure that the image is in the AP plane without rotation by moving the image intensifier in the mediolateral direction until the spinous processes project midway between the pedicles. **C,** Initial epidural needle placement at the L1-L2 interspace using a paramedian approach. The angle of entry into the epidural space must be less than 45 degrees relative to the plane of the epidural space to ensure that the lead can pass easily.

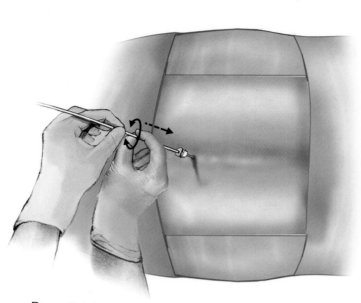

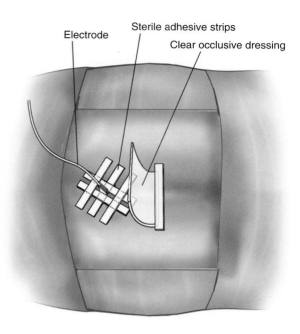

D   Slightly twist electrode to advance it in the spinal canal

E   Secure electrode with sterile adhesive strips, then tape a clear occlusive dressing on top

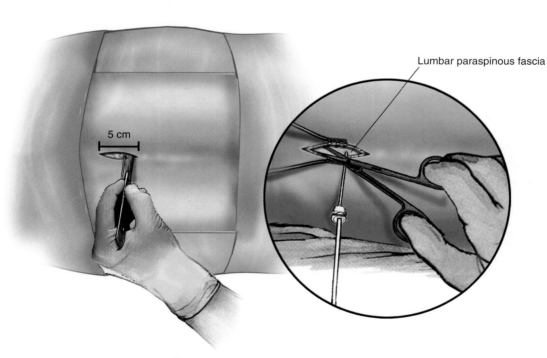

F   Incision and blunt dissection

Figure 51-1, cont'd. D, The electrode is advanced under continuous fluoroscopic guidance using a slight twisting motion to steer the catheter to the desired position just lateral to the midline on the side of the desired stimulation. **E,** For trial stimulation using a percutaneous lead, the lead is secured to the back using either sutures or sterile adhesive strips; a sterile occlusive dressing is then placed. **F,** A cephalocaudad incision is made through the skin and subcutaneous tissues, with the incision extending above and below the needle entry point. Using blunt dissection, the skin and subcutaneous tissues are further divided until the lumbar paravertebral fascia is exposed.

Continued

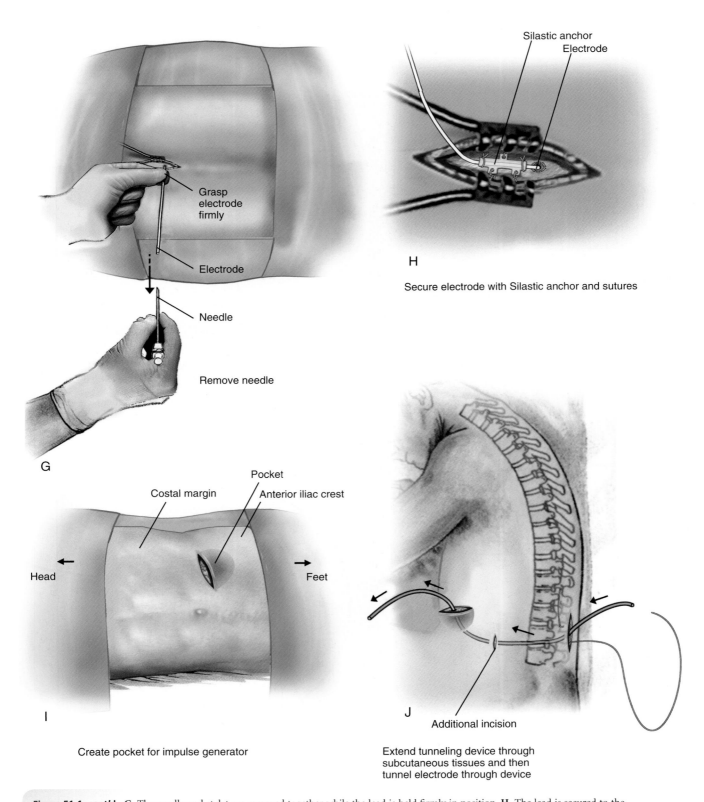

G

Grasp
electrode
firmly

Electrode

Needle

Remove needle

H

Silastic anchor
Electrode

Secure electrode with Silastic anchor and sutures

I

Costal margin

Pocket

Anterior iliac crest

Head

Feet

Create pocket for impulse generator

J

Additional incision

Extend tunneling device through
subcutaneous tissues and then
tunnel electrode through device

Figure 51-1, cont'd. **G,** The needle and stylet are removed together while the lead is held firmly in position. **H,** The lead is secured to the paravertebral fascia using an anchoring device provided by the manufacturer. **I,** A transverse incision is created in the abdominal wall midway between the umbilicus and the anterior axillary line or over the superolateral aspect of the buttock. A pocket of sufficient size to accommodate the impulse generator is then created using blunt dissection, which can be accomplished using the fingertips or surgical scissors and a repeated spreading (rather than cutting) motion. **J,** A tunneling device provided by the manufacturer is used to position the lead in the subcutaneous tissue between the paravertebral incision and the pocket.

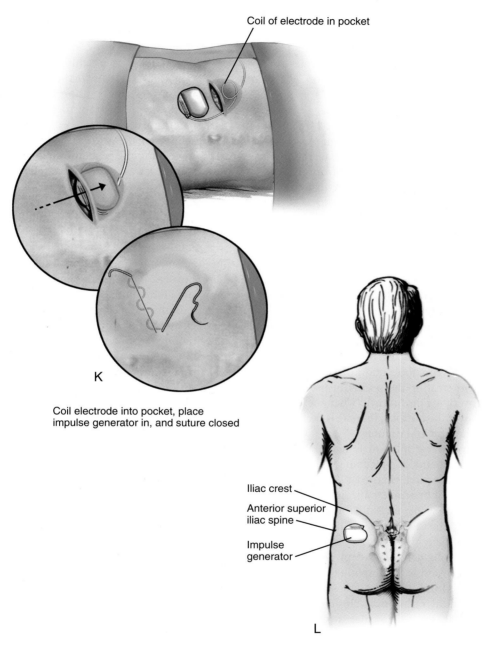

Coil of electrode in pocket

K

Coil electrode into pocket, place
impulse generator in, and suture closed

Iliac crest

Anterior superior
iliac spine

Impulse
generator

L

Alternative site for impulse generator
placement (upper buttock)

Figure 51-1, cont'd. K, After ensuring good hemostasis, the impulse generator is placed in the pocket, with any excess lead coiled loosely and inserted in the pocket, behind the impulse generator. The pocket and paravertebral incisions are then closed in two layers: a layer of interrupted absorbable sutures in the subcutaneous tissue overlying the impulse generator and lead, and a separate layer in the skin. **L,** The upper buttock, well lateral to the posterior superior iliac spine and sacral prominence, is also a common site for placement of the implanted pulse generator.

instructed in the use of the external pulse generator and scheduled to return in 5 to 7 days to assess his or her response and to remove the trial lead.

The procedure for initial lead placement for permanent implantation is identical to that for trial stimulation. Once the final lead is in position and the optimal pattern of stimulation confirmed, the lead is secured, a pocket for the impulse generator is created, and the lead is tunneled underneath the skin for connection to the impulse generator. After initial lead placement, the epidural needle is withdrawn slightly (about 1 to 2 cm) but left in place around the lead in the subcutaneous tissues to protect the lead during the subsequent incision and dissection. A 5- to 8-cm incision parallel to the axis of the spine is extended from cephalad to caudad to the needle, extending directly through the needle's skin entry point (Fig. 51-1F). The subcutaneous tissues are divided using blunt dissection until the lumbar paraspinous fascia is visible surrounding the needle shaft. The stylet is then removed from the lead and the needle is withdrawn, using care not to dislodge the electrode (Fig. 51-1G). The lead is then secured to the paraspinous fascia using a specific anchoring device supplied by the manufacturer (Fig. 51-1H).

If lead placement has been carried out in the prone position and the impulse generator is to be placed in the abdominal wall, the lead must be coiled underneath the skin, the paraspinous incision temporarily closed using staples, and a sterile occlusive dressing applied. The sterile drapes are then removed and the patient is repositioned in the lateral decubitus position with the side where the abdominal pocket is located facing upward. After repeat preparation of the skin and application of sterile drapes, attention is turned to creating the pocket in the patient's abdominal wall or overlying the buttock (when the impulse generator is placed over the buttock, this site is included in the initial skin preparation and draping).

An 8- to 10-cm transverse incision is made along the previously marked line and a subcutaneous pocket is created using blunt dissection (Fig. 51-1I). The pocket should always be created caudad to the incision; if the pocket is placed cephalad to the incision, the weight of the impulse generator on the suture line is likely to cause wound dehiscence. In many patients, the blunt dissection can be accomplished using gentle but firm pressure with the fingers. It is simpler and less traumatic to use a small surgical scissors to perform the blunt dissection, using repeated opening motions rather than closing or cutting motions that are likely to cut vascular structures and provoke marked bleeding. An alternative to blunt dissection is the use of a monopolar electrocautery device in the "cut" mode, an effective means to carry out the necessary dissection without excessive tissue trauma or blood loss. After the pocket has been created, the impulse generator is placed in the pocket to ensure that the pocket is large enough. The impulse generator should fit completely in the pocket without any part of the device extending into the incision. With the device in place, the wound margins must fall into close apposition. There should be no tension on the sutures during closure of the incision, lest the wound dehisce.

After the pocket creation is completed, a tunneling device is extended in the subcutaneous tissues between the paraspinous incision and the pocket, leaving a small tension-relief loop of lead in the subcutaneous area of the paraspinous dissection (Fig. 51-1J). The electrode is then advanced through the tunnel. Tunneling devices vary and are specific to each manufacturer. The means by which the electrode is connected to the impulse generator also varies by manufacturer; some devices use a lead extension that connects the impulse generator and the lead, and others use a one-piece lead that is connected directly to the impulse generator. After tunneling, the lead or lead extension is connected with the impulse generator. Any excess lead is coiled and placed behind the impulse generator in the pocket (Fig. 51-1K). This loop allows patient movement without placing tension on the distal electrode, causing it to be pulled from the epidural space. The skin incisions are then closed in two layers: a series of interrupted subcutaneous sutures to securely close the fascia overlying the impulse generator in the pocket and the electrode over the paraspinous fascia, followed by skin closure using sutures or staples (see Fig. 51-1K).

POTENTIAL PROBLEMS

Bleeding and infection are risks inherent to all open surgical procedures. Bleeding in the pocket can lead to a hematoma surrounding the impulse generator that may require surgical drainage. Bleeding along the subcutaneous tunneling track often causes significant bruising in the region but rarely requires treatment. Similar to other neuraxial techniques, bleeding in the epidural space can lead to significant neural compression. Signs of infection in the impulse generator pocket typically appear between 10 and 14 days after implantation but may occur at any time. Some practitioners have reported successful treatment of superficial infections of the incision overlying the pocket with oral antibiotics aimed at the offending organism and close observation alone. However, infections in the pocket or along the lead's subcutaneous course almost always require removal of all implanted hardware and treatment with parenteral antibiotics to eradicate the infection. Lead and deep tissue infections can extend to involve the neuraxis and result in epidural abscess formation, meningitis, or both.

There is a significant risk of dural puncture during initial localization of the epidural space using the loss-of-resistance technique. The epidural needle used for electrode placement is a Tuohy needle that has been modified by extending the orifice to allow the electrode to pass easily. This long bevel often results in equivocal loss of resistance; it is not uncommon to have minimal resistance to injection along the entire course of needle placement. To minimize the risk of dural puncture, the needle tip can be advanced under fluoroscopic guidance and first seated on the superior margin of the vertebral lamina (taking care to place additional local anesthetic during advancement). In this way, the depth of the lamina is certain and the needle need be advanced only a small distance over the lamina, through the ligamentum flavum, and into the epidural space. Loss of resistance is used only during the final few millimeters of needle advancement over the lamina. If dural puncture does occur, there is no clear consensus on how to proceed. Some practitioners abandon the lead placement and allow

1 to 2 weeks before any reattempt; this approach allows the practitioner to watch for and treat post–dural puncture headache, which is nearly certain to occur. Other practitioners proceed with lead placement through a more cephalad interspace; if post–dural puncture headache ensues and conservative treatment fails, an epidural blood patch is placed at the level of the dural puncture. Spinal cord and nerve root injury during initial lead placement have been reported. Placing the epidural needle and lead in the awake, lightly sedated patient able to report paresthesias should minimize the risk of direct neural injury.

The most frequent complication after spinal cord stimulator placement is lead migration. The first line of defense is to ensure that the lead is firmly secured to the paraspinous fascia. Suturing the lead to loose subcutaneous tissue or fat is not adequate. After surgery, the patient must be clearly instructed to avoid flexion/extension and rotation at the waist (lumbar leads) or flexion/extension and rotation of the neck (cervical leads) for at least 4 weeks after lead placement. Placing a soft cervical collar on those who have had a cervical lead placed provides a ready reminder to avoid movement. Lead fracture may also occur, often months or years after placement. Avoiding midline placement or tunneling the lead across the midline reduces the incidence of fracture caused by compression of the lead on bone. Lead fracture presents as a sudden loss of stimulation and is diagnosed by checking lead impedance using the spinal cord stimulator programmer.

Wound dehiscence and impulse generator migration are infrequent problems. Ensuring that the size of the pocket is sufficient to prevent tension on the suture line at the time of wound closure is essential for minimizing the risk of dehiscence. Subcutaneous collection of fluid surrounding the impulse generator (seroma formation) can be problematic and typically follows generator replacement. Percutaneous drainage of the sterile fluid collection is often successful in resolving the problem.

PEARLS

Routine administration of prophylactic antibiotics is warranted before spinal cord stimulator implantation because any infection that does occur may extend to involve the neuraxis. Appropriate agents include cefazolin 1 to 2 g intravenously (IV) 30 minutes before incision, clindamycin 900 mg IV 30 minutes before incision, or vancomycin 1 g IV over 60 minutes before incision. It is important to discuss the location of the impulse generator with the patient before surgery and mark the site using a skin marker with the patient in the sitting position. The operator should consider each patient's daily activities when selecting a location. For instance, a mechanic who spends much time leaning forward with his abdomen against a vehicle may be bothered by an impulse generator located in the abdominal wall.

Dural puncture is a significant risk during the procedure, and the particular needle used for placing the spinal cord stimulator lead often does not give a clear sign of loss of resistance during advancement. In such cases, the needle should be advanced using fluoroscopic guidance and the needle tip seated on the margin of the lamina immediately inferior to the interspace one is attempting to enter. In this way, the depth of the lamina is certain and loss of resistance is needed only during the final 3 to 5 mm of needle advancement, reducing the risk of dural puncture. If dural puncture does occur during lead placement, one should consider rescheduling the procedure or moving to a more cephalad interspace for lead placement. Post–dural puncture headache is a near certainty with the large-bore needle used for electrode placement, so the operator must be prepared to offer treatment as needed, including an epidural blood patch. Performing an epidural blood patch in the days immediately after spinal cord stimulator implantation has been described, but the risks associated with the approach are uncertain.

To minimize the risk of lead migration, a secure anchor for the lead is needed. The most important point during implantation is securing the lead to the paraspinous fascia. First, the incision must be extended deep enough to expose the fascia; securing the lead to loose subcutaneous tissue or fat is inadequate. Once the fascia is exposed, the lead anchor supplied by the manufacturer is placed over the lead and the anchor is advanced to the point where the lead enters the fascia. The lead anchor is securely fastened to the lead itself, first using sutures around the anchor and lead only. After this is accomplished, one should no longer be able to slide the anchor over the lead. Then, the lead and anchor are sutured securely to the fascia. Patients are advised to avoid bending or twisting for at least 4 weeks after implantation; a soft cervical collar can be placed for those with cervical leads for comfort and as an effective reminder to avoid movement.

It is also important to ensure that the size of the pocket created for the impulse generator is adequate to prevent tension on the suture line after wound closure. Similarly, one should use caution when placing the fascial closure sutures and know where the lead lies at all times to avoid damaging it with the suture needle.

It is good practice to obtain anteroposterior and lateral radiographs of the spine after successful lead placement. The radiographs can serve as a helpful reference when attempting to produce a similar pattern of stimulation during subsequent lead placement or when trying to determine if the lead has migrated. Loss of stimulation may signal lead migration or fracture. The operator should check lead impedance first to detect a lead fracture. Thereafter, radiography and comparison with films obtained at the time of initial lead placement are used to detect lead migration.

Impulse generator battery failure is inevitable and occurs over a broad range (about 1 to 4 years), depending on the stimulation parameters and frequency of use. Approaching battery end-of-life typically begins with intermittent malfunction of the device; the most common malfunction is the device shutting off on its own.

Bibliography

General

Benhamou D, Pequignot F, Auroy Y, et al. Factors associated with use of regional anaesthesia: a multivariate analysis in seven surgical procedures in France. *Eur J Anaesthesiol.* 2004;21:576-578.

Bernards CM, Hadzic A, Suresh S, Neal JM. Regional anesthesia in anesthetized or heavily sedated patients. *Reg Anesth Pain Med.* 2008;33:449-460.

Bonica JJ. *The Management of Pain.* 2nd ed. Philadelphia, Pa: Lea & Febiger; 1990.

Brown DL, ed. *Regional Anesthesia at Virginia Mason Medical Center: A Clinical Perspective. Problems in Anesthesia.* Vol 1, Issue 4. Philadelphia: JB Lippincott Co; 1987.

Brown DL, ed. *Perioperative Analgesia. Problems in Anesthesia.* Vol 2, Issue 3. Philadelphia, Pa: JB Lippincott Co; 1988.

Brown DL. Spinal, epidural and caudal anesthesia. In: Miller RD, ed. *Anesthesia.* 4th ed. New York, NY: Churchill Livingstone; 1994: 1505-1533.

Brown DL, ed. *Regional Anesthesia and Analgesia.* Philadelphia, Pa: WB Saunders Co; 1996.

Brull R, McCartney CJ, Chan VW, El-Beheiry H. Neurological complications after regional anesthesia: contemporary estimates of risk. *Anesth Analg.* 2007;104:965-974.

Cahill DR, Orland MJ, Miller GM. *Atlas of Human Cross-Sectional Anatomy: With CT and MR Images.* 3rd ed. New York, NY: Wiley-Liss; 1995.

Capdevila X, Ponrouch M, Choquet O. Continuous peripheral nerve blocks in clinical practice. *Curr Opin Anaesthesiol.* 2008;21:619-623.

Carron H, Korbon GA, Rowlingson JC. *Regional Anesthesia: Techniques and Clinical Applications.* Orlando, Fla: Grune & Stratton; 1984.

Chin KJ, Chan VW. Ultrasound-guided peripheral nerve blockade. *Curr Opin Anaesthesiol.* 2008;21:624-631.

Chin KJ, Perlas A, Chan VW, Brull R. Needle visualization in ultrasound-guided regional anesthesia: challenges and solutions. *Reg Anesth Pain Med.* 2008;33:532-544.

Christoforidis AJ. *Atlas of Axial, Sagittal, and Coronal Anatomy.* Philadelphia, Pa: WB Saunders Co; 1988.

Cousins M, Bridenbaugh PO, eds. *Neural Blockade.* 2nd ed. Philadelphia, Pa: JB Lippincott Co; 1988.

Covino BG, Scott DB. *Handbook of Epidural Anaesthesia and Analgesia.* Orlando, Fla: Grune & Stratton; 1985.

Eriksson E, ed. *Illustrated Handbook in Local Anaesthesia.* 2nd ed. Philadelphia, Pa: WB Saunders Co; 1980.

Gosling JA, Harris PF, Humpherson JR, et al. *Atlas of Human Anatomy with Integrated Text.* London, England: Gower Medical Publishing; 1985.

Grant JCB. *An Atlas of Anatomy.* 5th ed. Baltimore, Md: Williams & Wilkins; 1962.

Hahn MB, McQuillan PM, Sheplock GJ, eds. *Regional Anesthesia: An Atlas of Anatomy and Techniques.* St. Louis, Mo: Mosby; 1995.

Hanna MN, Jeffries MA, Hamzehzadeh S, et al. Survey of the utilization of regional and general anesthesia in a tertiary teaching hospital. *Reg Anesth Pain Med.* 2009;34:224-228.

Hanna MN, Murphy JD, Kumar K, Wu CL. Regional techniques and outcome: what is the evidence? *Curr Opin Anaesthesiol.* 2009;22: 672-677.

Hogan QH. Pathophysiology of peripheral nerve injury during regional anesthesia. *Reg Anesth Pain Med.* 2008;33:435-441.

Katz J. *Atlas of Regional Anesthesia.* Norwalk, Conn: Appleton-Century-Crofts; 1985.

Katz J, Renck H. *Handbook of Thoraco-Abdominal Nerve Block.* Orlando, Fla: Grune & Stratton; 1987.

Koscielniak-Nielsen ZJ. Ultrasound-guided peripheral nerve blocks: what are the benefits? *Acta Anaesthesiol Scand.* 2008;52:727-737.

Labat G. *Regional Anesthesia: Its Technique and Clinical Application.* Philadelphia, Pa: WB Saunders Co; 1923.

Lee LA, Posner KL, Domino KB, et al. Injuries associated with regional anesthesia in the 1980s and 1990s: a closed claims analysis. *Anesthesiology.* 2004;101:143-152.

Liu SS, Wu CL. The effect of analgesic technique on postoperative patient-reported outcomes including analgesia: a systematic review. *Anesth Analg.* 2007;105:789-808.

McMinn RMH, Hutchings RT. *Color Atlas of Human Anatomy.* Chicago, Ill: Year Book Medical Publishers; 1977.

Melloni JL, Dox I, Melloni HP, Melloni BJ. *Melloni's Illustrated Review of Human Anatomy.* Philadelphia, Pa: JB Lippincott Co; 1988.

Moore DC. *Regional Block.* 4th ed. Springfield, Ill: Charles C Thomas; 1965.

Moore DC. *Stellate Ganglion Block.* Springfield, Ill: Charles C Thomas; 1954.

Neal JM. Anatomy and pathophysiology of spinal cord injury associated with regional anesthesia and pain medicine. *Reg Anesth Pain Med.* 2008;33:423-434.

Neal JM, Bernards CM, Hadzic A, et al. ASRA practice advisory on neurologic complications in regional anesthesia and pain medicine. *Reg Anesth Pain Med.* 2008;33:404-415.

Raj PP. *Handbook of Regional Anesthesia.* New York, NY: Churchill Livingstone; 1985.

Sites BD, Brull R. Ultrasound guidance in peripheral regional anesthesia: philosophy, evidence-based medicine, and techniques. *Curr Opin Anaesthesiol.* 2006;19:630-639.

Sites BD, Brull R, Chan VW, et al. Artifacts and pitfall errors associated with ultrasound-guided regional anesthesia, I: understanding the basic principles of ultrasound physics and machine operations. *Reg Anesth Pain Med.* 2007;32:412-418.

Sites BD, Brull R, Chan VW, et al. Artifacts and pitfall errors associated with ultrasound-guided regional anesthesia, II: a pictorial approach to understanding and avoidance. *Reg Anesth Pain Med.* 2007;32: 419-433.

Sites BD, Chan VW, Neal JM, et al, American Society of Regional Anesthesia and Pain Medicine, European Society Of Regional Anaesthesia and Pain Therapy Joint Committee. The American Society of Regional Anesthesia and Pain Medicine and the European Society of Regional Anaesthesia and Pain Therapy Joint Committee recommendations for education and training in ultrasound-guided regional anesthesia. *Reg Anesth Pain Med.* 2009;34:40-46.

Sites BD, Neal JM, Chan V. Ultrasound in regional anesthesia: where should the "focus" be set? *Reg Anesth Pain Med.* 2009;34:531-533.

Thompson GE, Brown DL. The common nerve blocks. In: Nunn JF, Utting JE, Brown BR, eds. *General Anaesthesia.* 5th ed. London, England: Butterworth; 1989:1049-1085.

Tsui B. Ultrasound-guidance and nerve stimulation: implications for the future practice of regional anesthesia. *Can J Anaesth.* 2007;54: 165-170.

Tsui BC, Dillane D. Continuing medical education: ultrasound guidance for regional blockade—basic concepts. *Can J Anaesth.* 2008;55: 869-874.

Waldman SD, Winnie AP, eds. *Interventional Pain Management.* Philadelphia, Pa: WB Saunders Co; 1996.

Winnie AP. *Plexus Anesthesia, Volume I: Perivascular Techniques of Brachial Plexus Block.* Philadelphia, Pa: WB Saunders Co; 1983.

Woodburne RT. *Essentials of Human Anatomy.* 5th ed. New York, NY: Oxford University Press; 1973.

Introductory Chapter

Bashein G, Haschke RH, Ready LB. Electrical nerve location: numerical and electrophoretic comparison of insulated vs uninsulated needles. *Anesth Analg.* 1984;63:919-924.

Carpenter RL, Mackey DC. Local anesthetics. In: Barash PG, Cullen BF, Stoelting RK, eds. *Clinical Anesthesia.* Philadelphia, Pa: JB Lippincott Co; 1989.

DeJong R. Local anesthetic pharmacology. In: Brown DL, ed. *Regional Anesthesia and Analgesia.* Philadelphia, Pa: WB Saunders Co; 1996.

Heavner JE. Local anesthetics. *Curr Opin Anaesthesiol.* 2007;20:336-342.

Hiller DB, Gregorio GD, Ripper R, et al. Epinephrine impairs lipid resuscitation from bupivacaine overdose: a threshold effect. *Anesthesiology.* 2009;111:498-505.

Horton WG. Use of peripheral nerve stimulator. In: Brown DL, ed. *Regional Anesthesia at Virginia Mason Medical Center: A Clinical Perspective. Problems in Anesthesia.* Vol 1, Issue 4. Philadelphia, Pa: JB Lippincott Co; 1987:588-591.

McMahon D. Managing regional anesthesia equipment. In: Brown DL, ed. *Regional Anesthesia at Virginia Mason Medical Center: A Clinical Perspective. Problems in Anesthesia.* Vol 1, Issue 4. Philadelphia: JB Lippincott Co; 1987:592-601.

Rosenblatt MA, Abel M, Fischer GW, et al. Successful use of a 20% lipid emulsion to resuscitate a patient after a presumed bupivacaine-related cardiac arrest. *Anesthesiology.* 2006;105:217-218.

Rowlingson JC. Lipid rescue: a step forward in patient safety? Likely so! *Anesth Analg.* 2008;106:1333-1336.

Schafhalter-Zoppoth I, McCulloch CE, Gray AT. Ultrasound visibility of needles used for regional nerve block: an in vitro study. *Reg Anesth Pain Med.* 2004;29:480-488.

Schorr MR. Needles: some points to think about, part I. *Anesth Analg.* 1966;45:509-513.

Schorr MR. Needles: some points to think about, part II. *Anesth Analg.* 1966;45:514-526.

Weinberg G. Lipid rescue resuscitation from local anaesthetic cardiac toxicity. *Toxicol Rev.* 2006;25:139-145.

Weinberg G. The lipid resuscitation story: past and future. *Anaesthesia.* 2009;64:785-786.

Weinberg GL. Limits to lipid in the literature and lab: what we know, what we don't know. *Anesth Analg.* 2009;108:1062-1064.

Wildsmith JA. Treatment of severe local anaesthetic toxicity. *Anaesthesia.* 2008;63:778-779.

Zink W, Graf BM. The toxicity of local anesthetics: the place of ropivacaine and levobupivacaine. *Curr Opin Anaesthesiol.* 2008;21:645-650.

Upper Extremity Blocks

Ajar A, Hoeft M, Alsofrom GF, et al. Review of brachial plexus anatomy as seen on diagnostic imaging: clinical correlation with computed tomography-guided brachial plexus block. *Reg Anesth Pain Med.* 2007;32:79-83.

Benhamou D. Axillary plexus block using multiple nerve stimulation: a European view. *Reg Anesth Pain Med.* 2001;26:495-498.

Boezaart AP, Koorn R, Rosenquist RW. Paravertebral approach to the brachial plexus: an anatomic improvement in technique. *Reg Anesth Pain Med.* 2003;28:241-244.

Borene SC, Edwards JN, Boezaart AP. At the cords, the pinkie towards: interpreting infraclavicular motor responses to neurostimulation. *Reg Anesth Pain Med.* 2004;29:125-129.

Brown DL, Cahill DR, Bridenbaugh LD. Supraclavicular nerve block: anatomic analysis of a method to prevent pneumothorax. *Anesth Analg.* 1993;76:530-534.

Chan VW. Applying ultrasound imaging to interscalene brachial plexus block. *Reg Anesth Pain Med.* 2003;28:340-343.

Chan VW, Perlas A, McCartney CJ, et al. Ultrasound guidance improves success rate of axillary brachial plexus block. *Can J Anaesth.* 2007;54:176-182.

Chin KJ, Perlas A, Chan V, Brull R. Continuous infraclavicular plexus blockade. *Anesth Analg.* 2009;109:1347-1348.

Choyce A, Chan VW, Middleton WJ, et al. What is the relationship between paresthesia and nerve stimulation for axillary brachial plexus block? *Reg Anesth Pain Med.* 2001;26:100-104.

DeJong RH. Axillary block of the brachial plexus. *Anesthesiology.* 1961;22:215-225.

Desroches J. The infraclavicular brachial plexus block by the coracoid approach is clinically effective: an observational study of 150 patients. *Can J Anaesth.* 2003;50:253-257.

De Tran QH, Clemente A, Doan J, Finlayson RJ. Brachial plexus blocks: a review of approaches and techniques. *Can J Anaesth.* 2007;54:662-674.

Finucane BT, Yilling F. Safety of supplementing axillary brachial plexus blocks. *Anesthesiology.* 1989;70:401-403.

Grice SC, Morell RC, Balestrieri FJ, et al. Intravenous regional anesthesia: evaluation and prevention of leakage under the tourniquet. *Anesthesiology.* 1986;65:316-320.

Hadzic A, Arliss J, Kerimoglu B, et al. A comparison of infraclavicular nerve block versus general anesthesia for hand and wrist day-case surgeries. *Anesthesiology.* 2004;101:127-132.

Ilfeld BM, Le LT, Ramjohn J, et al, PAINfRETM Investigators. The effects of local anesthetic concentration and dose on continuous infraclavicular nerve blocks: a multicenter, randomized, observer-masked, controlled study. *Anesth Analg.* 2009;108:345-350.

Klaastad O, Lilleas FG, Rotnes JS, et al. A magnetic resonance imaging study of modifications to the infraclavicular brachial plexus block. *Anesth Analg.* 2000;91:929-933.

Klaastad O, Sauter AR, Dodgson MS. Brachial plexus block with or without ultrasound guidance. *Curr Opin Anaesthesiol.* 2009;22:655-660.

Koscielniak-Nielsen ZJ, Frederiksen BS, Rasmussen H, Hesselbjerg L. A comparison of ultrasound-guided supraclavicular and infraclavicular blocks for upper extremity surgery. *Acta Anaesthesiol Scand.* 2009;53:620-626.

Lavoie J, Martin R, Tetrault JP, et al. Axillary plexus block using a peripheral nerve stimulator: single or multiple injections. *Can J Anaesth.* 1992;39:583-586.

Lillie PE, Glynn CJ, Fenwick DG. Site of action of intravenous regional anesthesia. *Anesthesiology.* 1984;61:507-510.

Lo N, Brull R, Perlas A, et al. Evolution of ultrasound guided axillary brachial plexus blockade: retrospective analysis of 662 blocks. *Can J Anaesth.* 2008;55:408-413.

Mariano ER, Loland VJ, Ilfeld BM. Interscalene perineural catheter placement using an ultrasound-guided posterior approach. *Reg Anesth Pain Med.* 2009;34:60-63.

McCartney CJ, Xu D, Constantinescu C, et al. Ultrasound examination of peripheral nerves in the forearm. *Reg Anesth Pain Med.* 2007;32:434-439.

Moore DC. *Regional Block.* 4th ed. Springfield, Ill: Charles C Thomas; 1965.

Neal JM, Hebl JR, Gerancher JC, Hogan QH. Brachial plexus anesthesia: essentials of our current understanding. *Reg Anesth Pain Med.* 2002;27:402-428.

Neal JM, Gerancher JC, Hebl JR, et al. Upper extremity regional anesthesia: essentials of our current understanding. *Reg Anesth Pain Med.* 2009;34:134-170.

Partridge BL, Katz J, Benirschke K. Functional anatomy of the brachial plexus sheath: implications for anesthesia. *Anesthesiology.* 1987;66:743-747.

Pere P, Pitkanen M, Tuominen M, et al. Clinical and radiologic comparison of perivascular and transarterial techniques of axillary brachial plexus block. *Br J Anaesth.* 1993;70:276-279.

Perlas A, Chan VW, Simons M. Brachial plexus examination and localization using ultrasound and electrical stimulation: a volunteer study. *Anesthesiology.* 2003;99:429-435.

Perlas A, Lobo G, Lo N, et al. Ultrasound-guided supraclavicular block: outcome of 510 consecutive cases. *Reg Anesth Pain Med.* 2009;34:171-176.

Peterson DO. Shoulder block anesthesia for shoulder reconstruction surgery. *Anesth Analg.* 1985;64:373-375.

Sharrock NE, Bruce G. An improved technique for locating the interscalene groove. *Anesthesiology.* 1976;44:431-433.

Soares LG, Brull R, Lai J, Chan VW. Eight ball, corner pocket: the optimal needle position for ultrasound-guided supraclavicular block. *Reg Anesth Pain Med.* 2007;32:94-95.

Sukhani R, Garcia CJ, Munhall RJ, et al. Lidocaine distribution following intravenous regional anesthesia with different tourniquet inflation techniques. *Anesth Analg.* 1989;68:633-637.

Thompson GE, Rorie DK. Functional anatomy of the brachial plexus sheaths. *Anesthesiology.* 1983;59:117-122.

van Geffen GJ, Moayeri N, Bruhn J, et al. Correlation between ultrasound imaging, cross-sectional anatomy, and histology of the brachial plexus: a review. *Reg Anesth Pain Med.* 2009;34:490-497.

Vester-Andersen T, Christiansen C, Hansen A, et al. Interscalene brachial plexus block: area of analgesia, complications and blood concentrations of local anesthetics. *Acta Anaesthesiol Scand.* 1981;25:81-84.

Vester-Andersen T, Christiansen C, Sorensen M, Eriksen C. Perivascular axillary block I: blockade following 40 ml 1% mepivacaine with adrenaline. *Acta Anaesthesiol Scand.* 1982;26:519-523.

Vester-Andersen T, Christiansen C, Sorensen M, et al. Perivascular axillary block II: influence of volume of local anaesthetic on neural blockade. *Acta Anaesthesiol Scand.* 1983;27:95-98.

Vester-Andersen T, Eriksen C, Christiansen C. Perivascular axillary block III: blockade following 40 ml of 0.5%, 1% or 1.5% mepivacaine with adrenaline. *Acta Anaesthesiol Scand.* 1984;28:95-98.

Vester-Andersen T, Husum B, Lindeburg T, et al. Perivascular axillary block IV: blockade following 40, 50 or 60 ml of mepivacaine 1% with adrenaline. *Acta Anaesthesiol Scand.* 1984;28:99-105.

Vester-Andersen T, Husum B, Lindeburg T, et al. Perivascular axillary block V: blockade following 60 ml of mepivacaine 1% injected as a bolus or as 30 + 30 ml with a 20-min interval. *Acta Anaesthesiol Scand.* 1984;28:612-616.

Vester-Andersen T, Husum B, Zaric D, Eriksen C. Perivascular axillary block VII: the effect of a supplementary dose of 20 ml mepivacaine 1% with adrenaline to patients with incomplete sensory blockade. *Acta Anaesthesiol Scand.* 1986;30:231-234.

Wehling MJ, Koorn R, Leddell C, Boezaart AP. Electrical nerve stimulation using a stimulating catheter: what is the lower limit? *Reg Anesth Pain Med.* 2004;29:230-233.

Williams SR, Chouinard P, Arcand G, et al. Ultrasound guidance speeds execution and improves the quality of supraclavicular block. *Anesth Analg.* 2003;97:1518-1523.

Winnie AP. *Plexus Anesthesia, Volume I: Perivascular Techniques of Brachial Plexus Block.* Philadelphia, Pa: WB Saunders Co; 1983.

Winnie AP. Interscalene brachial plexus block. *Anesth Analg.* 1970;49:455-466.

Lower Extremity Blocks

Beck GP. Anterior approach to sciatic nerve block. *Anesthesiology.* 1963;24:222-224.

Borgeat A, Blumenthal S, Karovic D, et al. Clinical evaluation of a modified posterior anatomical approach to performing the popliteal block. *Reg Anesth Pain Med.* 2004;29:290-296.

Bridenbaugh PO. The lower extremity: somatic block. In: Cousins M, Bridenbaugh PO, eds. *Neural Blockade.* 2nd ed. Philadelphia, Pa: JB Lippincott Co; 1988:417-442.

Brown TCK, Dickens DRV. A new approach to lateral cutaneous nerve of thigh block. *Anaesth Intensive Care.* 1986;14:126-127.

Capdevila X, Biboulet P, Morau D, et al. Continuous three-in-one block for postoperative pain after lower limb orthopedic surgery: where do the catheters go? *Anesth Analg.* 2002;94:1001-1006.

Capdevila X, Macaire P, Dadure C, et al. Continuous psoas compartment block for postoperative analgesia after total hip arthroplasty: new landmarks, technical guidelines, and clinical evaluation. *Anesth Analg.* 2002;94:1606-1613.

Chayen D, Nathan H, Clayen M. The psoas compartment block. *Anesthesiology.* 1976;45:95-99.

Choquet O, Capdevila X, Bennourine K, et al. A new inguinal approach for the obturator nerve block: anatomical and randomized clinical studies. *Anesthesiology.* 2005;103:1238-1245.

Dalens B, Tanguy A, Vanneuville G. Sciatic nerve block in children: comparison of the posterior, anterior, and lateral approaches in 180 pediatric patients. *Anesth Analg.* 1990;70:131-137.

Dalens B, Tanguy A, Vanneuville G. Lumbar plexus block in children. A comparison of two procedures in 50 patients. *Anesth Analg.* 1988;67:750-758.

Dalens B, Tanguy A, Vanneuville G. Lumbar plexus blocks and lumbar plexus nerve blocks [letter]. *Anesth Analg.* 1989;69:850-857.

Hopkins PM, Ellis FR, Halsall PJ. Evaluation of local anaesthetic blockade of the lateral femoral cutaneous nerve. *Anaesthesia.* 1991;46:95-96.

Ilfeld BM, Loland VJ, Gerancher JC, et al, PAINfRETM Investigators. The effects of varying local anesthetic concentration and volume on continuous popliteal sciatic nerve blocks: a dual-center, randomized, controlled study. *Anesth Analg.* 2008;107:701-707.

Ilfeld BM, Morey TE, Wang RD, Enneking FK. Continuous popliteal sciatic nerve block for postoperative pain control at home: a randomized, double-blinded, placebo-controlled study. *Anesthesiology.* 2002;97:959-965.

Labat G. *Regional Anesthesia: Its Technique and Clinical Application.* Philadelphia, Pa: WB Saunders Co; 1923.

McLeod DH, Wong DHW, Claridge RJ. Lateral popliteal sciatic nerve block compared with subcutaneous infiltration for analgesia following foot surgery. *Can J Anaesth.* 1994;41:673-676.

McNicol LR. Sciatic nerve block for children: anterior approach for postoperative pain relief. *Anaesthesia.* 1985;40:410-414.

Moore DC. *Regional Block.* 4th ed. Springfield, Ill: Charles C Thomas; 1965.

Neal JM. Assessment of lower extremity nerve block: reprise of the Four P's acronym. *Reg Anesth Pain Med.* 2002;27:618-620.

Parkinson SK, Mueller JB, Little WL, Bailey SL. Extent of blockade with various approaches to the lumbar plexus. *Anesth Analg.* 1989;68:243-248.

Perlas A, Brull R, Chan VW, et al. Ultrasound guidance improves the success of sciatic nerve block at the popliteal fossa. *Reg Anesth Pain Med.* 2008;33:259-265.

Redborg KE, Sites BD, Chinn CD, et al. Ultrasound improves the success rate of a sural nerve block at the ankle. *Reg Anesth Pain Med.* 2009;34:24-28.

Rorie DK, Byer DE, Nelson DO, et al. Assessment of block of the sciatic nerve in the popliteal fossa. *Anesth Analg.* 1980;59:371-376.

Schurman DJ. Ankle-block anesthesia for foot surgery. *Anesthesiology.* 1976;44:348-352.

Sinha A, Chan VW. Ultrasound imaging for popliteal sciatic nerve block. *Reg Anesth Pain Med.* 2004;29:130-134.

Sites BD, Brull R. Ultrasound guidance in peripheral regional anesthesia: philosophy, evidence-based medicine, and techniques. *Curr Opin Anaesthesiol.* 2006;19:630-639.

Tsui BC, Özelsel T. Ultrasound-guided transsartorial perifemoral artery approach for saphenous nerve block. *Reg Anesth Pain Med.* 2009;34:177-178.

Tumber PS, Bhatia A, Chan VW. Ultrasound-guided lateral femoral cutaneous nerve block for meralgia paresthetica. *Anesth Analg.* 2008;106:1021-1022.

van Geffen GJ, van den Broek E, Braak GJ, et al. A prospective randomised controlled trial of ultrasound guided versus nerve stimulation guided distal sciatic nerve block at the popliteal fossa. *Anaesth Intensive Care.* 2009;37:32-37.

Vloka JD, Hadzic A, April E, Thys DM. The division of the sciatic nerve in the popliteal fossa: anatomical implications for popliteal nerve blockade. *Anesth Analg.* 2001;92:215-217.

Vloka JD, Hadzic A, April E, Thys DM. Anterior approach to the sciatic nerve block: the effects of leg rotation. *Anesth Analg.* 2001;92:460-462.

Winnie AP, Ramamurthy S, Durrani Z. The inguinal paravascular technic of lumbar plexus anesthesia: the "3-in-1" block. *Anesth Analg.* 1973;52:989-996.

Zaric D, Boysen K, Christiansen J, et al. Continuous popliteal sciatic nerve block for outpatient foot surgery: a randomized, controlled trial. *Acta Anaesthesiol Scand.* 2004;48:337-341.

Head and Neck Blocks

Anthony M. Headache and the greater occipital nerve. *Clin Neurol Neurosurg.* 1992;94:297-301.

Barton S, Williams JD. Glossopharyngeal nerve block. *Arch Otolaryngol.* 1971;93:186-188.

Bedder MD, Lindsay DL. Glossopharyngeal nerve block using ultrasound guidance: a case report of a new technique. *Reg Anesth.* 1989;14:304-307.

Bovim G, Sand T. Cervicogenic headache, migraine without aura and tension-type headache: diagnostic blockade of greater occipital and supra-orbital nerves. *Pain.* 1992;51:43-48.

Eriksson E, ed. *Illustrated Handbook in Local Anaesthesia.* 2nd ed. Philadelphia, Pa: WB Saunders Co; 1980.

Feitl ME, Krupin T. Neural blockade for ophthalmologic surgery. In: Cousins M, Bridenbaugh PO, eds. *Neural Blockade.* 2nd ed. Philadelphia, Pa: JB Lippincott Co; 1988:577-592.

Gotta AW, Sullivan CA. Anaesthesia of the upper airway using topical anaesthetic and superior laryngeal nerve block. *Br J Anaesth.* 1981;53:1055-1057.

Guntamukkala M, Hardy PAJ. Spread of injectate after stellate ganglion block in man: an anatomical study. *Br J Anaesth.* 1991;66:643-644.

Hamilton RC. Techniques of orbital regional anaesthesia. *Br J Anaesth.* 1995;75:88-92.

Hogan QH, Erickson SJ, Abram SE. Computerized tomography-guided stellate ganglion blockade. *Anesthesiology.* 1992;77:596-599.

Johnson RW. Anatomy for ophthalmic anaesthesia. *Br J Anaesth.* 1995;75:80-87.

Kroll DA, Knight PR, Mullin V. Electrocardiographic changes in patients with stellate ganglion blockade. *Reg Anesth.* 1982;7:157-159.

Lee LA, Posner KL, Cheney FW, et al. Complications associated with eye blocks and peripheral nerve blocks: an American Society of Anesthesiologists closed claims analysis. *Reg Anesth Pain Med.* 2008;33:416-422.

Macintosh RR, Ostlere M. *Local Analgesia: Head and Neck.* Edinburgh, Scotland: E & S Livingstone; 1955.

Moore DC. *Stellate Ganglion Block.* Springfield, Ill: Charles C Thomas; 1954.

Murphy TM. Somatic blockade of head and neck. In: Cousins M, Bridenbaugh PO, eds. *Neural Blockade.* 2nd ed. Philadelphia, Pa: JB Lippincott Co; 1988:533-558.

Slappendel R, Thijssen HOM, Crul BJP, Merx JL. The stellate ganglion in magnetic resonance imaging: a quantification of anatomic variability. *Anesthesiology.* 1995;83:424-426.

Tsui BC. Ultrasound imaging to localize foramina for superficial trigeminal nerve block. *Can J Anaesth.* 2009;56:704-706.

Voronov P, Suresh S. Head and neck blocks in children. *Curr Opin Anaesthesiol.* 2008;21:317-322.

Wang BC, Bogart B, Hillman DE, Turndorf H. Subarachnoid injection: a potential complication of retrobulbar block. *Anesthesiology.* 1989;71:845-847.

Winnie AP, Ramamuthy S, Durrani Z, Radonjic R. Interscalene cervical plexus block: a single injection technique. *Anesth Analg.* 1975;54:370-375.

Wong DHW. Regional anaesthesia for intraocular surgery. *Can J Anaesth.* 1993;40:635-657.

Truncal Blocks

Amid PK, Shulman AG, Lichtenstein IL. Local anesthesia for inguinal hernia repair: step-by-step procedure. *Ann Surg.* 1994;220:735-737.

Ben-David B, Lee E. The falling column: a new technique for interpleural catheter placement [letter]. *Anesth Analg.* 1990;71:212.

Boezaart AP, Koorn R, Rosenquist RW. Paravertebral approach to the brachial plexus: an anatomic improvement in technique. *Reg Anesth Pain Med*. 2003;28:241-244.

Boezaart AP, De Beer JF, Nell ML. Early experience with continuous cervical paravertebral block using a stimulating catheter. *Reg Anesth Pain Med*. 2003;28:406-413.

Boezaart AP, Raw RM. Continuous thoracic paravertebral block for major breast surgery. *Reg Anesth Pain Med*. 2006;31:470-476.

Boezaart AP, Lucas SD, Elliott CE. Paravertebral block: cervical, thoracic, lumbar, and sacral. *Curr Opin Anaesthesiol*. 2009;22:637-643.

Bonnet F, Berger J, Aveline C. Transversus abdominis plane block: what is its role in postoperative analgesia? *Br J Anaesth*. 2009;103:468-470.

Bugedo GJ, Carcamo CR, Mertens RA, et al. Preoperative percutaneous ilioinguinal and iliohypogastric nerve block with 0.5% bupivacaine for post-herniorrhaphy pain management in adults. *Reg Anesth*. 1990; 15:130-133.

Capdevila X, Macaire P, Dadure C, et al. Continuous psoas compartment block for postoperative analgesia after total hip arthroplasty: new landmarks, technical guidelines, and clinical evaluation. *Anesth Analg*. 2002;94:1606-1613.

Conacher ID. Resin injection of thoracic paravertebral spaces. *Br J Anaesth*. 1988;61:657-661.

Covino BG. Interpleural regional anesthesia [editorial]. *Anesth Analg*. 1987;67:427-429.

Crossley AWA, Hosie HE. Radiographic study of intercostal nerve blockade in healthy volunteers. *Br J Anaesth*. 1987;59:149-154.

Kairaluoma PM, Bachmann MS, Korpinen AK, et al. Single-injection paravertebral block before general anesthesia enhances analgesia after breast cancer surgery with and without associated lymph node biopsy. *Anesth Analg*. 2004;99:1837-1843.

Kairaluoma PM, Bachmann MS, Rosenberg PH, Pere PJ. Preincisional paravertebral block reduces the prevalence of chronic pain after breast surgery. *Anesth Analg*. 2006;103:703-708.

Karmakar MK. Thoracic paravertebral block. *Anesthesiology*. 2001;95: 771-780.

Karmakar MK, Critchley LA, Ho AM, et al. Continuous thoracic paravertebral infusion of bupivacaine for pain management in patients with multiple fractured ribs. *Chest*. 2003;123:424-431.

Katz J, Renck H. *Handbook of Thoraco-Abdominal Nerve Block*. Orlando, Fla: Grune & Stratton; 1987.

Klein SM, Bergh A, Steele SM, Georgiade GS, Greengrass RA. Thoracic paravertebral block for breast surgery. *Anesth Analg*. 2000;90: 1402-1405.

Klein SM, Greengrass RA, Weltz C, Warner DS. Paravertebral somatic nerve block for outpatient inguinal herniorrhaphy: an expanded case report of 22 patients. *Reg Anesth Pain Med*. 1998;23:306-310.

Jankovic ZB, du Feu FM, McConnell P. An anatomical study of the transversus abdominis plane block: location of the lumbar triangle of Petit and adjacent nerves. *Anesth Analg*. 2009;109:981-985.

Joshi GP, Bonnet F, Shah R, et al. A systematic review of randomized trials evaluating regional techniques for postthoracotomy analgesia. *Anesth Analg*. 2008;107:1026-1040.

Magee DJ. *Orthopedic Physical Assessment*. Philadelphia, Pa: WB Saunders Co; 1992:319-323.

Moore DC. Intercostal nerve block: Spread of India ink injected to the rib's costal groove. *Br J Anaesth*. 1981;53:325-329.

Moore DC, Bush WH, Scurlock JE. Intercostal nerve block: a roentgenographic anatomic study of technique and absorption in humans. *Anesth Analg*. 1979;59:815-825.

Mulroy MF. Intercostal block at the mid-axillary line. *Reg Anesth*. 1985;10: A39.

Murphy DF. Interpleural analgesia. *Br J Anaesth*. 1993;71:426-434.

Naja MZ, Ziade MF, El Rajab M, et al. Varying anatomical injection points within the thoracic paravertebral space: effect on spread of solution and nerve blockade. *Anaesthesia*. 2004;59:459-463.

Richardson J, Sabanathan S. Thoracic paravertebral analgesia. *Acta Anaesthesiol Scand*. 1995;39:1005-1015.

Richardson J, Sabanathan S, Jones J, et al. A prospective, randomized comparison of preoperative and continuous balanced epidural or paravertebral bupivacaine on post-thoracotomy pain, pulmonary function and stress responses. *Br J Anaesth*. 1999;83:387-392.

Rocco A, Reiestad F, Gudman J, McKay W. Intrapleural administration of local anesthetics for pain relief in patients with multiple rib fractures. *Reg Anesth*. 1987;12:10-14.

Stromskag KE, Hauge O, Steen PA. Distribution of local anesthetics injected into the interpleural space, studied by computerized tomography. *Acta Anaesthesiol Scand*. 1990;34:323-326.

Suresh S, Chan VW. Ultrasound guided transversus abdominis plane block in infants, children and adolescents: a simple procedural guidance for their performance. *Paediatr Anaesth*. 2009;19:296-299.

Thompson GE, Brown DL. The common nerve blocks. In: Nunn JF, Utting JE, Brown BR, eds. *General Anaesthesia*. 5th ed. London, England: Butterworth; 1989:1049-1085.

Thompson GE, Moore DC. Celiac plexus, intercostal, and minor peripheral blockade. In: Cousins M, Bridenbaugh PO, eds. *Neural Blockade*. 2nd ed. Philadelphia, Pa: JB Lippincott Co; 1988:503-532.

Tverskoy M, Cozacov C, Ayache M, et al. Postoperative pain after inguinal herniorrhaphy with different types of anesthesia. *Anesth Analg*. 1990;70:29-35.

Weltz CR, Greengrass RA, Lyerly HK. Ambulatory surgical management of breast carcinoma using paravertebral block. *Ann Surg*. 1995; 222:19-26.

Chronic Pain

Artuso JD, Stevens RA, Lineberry PJ. Postdural puncture headache after lumbar sympathetic block: a report of two cases. *Reg Anesth*. 1991; 16:288-291.

Boswell MV, Trescot AM, Datta S, et al. American Society of Interventional Pain Physicians. Interventional techniques: evidence-based practice guidelines in the management of chronic spinal pain. *Pain Physician*. 2007;10:7-111.

Botwin KP, Gruber RD, Bouchlas CG, et al. Fluoroscopically guided lumbar transforaminal epidural steroid injections in degenerative lumbar stenosis: an outcome study. *Am J Phys Med Rehabil*. 2002; 81:898-905.

Brown DL. Neurolytic celiac plexus block in your practice. In: Brown DL, ed. *Regional Anesthesia at Virginia Mason Medical Center: A Clinical Perspective. Problems in Anesthesia*. Vol 1, Issue 4. Philadelphia, Pa: JB Lippincott Co; 1987:612-621.

Brown DL, Rorie DK. Altered reactivity of isolated segmental lumbar arteries of dogs following exposure to ethanol and phenol. *Pain*. 1994;56:139-143.

Burton AW, Hassenbusch SJ 3rd, Warneke C, et al. Complex regional pain syndrome (CRPS): survey of current practices. *Pain Pract*. 2004; 4:74-83.

Burton AW, Fanciullo GJ, Beasley RD, Fisch MJ. Chronic pain in the cancer survivor: a new frontier. *Pain Med*. 2007;8:189-198.

Burton AW. Celiac plexus blocks: wider application warranted for treating pancreatic cancer pain. *J Support Oncol*. 2009;7:88-89.

Cameron T. Safety and efficacy of spinal cord stimulation for the treatment of chronic pain: a 20-year literature review. *J Neurosurg Spine*. 2004;100:254-267.

Carette S, Marcoux S, Truchon R, et al. A controlled trial of corticosteroid injections into facet joints for chronic low back pain. *N Engl J Med*. 1991;325:1002-1007.

Carter ML. Spinal cord stimulation in chronic pain: a review of the evidence. *Anaesth Intensive Care*. 2004;32:11-21.

Cherry DA, Rao DM. Lumbar sympathetic and coeliac plexus blocks: an anatomical study in cadavers. *Br J Anaesth*. 1982;54:1037.

Chou R, Atlas SJ, Stanos SP, Rosenquist RW. Nonsurgical interventional therapies for low back pain: a review of the evidence for an American Pain Society clinical practice guideline. *Spine (Phila Pa 1976)*. 2009; 34:1078-1093.

Chou R, Loeser JD, Owens DK, et al, American Pain Society Low Back Pain Guideline Panel. Interventional therapies, surgery, and interdisciplinary rehabilitation for low back pain: an evidence-based clinical practice guideline from the American Pain Society. *Spine (Phila Pa 1976)*. 2009;34:1066-1077.

Davies DD. Incidence of major complications of neurolytic coeliac plexus block. *J R Soc Med*. 1993;86:264-266.

Destouset JM, Gilula LA, Murphy WA, et al. Lumbar facet injections: Indications, technique, clinical correlation, and preliminary results. *Radiology*. 1982;145:321.

Fukui S, Ohseto K, Shiotani M, et al. Referred pain distribution of the cervical zygapophyseal joints and cervical dorsal rami. *Pain*. 1996;68: 79-83.

Furman MB, O'Brien EM. Is it really possible to do a selective nerve root block? *Pain*. 2000;85:526.

Grabow TS, Tella PK, Raja SN. Spinal cord stimulation for complex regional pain syndrome: an evidence-based medicine review of the literature. *Clin J Pain*. 2003;19:371-383.

Harden RN, Bruehl S, Stanton-Hicks M, Wilson PR. Proposed new diagnostic criteria for complex regional pain syndrome. *Pain Med*. 2007;8: 326-331.

Hassenbusch S, Burchiel K, Coffey RJ, et al. Management of intrathecal catheter-tip inflammatory masses: a consensus statement. *Pain Med*. 2002;3:313-323.

Hassenbusch SJ, Portenoy RK, Cousins M, et al. Polyanalgesic Consensus Conference 2003: an update on the management of pain by intraspinal drug delivery—report of an expert panel. *J Pain Symptom Manage*. 2004;27:540-563.

Ischia S, Luzzani A, Ischia A, Faggion S. A new approach to neurolytic block of the coeliac plexus: the transaortic technique. *Pain*. 1983;16: 333-341.

Karppinen J, Malmivaara A, Kurunlahti M, et al. Periradicular infiltration for sciatica: a randomized controlled trial. *Spine (Phila Pa 1976)*. 2001;26:1059-1067.

Lutz G, Vad V, Wisneski R. Fluoroscopic transforaminal lumbar epidural steroids: an outcome study. *Arch Phys Med Rehabil*. 1998;79: 1362-1366.

Merrill DG, Rathmell JP, Rowlingson JC. Epidural steroid injections. *Anesth Analg*. 2003;96:907-908.

Moore DC, Bush WH, Burnett LL. Celiac plexus block: a roentgenographic anatomic study of technique and spread of solution in patients and corpses. *Anesth Analg*. 1981;60:369-379.

Plancarte R, Amescua C, Patt RB, Aldrete JA. Superior hypogastric plexus block for pelvic cancer pain. *Anesthesiology*. 1990;73:236-239.

Rathmell JP. The promise of an effective treatment for sacroiliac-related low back pain. *Anesthesiology*. 2008;109:167-168.

Rathmell JP. Toward improving the safety of transforaminal injection. *Anesth Analg*. 2009;109:8-10.

Rathmell JP, Aprill C, Bugduk N. Cervical transforaminal injection of steroids. *Anesthesiology*. 2004;100:1595-1600.

Riew KD, Yin Y, Gilula L, et al. The effect of nerve-root injections on the need for operative treatment of lumbar radicular pain: a prospective, randomized, controlled, double-blind study. *J Bone Joint Surg Am*. 2000;82:1589-1593.

Schwarzer AC, Aprill CN, Bogduk N. The sacroiliac joint in chronic low back pain. *Spine (Phila Pa 1976)*. 1995;20:31-37.

Simpson BA. Spinal-cord stimulation for reflex sympathetic dystrophy. *Lancet Neurol*. 2004;3:142.

Smith TJ, Staats PS, Deer T, et al, Implantable Drug Delivery Systems Study Group. Randomized clinical trial of an implantable drug delivery system compared with comprehensive medical management for refractory cancer pain: impact on pain, drug-related toxicity, and survival. *J Clin Oncol*. 2002;20:4040-4049.

Staal JB, de Bie RA, de Vet HC, et al. Injection therapy for subacute and chronic low back pain: an updated Cochrane review. *Spine (Phila Pa 1976)*. 2009;34:49-59.

Taylor RS, Taylor RJ, Van Buyten JP, et al. The cost effectiveness of spinal cord stimulation in the treatment of pain: a systematic review of the literature. *J Pain Symptom Manage*. 2004;27:370-378.

Thimineur MA, Kravitz E, Vodapally MS. Intrathecal opioid treatment for chronic non-malignant pain: a 3-year prospective study. *Pain*. 2004;109:242-249.

Turner JA, Loeser JD, Deyo RA, Sanders SB. Spinal cord stimulation for patients with failed back surgery syndrome or complex regional pain syndrome: a systematic review of effectiveness and complications. *Pain*. 2004;108:137-147.

Ubbink DT, Vermeulen H, Spincemaille GH, et al. Systematic review and meta-analysis of controlled trials assessing spinal cord stimulation for inoperable critical leg ischaemia. *Br J Surg*. 2004;91:948-955.

Umeda S, Arai T, Hatano Y, et al. Cadaver anatomic analysis of the best site for chemical lumbar sympathectomy. *Anesth Analg*. 1987;66: 643-646.

Vad V, Bhat A, Lutz G, Cammisa F. Transforaminal epidural steroid injections in lumbosacral radiculopathy: a prospective randomized study. *Spine (Phila Pa 1976)*. 2002;27:11-16.

Ward EM, Rorie DK, Nauss LA, Bahn RC. The celiac ganglia in man: normal anatomic variations. *Anesth Analg*. 1979;58:461-465.

Weber JG, Brown DL, Stephens DH, Wong GY. Celiac plexus block: retrocrural computed tomographic anatomy in patients with and without pancreatic cancer. *Reg Anesth*. 1996;21:407-413.

Wulf H, Gleim M, Schele HA. Plasma concentrations of bupivacaine after lumbar sympathetic block. *Anesth Analg*. 1994;79:918-920.

Yahia LH, Garzon S. Structure of the capsular ligaments of the facet joints. *Ann Anat*. 1993;175:185-188.

Neuraxial Block

Asato F, Goto F. Radiograph findings of unilateral epidural block. *Anesth Analg*. 1996;83:519-522.

Benhamou D, Wong C. Neuraxial anesthesia for cesarean delivery: what criteria define the "optimal" technique? *Anesth Analg*. 2009;109: 1370-1373.

Blomberg RG. A method for epiduroscopy and spinaloscopy: presentation of preliminary results. *Acta Anaesthesiol Scand*. 1985;29:113-116.

Blomberg RG. The dorsomedian connective tissue band in the lumbar epidural space of humans: an anatomic study using epiduroscopy in autopsy cases. *Anesth Analg*. 1986;65:747-752.

Blomberg RG. The lumbar subdural extra-arachnoid space in humans: an anatomical study using spinaloscopy in autopsy cases. *Anesth Analg*. 1987;66:177-180.

Blomberg RG. Fibrous structures in the subarachnoid space: a study with spinaloscopy in autopsy subjects. *Anesth Analg*. 1995;80:875-879.

Blomberg RG, Olsson SS. The lumbar epidural space in patients examined with epiduroscopy. *Anesth Analg*. 1989;68:157-160.

Bodily MN, Carpenter RL, Owens BD. Lidocaine 0.5% spinal anaesthesia: a hypobaric solution for short-stay perirectal surgery. *Can J Anaesth*. 1992;39:770-773.

Borges BC, Wieczoreck P, Balki M, Carvalho JC. Sonoanatomy of the lumbar spine of pregnant women at term. *Reg Anesth Pain Med*. 2009;34:581-585.

Bridenbaugh PO, Greene NM. Spinal (subarachnoid) neural blockade. In: Cousins M, Bridenbaugh PO, eds. *Neural Blockade*. 2nd ed. Philadelphia, Pa: JB Lippincott Co; 1988:213-251.

Bromage PR. *Epidural Anesthesia*. Philadelphia, Pa: WB Saunders Co; 1978.

Brown DL, Wedel DJ. Spinal, epidural and caudal anesthesia. In: Miller RD, ed. *Anesthesia*. 3rd ed. New York, NY: Churchill Livingstone; 1990:1377-1405.

Brown EM, Elman DS. Postoperative backache. *Anesth Analg*. 1961; 40:683-685.

Butler BD, Warters RD, Elk JR, et al. Loss of resistance technique for locating the epidural space: evaluation of glass and plastic syringes. *Can J Anaesth*. 1990;37:438-439.

Caldwell C, Nielsen C, Baltz T, et al. Comparison of high-dose epinephrine and phenylephrine in spinal anesthesia with tetracaine. *Anesthesiology*. 1985;62:804-807.

Choi S, Brull R. Neuraxial techniques in obstetric and non-obstetric patients with common bleeding diatheses. *Anesth Analg*. 2009;109: 648-660.

Concepcion M, Maddi R, Francis D, et al. Vasoconstrictors in spinal anesthesia with tetracaine: a comparison of epinephrine and phenylephrine. *Anesth Analg*. 1984;63:134-138.

Cousins MJ, Bromage PR. Epidural neural blockade. In: Cousins M, Bridenbaugh PO, eds. *Neural Blockade*. 2nd ed. Philadelphia, Pa: JB Lippincott Co; 1988:253-360.

Covino BG, Scott DB. *Handbook of Epidural Anaesthesia and Analgesia*. Orlando, Fla: Grune & Stratton; 1985.

DiGiovanni AJ, Dunbar BS. Epidural injections of autologous blood for post-lumbar puncture headache. *Anesth Analg*. 1970;49:268-271.

Felsby S, Juelsgaard P. Combined spinal and epidural anesthesia. *Anesth Analg*. 1995;80:821-826.

Fettes PD, Jansson JR, Wildsmith JA. Failed spinal anaesthesia: mechanisms, management, and prevention. *Br J Anaesth*. 2009;102: 739-748.

Gallart L, Blanco D, Samso E, Vidal F. Clinical and radiologic evidence of the epidural plica mediana dorsalis. *Anesth Analg*. 1990;71:698-701.

Gormley JB. Treatment of postspinal headache. *Anesthesiology*. 1960; 21:565-566.

Greene NM. Distribution of local anesthetic solutions within the subarachnoid space. *Anesth Analg*. 1985;64:715-730.

Greene NM. Uptake and elimination of local anesthetics during spinal anesthesia. *Anesth Analg*. 1983;62:1013-1024.

Greene NM. *Physiology of Spinal Anesthesia*. 3rd ed. Baltimore, Md: Williams & Wilkins; 1981.

Halpern SH, Carvalho B. Patient-controlled epidural analgesia for labor. *Anesth Analg*. 2009;108:921-928.

Harbers JBM, Stienstra R, Gielen MJM, Cromheecke GJ. A double blind comparison of lidocaine 2% with or without glucose for spinal anesthesia. *Acta Anaesthesiol Scand*. 1995;39:881-884.

Hardy PAJ. Can epidural catheters penetrate dura mater? An anatomical study. *Anaesthesia*. 1986;41:1146-1147.

Harrison GR, Clowes NWB. The depth of the lumbar epidural space from the skin. *Anaesthesia*. 1985;40:685-687.

Hirabayashi Y, Shimizu R, Saitoh K, et al. Anatomical configuration of the spinal column in the supine position, I: A study using magnetic resonance imaging. *Br J Anaesth*. 1995;75:3-5.

Hogan Q. Size of human lower thoracic and lumbosacral nerve roots. *Anesthesiology*. 1996;85:37-42.

Hogan QH. Lumbar epidural anatomy: a new look by cryomicrotome section. *Anesthesiology*. 1991;75:767-775.

Horlocker TT, Wedel DJ. Density, specific gravity, and baricity of spinal anesthetic solutions at body temperature. *Anesth Analg*. 1993;76: 1015-1018.

Horlocker TT. Complications of spinal and epidural anesthesia. *Anesthesiol Clin North Am*. 2000;18:461-485.

Horlocker TT, Wedel DJ. Neuraxial block and low-molecular-weight heparin: balancing perioperative analgesia and thromboprophylaxis. *Reg Anesth Pain Med*. 1998;23(suppl 2):164-177.

Hynson JM, Katz JA, Bueff HU. Epidural hematoma associated with enoxaparin. *Anesth Analg*. 1996;82:1072-1075.

Kane RE. Neurologic deficits following epidural or spinal anesthesia. *Anesth Analg*. 1981;60:150-161.

Kozody R, Palahniuk RJ, Wade JG, Cumming MO. The effect of subarachnoid epinephrine and phenylephrine on spinal cord blood flow. *Can Anaesth Soc J*. 1984;31:503-508.

Leicht CH, Carlson SA. Prolongation of lidocaine spinal anesthesia with epinephrine and phenylephrine. *Anesth Analg*. 1986;65:365-369.

Lui S, Chiui AA, Carpenter RL, et al. Fentanyl prolongs lidocaine spinal anesthesia without prolonging recovery. *Anesth Analg.* 1995;80: 730-734.

Lui S, Kopacz DJ, Carpenter RL. Quantitative assessment of differential sensory nerve block after lidocaine spinal anesthesia. *Anesthesiology.* 1995;82:60-63.

Lui S, Pollock JE, Mulroy MF, et al. Comparison of 5% with dextrose, 1.5% with dextrose, and 1.5% dextrose-free lidocaine solutions for spinal anesthesia in human volunteers. *Anesth Analg.* 1995;81: 697-702.

Lui S, Ware PD, Allen HW, et al. Dose-response characteristics of spinal bupivacaine in volunteers: clinical implications for ambulatory anesthesia. *Anesthesiology.* 1996;85:729-736.

Lui SS, McDonald SB. Current issues in spinal anesthesia. *Anesthesiology.* 2001;94:888-906.

Lund PC. Reflections upon the historical aspects of spinal anesthesia. *Reg Anesth.* 1983;8:89-98.

Marinacci AA. Neurologic aspects of complications of spinal anesthesia. *LA Neurol Soc Bull.* 1960;25:170-192.

Meiklejohn BH. Distance from skin to the lumbar epidural space in obstetric population. *Reg Anesth.* 1990;15:134-136.

Moore DC. *Regional Block.* 4th ed. Springfield, Ill: Charles C Thomas; 1965.

Moore DC. Spinal anesthesia: Bupivacaine compared with tetracaine. *Anesth Analg.* 1980;59:743-750.

Moore DC, Bridenbaugh LD. Spinal (subarachnoid) block: a review of 11,574 cases. *JAMA.* 1966;195:907-912.

Moore DC, Bridenbaugh LD, Bagdi PA, et al. The present status of spinal (subarachnoid) and epidural (peridural) block. *Anesth Analg.* 1968;47:40-49.

Moore DC, Chadwick HS, Ready LB. Epinephrine prolongs lidocaine spinal: pain in the operative site the most accurate method of determining local anesthetic duration. *Anesthesiology.* 1987;67:416-418.

Parkinson D. Human spinal arachnoid septa, trabeculae, and "rogue strands." *Am J Anat.* 1991;192:498-509.

Patin DJ, Eckstein EC, Harum K, Pallares VS. Anatomic and biomechanical properties of human lumbar dura mater. *Anesth Analg.* 1993; 76:535-540.

Puolakka R, Haasio J, Pitkanen MT, et al. Technical aspects and postoperative sequelae of spinal and epidural anesthesia: a prospective study of 3,230 orthopedic patients. *Reg Anesth Pain Med.* 2000;25:488-497.

Reynolds AF, Roberts PA, Pollay M, Stratemeier PH. Quantitative anatomy of the thoracolumbar epidural space. *Neurosurgery.* 1985; 17:905-907.

Rigler ML, Drasner K, Krejcie TC, et al. Cauda equina syndrome after continuous spinal anesthesia. *Anesth Analg.* 1991;72:275-281.

Ruppen W, Steiner LA, Drewe J, et al. Bupivacaine concentrations in the lumbar cerebrospinal fluid of patients during spinal anaesthesia. *Br J Anaesth.* 2009;102:832-838.

Savolaine ER, Pandya JB, Greenblatt SH, Conover SR. Anatomy of the human lumbar epidural space: new insights using CT-epidurography. *Anesthesiology.* 1988;68:217-220.

Schug SA, Saunders D, Kurowski I, Paech MJ. Neuraxial drug administration: a review of treatment options for anaesthesia and analgesia. *CNS Drugs.* 2006;20:917-933.

Smith TC. The lumbar spine and subarachnoid block. *Anesthesiology.* 1968;29:60-64.

Steiner LA, Hauenstein L, Ruppen W, et al. Bupivacaine concentrations in lumbar cerebrospinal fluid in patients with failed spinal anaesthesia. *Br J Anaesth.* 2009;102:839-844.

Sternlo JE, Hybbinette CH. Spinal subdural bleeding after attempted epidural and subsequent spinal anesthesia in a patient on thromboprophylaxis with low molecular weight heparin. *Acta Anaesthesiol Scand.* 1995;39:557-559.

Tarkkila PJ. Incidence and causes of failed spinal anesthetics in a university hospital: a prospective study. *Reg Anesth.* 1991;16:48-51.

Taylor JA. Lumbosacral subarachnoid tap. *J Urol.* 1940;43:561-564.

Trotter M. Variations of the sacral canal: their significance in the administration of caudal anesthesia. *Anesth Analg.* 1947;26:192-202.

Tuominen M. Bupivacaine spinal anaesthesia. *Acta Anaesthesiol Scand.* 1991;35:1-10.

Urmey WF, Stanton J, Peterson M, Sharrock NE. Combined spinal-epidural anesthesia for outpatient surgery. *Anesthesiology.* 1995;83: 528-534.

Vandam LD, Dripps RD. A long-term follow-up of patients who received 10,098 spinal anesthetics, II: Incidence and analyses of minor sensory neurologic defects. *Surgery.* 1955;38:463-469.

VandePol C. Enoxaparin and epidural analgesia [letter]. *Anesthesiology.* 1996;85:433-434.

Weitz SR, Chan V. Enoxaparin and epidural analgesia [letter]. *Anesthesiology.* 1996;85:432-433.

Westbrook JL, Renowden SA, Carrie LES. Study of the anatomy of the extradural region using magnetic resonance imaging. *Br J Anaesth.* 1993;71:495-498.

Willis RJ. Caudal epidural block. In: Cousins M, Bridenbaugh PO, eds. *Neural Blockade.* 2nd ed. Philadelphia, Pa: JB Lippincott Co; 1988: 361-383.

Zaric D, Pace NL. Transient neurologic symptoms (TNS) following spinal anaesthesia with lidocaine versus other local anaesthetics. Cochrane Database Syst Rev. 2009;15(2):CD003006.

Zarzur E. Anatomic studies of the human lumbar ligamentum flavum. *Anesth Analg.* 1984;63:499-502.

Index

Note: Page numbers followed by b and f indicate boxes and figures, respectively.

A

Abdominal aorta, anatomy of, in superior hypogastric plexus block, 351f
Abdominal pain, celiac plexus block for, 340
Abdominal wall incisions, transversus abdominis plane block for, 256
Abdominal wall pocket, for spinal drug delivery system, 367, 368f-371f
Accessory nerve, anatomy of
  in cervical plexus block, 179, 179f
  in glossopharyngeal block, 199f, 201f
Accessory phrenic nerve, anatomy of, in supraclavicular block, 37f
Adductor muscles, cross section of, 96f
Airway block
  anatomy for, 191-193, 192f-196f
  glossopharyngeal, 197-201, 199f-201f
  magnetic resonance imaging in, 193, 196f
  superior laryngeal, 203-205, 204f-205f
  translaryngeal, 207-209, 208f-209f
Alcohol
  for celiac plexus neurolysis, 340
  for superior hypogastric plexus neurolysis, 350
American Society of Regional Anesthesiologists (ASRA), ultrasonography-guided nerve block recommendations of, 10b
Amino amides, 5-6, 6f
Amino esters, 4-5, 4f-5f
Anesthetics, local. See Local anesthetics.
Ankle block, 135-138
  anatomy for, 136-137, 136f-137f
  local anesthetics for, 136
  needle puncture for, 137-138, 137f
  patient selection for, 136
  problems with, 138
Ansa cervicalis complex, anatomy of, in cervical plexus block, 179, 179f
Ansa subclavia, anatomy of, in stellate block, 184f-185f
Anterior scalene muscle, anatomy of
  in cervical paravertebral block, 248f
  in infraclavicular block, 61f-63f
  in interscalene block, 42f-44f, 43, 46f-47f
  in stellate block, 185f-187f
  in supraclavicular block, 37f-38f, 51f, 53f-55f
Anterior spinal artery, anatomy of, 267f
Anterior superior iliac spine, anatomy of
  in femoral block, 114f-115f
  in inguinal block, 240-241, 241f-243f
  in lateral femoral cutaneous block, 122f-123f
  in sciatic block, 108f
Anterior vagal trunk, anatomy of, in celiac plexus block, 341f-343f
Anterocrural needle puncture, for celiac plexus block, 346, 347f
Antibiotics
  with spinal cord stimulator implantation, 383
  with spinal drug delivery system, 373
Anticoagulants, with epidural block, 297-298

Antiplatelet drugs, epidural block and, 297-298
Aorta
  anatomy of
    in celiac plexus block, 340, 342f-344f, 346f-347f
    in interpleural block, 228f
    in lumbar somatic block, 234f
    in stellate block, 185f
    in superior hypogastric plexus block, 351f
  puncture of
    with celiac plexus block, 348
    with lumbar sympathetic block, 338, 338f
Aortic plexus, intermesenteric, anatomy of, in lumbar sympathetic block, 336f
Arachnoid mater, anatomy of, 266-269, 267f-268f
  in epidural block, 287f
  in facet block, 319f
  in spinal block, 273f, 280f
Arm
  dermatomes of, 34f-35f
  innervation of
    with pronation, 34f
    with supination, 34f
  osteotomes of, 35f
Arm sling, during continuous brachial plexus block, 27
Auricular nerve, anatomy of, 142f-143f, 146f
  in cervical plexus block, 178f-179f, 179, 181f
  in occipital block, 148f
Auriculotemporal nerve, anatomy of, in mandibular block, 164
Axilla
  anatomy of, in infraclavicular block, 60-64, 61f-63f
  proximal, anatomy of, in infraclavicular block, 39, 39f
Axillary artery, anatomy of
  in axillary block, 68-70, 70f
  in infraclavicular block, 39f, 63f
Axillary block, 67-72
  anatomy for, 68, 69f
  continuous catheter technique for, 71-72, 71f
  local anesthetics for, 68, 72
  needle for, 7f
  needle puncture for, 68-71, 70f-71f
  neuropathy with, 71
  patient selection for, 68
  position for, 68, 69f
  problems with, 71
  systemic toxicity with, 71
  ultrasonography-guided, 71-72, 72f
Axillary nerve, anatomy of, 33f
  in infraclavicular block, 62f-63f
  in pronated arm, 34f
  in supinated arm, 34f
Axillary sheath, anatomy of, in infraclavicular block, 60
Axillary vein, anatomy of, in infraclavicular block, 39f
AXIS block, versus supraclavicular block, 56

B

Back pain
  low
    sacroiliac block for, 328
    spinal cord stimulation for, 376
  with spinal block, 284
Battery failure, spinal cord stimulation and, 383
Betamethasone
  for cervical nerve root block, 360
  for lumbar nerve root block, 361
Bicarbonate, local anesthetic with, for epidural block, 286
Biceps femoris muscle
  anatomy of, in popliteal block, 130f
  cross section of, 96f
Biceps muscle and tendon, anatomy of, in elbow nerve block, 74-75, 74f-75f
Bier block, 82, 82f
Bladder, anatomy of, in superior hypogastric plexus block, 351f
Bleeding
  with spinal cord stimulator implantation, 382
  with spinal drug delivery system, 373
Brachial artery, anatomy of
  in axillary block, 71f
  in elbow nerve block, 74-75, 74f-75f
Brachial cutaneous nerve, anatomy of
  in pronated arm, 34f
  in supinated arm, 34f
Brachial plexus
  anatomy of, 32, 33f
    dermatomes in, 34f-35f
    at first rib, 38-39, 38f
    in infraclavicular block, 39, 39f, 60, 62f-63f, 65f
    in interscalene block, 43f-44f
    osteotomes in, 35f
    peripheral nerves in, 32-37, 33f-34f
    prevertebral fascia in, 32
    in supraclavicular block, 37-39, 37f-38f, 51f, 53f-57f
    variation in, 47-48, 47f
  cords of, 32, 33f
  divisions of, 32, 33f
  roots of, 32, 33f
  trunks of, 32, 33f
Brachial plexus block
  anatomy for, 31-39
  axillary, 67-72. See also Axillary block.
  continuous, nerve protection during, 27
  infraclavicular, 59-66. See also Infraclavicular block.
  interscalene, 41-48. See also Interscalene block.
  "push, pull, pinch, pinch" mnemonic in, 36f
  supraclavicular, 49-57. See also Supraclavicular block.
Brachioradialis muscle, anatomy of, in elbow nerve block, 75f
Breast block, 217-220, 219f-220f
Bromage needle–syringe grip, in thoracic epidural block, 291-294, 294f

Buccal nerve, anatomy of, in mandibular block, 164
Bupivacaine, 4f, 6, 6f
  for ankle block, 136
  for axillary block, 68
  for breast block, 218
  cardiotoxicity of, 6
  for celiac plexus block, 340
  for cervical paravertebral block, 247
  for cervical plexus block, 178
  for elbow nerve block, 74
  for epidural block, 286
  for facet block, 316
  for femoral block, 112
  for infraclavicular block, 60
  for inguinal block, 240
  for intercostal block, 222
  for interpleural block, 228
  for interscalene block, 42-43, 45
  for lateral femoral cutaneous block, 124
  for obturator block, 127
  for popliteal block, 130
  for sacroiliac block, 328-330
  for sciatic block, 102
  for spinal block, 272
  for stellate block, 185
  for superior hypogastric plexus block, 350
  for supraclavicular block, 50
  for transversus abdominis plane block, 256

C

Calcaneal nerve, anatomy of, 93f-94f
  in ankle block, 136f
Calcaneus, cross section of, 96f
Cancer pain, 311-313, 312f. *See also* Pain, chronic.
Cardiac plexus, anatomy of, 340
Carotid artery, anatomy of
  in cervical plexus block, 180f
  in glossopharyngeal block, 199f, 201f
Carotid sheath, anatomy of, in stellate block, 186f-187f
Catheter
  for continuous nerve block
    fixation of, 20-26, 24f-26f
    removal of, 27
    tunneling techniques with, 20, 24f-25f
  epidural, 8, 8f, 298, 299f
    permanent, for spinal drug delivery system, 367-373, 372f
  intrathecal, 365-373, 368f-372f. *See also* Spinal drug delivery system.
Cauda equina, anatomy of, 268f-269f
  in spinal block, 273f, 280f
Cauda equina syndrome, with spinal block, 284
Caudal block, 301-307
  anatomy for, 269-270, 270f, 302-306, 302f-303f
  circle of errors in, 306, 306f
  ineffective, 306, 306f
  local anesthetics for, 302
  needle puncture for, 304-306, 305f
  palpation technique in, 307, 307f
  patient selection for, 302
  position for, 303-304, 304f
  problems with, 306, 306f
Cecum, anatomy of, in superior hypogastric plexus block, 352f
Cefazolin
  with spinal cord stimulator implantation, 383
  with spinal drug delivery system, 373
Celiac artery, anatomy of, in celiac plexus block, 342f, 344f
Celiac plexus
  anatomy of, 340, 341f-345f
  neurolysis of, 340

Celiac plexus block, 339-348
  anatomy for, 340, 341f-345f
  magnetic resonance imaging in, 344f
  needle puncture for
    anterocrural, 346, 347f
    retrocrural, 340-346, 345f-347f
  patient selection for, 340
  pharmacologic agents for, 340
  position for, 340
  problems with, 348
  surface markings for, 340, 345f
Cerebrospinal fluid aspiration
  in intrathecal catheter placement, 367
  in spinal block, 280, 281f
Cervical epidural block
  anatomy for, 286-287, 295f
  needle puncture for, 294, 295f-296f
Cervical facet block, needle puncture for, 321, 324f-325f
Cervical facet joints, anatomy of, 316, 317f-318f, 320f
Cervical facet pain syndrome, 316
Cervical ganglion, anatomy of, in stellate block, 184f-185f, 185-186
Cervical paravertebral block, continuous, 246-250, 246f, 248f-249f
Cervical plexus, anatomy of, 178-182, 178f-180f
Cervical plexus block, 177-182
  anatomy for, 178-182, 178f-180f
  deep, 180, 181f, 182
  local anesthetics for, 178
  needle puncture for, 180-182, 181f
  patient selection for, 178
  phrenic nerve block with, 182
  problems with, 182
  superficial, 180-182, 181f
Cervical sympathetic ganglion, anatomy of, in airway block, 193f-194f
Cervical sympathetic trunk, anatomy of, in stellate block, 184f-185f, 185-186
Cervical transforaminal injection, 358-361, 359f-360f
Cervical vertebral body, sixth, anatomy of, in cervical paravertebral block, 248f
Cervical vertebral tubercle, sixth, palpation of, in stellate block, 186, 186f, 188
Cervicothoracic ganglion. *See* Stellate ganglion.
Chassaignac's tubercle, anatomy of
  in cervical plexus block, 180, 181f
  in infraclavicular block, 64f
  in stellate block, 185f-186f
Chloroprocaine, 4f-5f, 5
  for epidural block, 286
Ciliary ganglion, anatomy of, in retrobulbar (peribulbar) block, 172-173, 172f, 174f, 176f
Ciliary nerve, anatomy of, in retrobulbar (peribulbar) block, 172-173, 176f
Clavicle, anatomy of
  in cervical plexus block, 181f
  in infraclavicular block, 39f, 61f-63f
  in interscalene block, 43f-44f
  in stellate block, 185f
  in supraclavicular block, 37f-38f, 51f, 53f-55f
Clindamycin
  with spinal cord stimulator implantation, 383
  with spinal drug delivery system, 373
Cluneal nerve, anatomy of, 93f-94f
Coaxial technique, for transforaminal injection, 363
Cocaine, 4, 4f
Coccyx, anatomy of
  in neuraxial block, 270f
  in sacroiliac block, 330f-331f
Colon, anatomy of, in lumbar sympathetic block, 336f
Common hepatic artery, anatomy of, in celiac plexus block, 343f

Common peroneal nerve, anatomy of, 91f
  in ankle block, 136f
  in popliteal block, 130-131, 130f-131f, 133, 134f
Complex regional pain syndrome, spinal cord stimulation for, 376
Continuous nerve block, 17-27
  catheter fixation for, 20-26, 24f-26f
  catheter removal after, 27
  local anesthetics for, 20
  nerve protection during, 27
  nonstimulating catheter technique for, 18-20, 19f
  stimulating catheter technique for, 18, 20, 21f-23f
  tip localization in, 20
Conus medullaris, anatomy of, 264, 268f
Coracobrachialis muscle, anatomy of, in axillary block, 72f
Coracoid process, anatomy of
  in axillary block, 71f
  in infraclavicular block, 39f
Corticosteroids
  for cervical nerve root block, 358, 360
  for lumbar nerve root block, 361
Costal margin, in transversus abdominis plane block, 257f
Costotransverse joint, anatomy of, in thoracic paravertebral block, 251f
Costotransverse ligament, anatomy of, in thoracic paravertebral block, 251f
Costovertebral joint, anatomy of, in thoracic paravertebral block, 251f
Crawford needle, 8f
  for lumbar epidural block, 287
Cricoid cartilage, anatomy of
  in airway block, 194f-196f
  in cervical plexus block, 181f
  in interscalene block, 42-43, 42f-45f
  in stellate block, 186f-187f
  in superior laryngeal block, 204f-205f
  in supraclavicular block, 51f
  in translaryngeal block, 208f
Cricothyroid membrane, anatomy of
  in airway block, 194f-195f
  in translaryngeal block, 208f-209f
Cutaneous nerve
  brachial, anatomy of
    in pronated arm, 34f
    in supinated arm, 34f
  lateral femoral. *See* Lateral femoral cutaneous nerve.
  median, anatomy of, 33f
  posterior, anatomy of, in sciatic block, 104f
  posterior femoral, anatomy of, 93f-94f

D

Deep cervical plexus block, 180, 181f, 182
Deep peroneal nerve, anatomy of, 91f, 93f-94f
  in ankle block, 136-137, 136f
Deep peroneal nerve block, at ankle, 137f, 138
Dentate ligaments, anatomy of, 266-269
Dermatomes
  in breast block, 219f
  of lower extremity, 94f
  in lumbar somatic block, 235f
  in truncal anatomy, 215f
  of upper extremity, 34f-35f
Descending genicular artery, anatomy of, in popliteal block, 132f
Dexamethasone
  for cervical nerve root block, 360
  for lumbar nerve root block, 361
Dextrose, for hydrodissection, 20
Diaphragm, anatomy of, in celiac plexus block, 341f-342f, 344f-347f
Digital nerve block, 78-79, 79f

Distal trigeminal block, 167-168, 169f-170f
Distal upper extremity block, 73-79
   at digits, 78-79, 79f
   at elbow, 74-78, 74f-76f
   problems with, 77
   at wrist, 77, 77f-78f
Doppler shift, 12-13
Dorsal digital nerve, anatomy of, in digital nerve
   block, 79f
Dorsomedian connective tissue band, 269
Doughnut sign, in ultrasonography-guided nerve
   block, 18-20
Drugs for regional anesthesia, 4-7. See also Local
   anesthetics; Vasoconstrictors.
Dura mater, anatomy of, 266-269, 267f-268f
   in epidural block, 287f-288f, 291f-292f, 295f-296f
   in facet block, 319f
   in interscalene block, 46f
   in spinal block, 273f, 280f
Dural puncture
   headache after, 272, 276, 284
     with epidural block, 298
     with spinal block, 272, 276, 284
   with lumbar sympathetic block, 338
   with spinal cord stimulator implantation, 382-383
Dural sac, anatomy of, 268f
Dysesthesias, with sciatic block, 109
   Dyspnea, with high spinal block, 284

E
Elbow nerve block, 74-78, 74f-76f
Elbow surgery
   axillary block for, 68
   cervical paravertebral block for, 247
Eleventh cranial nerve. See Accessory nerve.
Epidural block, 285-298
   anatomy for, 286-294, 287f-289f
   anticoagulation with, 297-298
   catheter in, 298, 299f
   cervical
     anatomy for, 286-287, 295f
     needle puncture for, 294, 295f-296f
   headache with, 298
   hematoma with, 297-298
   incorrect injection sites in, 297, 297f
   local anesthetics for, 286
   lumbar
     anatomy of, 286-287
     needle puncture for, 287-291, 290f
   with lumbar somatic block, 237
   neurologic injury with, 297
   patient selection for, 286
   position for, 287
   problems with, 297-298, 297f
   with spinal block, 284
   thoracic
     anatomy of, 286-287, 288f
     needle puncture for, 291-294, 291f-294f
   unilateral, 269
Epidural blood patching, for post–dural puncture
   headache, 284
Epidural catheter, 8, 8f, 298, 299f
   permanent, for spinal drug delivery system,
     367-373, 372f
Epidural needles, 8, 8f
Epidural space, 268f-269f, 269
   anatomy of
     in epidural block, 287f-288f
     in spinal block, 273f
   spinal cord stimulator lead placement in, 377-383,
     378f-381f
Epiglottis, anatomy of
   in airway block, 194f-195f
   in translaryngeal block, 208f

Epinephrine, 6-7, 6f
   for digital nerve block, 79
   for epidural block, 286
   for infraclavicular block, 60
   for spinal block, 272
   for stellate block, 185
Epiradicular vein injection, with transforaminal
   injection, 361, 363
Erector spinae muscle, anatomy of, in lumbar
   paravertebral block, 253f
Esmarch bandage, venous exsanguination with,
   82-85, 84f
Esophagus, anatomy of
   in celiac plexus block, 342f-343f
   in interpleural block, 228f
Etidocaine, 4f, 6, 6f
Exsanguination, venous, in intravenous regional
   block, 82-85, 84f
Extensor digitorum longus tendon, cross section of,
   96f
Extensor hallucis longus tendon, cross section of,
   96f
External jugular vein, anatomy of
   in cervical plexus block, 180f
   in interscalene block, 42-43, 42f-43f
   in supraclavicular block, 51f
External laryngeal nerve, anatomy of, in airway
   block, 192-193, 193f-194f
External oblique muscle, anatomy of
   in inguinal block, 242f
   in transversus abdominis plane block, 256,
     257f-260f
Eye complications, with maxillary block, 160

F
Face, sensory innervation of, 142-143, 142f-143f
Facet block, 315-326
   anatomy for, 316, 317f-320f
   fluoroscopy in, 316, 321, 323f-325f, 326
   local anesthetics for, 316
   needle puncture for, 321, 323f-325f
   patient selection for, 316
   position for, 316-321, 321f-322f
Facet joints
   anatomy of, 264, 265f
   cervical, anatomy of, 316, 317f-318f, 320f
   lumbar, anatomy of, 316, 317f-319f
   thoracic, anatomy of, 316, 317f
Facial neuralgia, diagnosis of, maxillary block for,
   158
Falling column technique, in interpleural block, 230
Fascia iliaca, anatomy of, in femoral block, 117, 118f
Fascia lata, anatomy of, in lateral femoral cutaneous
   block, 124f
Femoral artery, anatomy of, in femoral block,
   114f-115f, 118f
Femoral block, 111-119
   continuous catheter technique for, 112, 117f
   local anesthetics for, 112
   needle puncture for, 112, 115f-116f
   patient selection for, 112
   position for, 112
   problems with, 112
   ultrasonography-guided, 117-119, 118f
Femoral cutaneous nerve
   lateral. See Lateral femoral cutaneous nerve.
   posterior, anatomy of, 93f-94f
Femoral nerve, anatomy of, 90f-94f, 93
   in femoral block, 112, 113f-114f, 118f, 119
   in inguinal block, 240f
   in lumbar plexus block, 98f
   in sciatic block, 103f-105f
Femoral neurovascular bundle, cross section of, 96f
Femoral vein, anatomy of, in femoral block, 114f

Femur
   cross section of, 96f
   greater trochanter of, anatomy of, in sciatic block,
     104f, 106f-108f, 110f
Fentanyl, in spinal block, 284
Fifth cranial nerve. See Trigeminal nerve.
Filum terminale, anatomy of, 266-269, 268f-269f
Flamingo test, of sacroiliac joint, 328, 328f-329f
Flexor carpi radialis tendon, anatomy of, in wrist
   nerve block, 77f-78f
Flexor digitorum longus tendon, cross section of, 96f
Flexor hallucis longus muscle and tendon, cross
   section of, 96f
Fluoroscopy
   in cervical transforaminal injection, 358, 359f-360f,
     360
   in facet block, 316, 321, 323f-325f, 326
   in intrathecal catheter placement, 367, 368f-371f
   in lumbar transforaminal injection, 360, 362f
   in sacroiliac block, 332-334, 334f
   in superior hypogastric plexus block, 350-354, 356
Foramen ovale, anatomy of, 143-144, 144f
   in mandibular block, 162f
   in trigeminal (gasserian) ganglion block, 152,
     152f-153f, 156f
Foramen rotundum, anatomy of, 143-144, 144f
   in trigeminal (gasserian) ganglion block, 152f-153f
Forearm surgery
   axillary block for, 68
   interscalene block for, 43

G
Gaenslen's test, of sacroiliac joint, 328, 328f-329f
Gag reflex, elimination of, glossopharyngeal block
   for, 198
Gasserian ganglion block. See Trigeminal (gasserian)
   ganglion block.
Gastric artery, anatomy of, in celiac plexus block,
   343f
Gastrocnemius muscle, anatomy of, in popliteal
   block, 130f
Gemmelus muscle, anatomy of, in sciatic block, 110f
Genicular artery, anatomy of, in popliteal block, 132f
Geniohyoid muscle, anatomy of, in stellate block,
   185f
Genitofemoral nerve, anatomy of, 90f-94f, 92
   in inguinal block, 240-241, 240f-242f
   in lateral femoral cutaneous block, 122f
   in lumbar somatic block, 234f
   in lumbar sympathetic block, 336f
Glossopharyngeal block, 197-201
   anatomy for, 198
   intraoral approach to, 198, 200f, 201
   local anesthetics for, 198
   needle for, 201
   patient selection for, 198
   peristyloid approach to, 198, 201f
   position for, 198
   problems with, 201
Glossopharyngeal nerve, anatomy of
   in airway block, 192, 192f, 196f
   in glossopharyngeal block, 198, 201f
Gluteus maximus muscle
   anatomy of
     in inguinal block, 242f
     in lateral femoral cutaneous block, 124f
     in lumbar somatic block, 233f-234f
     in sciatic block, 110f
   cross section of, 96f
Gluteus medius muscle, anatomy of
   in inguinal block, 242f
   in lateral femoral cutaneous block, 124f
Gluteus minimus muscle, anatomy of, in lateral
   femoral cutaneous block, 124f

Gracilis muscle, anatomy of, in popliteal block, 132f
Gravity, venous exsanguination by, 82-85, 84f
Greater auricular nerve, anatomy of, 142f-143f, 146f
    in cervical plexus block, 178f-179f, 179, 181f
    in occipital block, 148f
Greater occipital nerve, anatomy of, 142-143,
        142f-143f
    in occipital block, 148, 148f
Greater saphenous vein, cross section of, 96f
Greene needle, 8f
    for spinal block, 276
Groin pain relief, after sacroiliac block, 334

H

Hamstrings muscle, continuous block involving, leg
        splints during, 27
Hand surgery
    axillary block for, 68
    interscalene block for, 43
    supraclavicular block for, 55-56
Hanging-drop technique
    in epidural block, 287, 290f
    in interpleural block, 230
Head and neck block
    anatomy for, 141-144
        coronal, 143-144, 145f
        innervation and, 142-144, 142f-143f
        intracranial, 143-144, 144f
        superficial neural relationships in, 146f
    indications for, 142
Headache, post–dural puncture, 272, 276, 284
    with epidural block, 298
    with spinal block, 272, 276, 284
Hematoma
    with epidural block, 297-298
    with inguinal block, 243
    with mandibular block, 165
    with maxillary block, 160
    with retrobulbar (peribulbar) block, 176
    with superior hypogastric plexus block, 356
    with supraclavicular block, 55
Heparin, low-molecular-weight, epidural block and,
        297-298
Hepatic artery, anatomy of, in celiac plexus block,
        343f
Herniorrhaphy, inguinal
    inguinal block for, 240
    lumbar somatic block for, 232
Hip pain, diagnosis of, obturator block for, 126
Horner's syndrome, with cervical paravertebral
        block, 249
Humerus
    anatomy of
        in axillary block, 70f
        in elbow nerve block, 74f
        medial epicondyle of, in elbow nerve block, 75f-76f
Hustead needle, 8f
Hydrodissection, in ultrasonography-guided nerve
        block, 18-20
Hyoid bone
    anatomy of
        in airway block, 194f-195f
        in stellate block, 185f
        in superior laryngeal block, 204f-205f
        in translaryngeal block, 208f-209f
    displacement of, in superior laryngeal block,
        204-205, 205f
"Hypodermic" block needle, 7f
Hypogastric nerves, anatomy of, in superior
        hypogastric plexus block, 350, 351f-354f
Hypogastric plexus
    anatomy of, 340
    inferior, anatomy of, 350
    superior. See Superior hypogastric plexus.

Hypoglossal nerve, anatomy of, in glossopharyngeal
        block, 199f, 201f
Hypoglossus muscle, anatomy of, in stellate block,
        185f

I

Iliac artery, anatomy of, in superior hypogastric
        plexus block, 356f
Iliac crest, anatomy of
    in epidural block, 289f
    in lumbar paravertebral block, 254f
    in sacroiliac block, 330f-331f
    in superior hypogastric plexus block, 355f
    in transversus abdominis plane block, 257f, 260f
Iliac muscle, anatomy of
    in celiac plexus block, 341f
    in femoral block, 113f
    in inguinal block, 241f-242f
    in lateral femoral cutaneous block, 122f
    in lumbar plexus block, 98f
    in obturator block, 126f
    in superior hypogastric plexus block, 351f
Iliac spine
    anterior superior, anatomy of
        in femoral block, 114f-115f
        in inguinal block, 240-241, 241f-243f
        in lateral femoral cutaneous block, 122f-123f
        in sciatic block, 108f
    posterior superior, anatomy of
        in caudal block, 302-303, 302f-303f
        in epidural block, 289f
        in sacroiliac block, 330f-331f
        in sciatic block, 106f-107f
Iliac vein, anatomy of, in superior hypogastric plexus
        block, 356f
Iliacus muscle. See Iliac muscle.
Iliohypogastric nerve, anatomy of, 90f-91f, 92,
        93f-94f
    in inguinal block, 240-241, 241f-242f
    in lateral femoral cutaneous block, 122f
Ilioinguinal nerve, anatomy of, 90f-92f, 92
    in inguinal block, 240-241, 240f-242f
    in lateral femoral cutaneous block, 122f
Iliopsoas muscle
    anatomy of
        in femoral block, 118f
        in lateral femoral cutaneous block, 124f
    cross section of, 96f
Ilium, anatomy of
    in celiac plexus block, 341f
    in inguinal block, 242f
    in lateral femoral cutaneous block, 124f
    in lumbar somatic block, 233f-234f
Infection
    with spinal cord stimulator implantation, 382
    with spinal drug delivery system, 373
Inferior alveolar nerve, anatomy of, in mandibular
        block, 164
Inferior articular process, anatomy of, in epidural
        block, 292f
Inferior cervical ganglion, anatomy of, in stellate
        block, 184f
Inferior ganglion of vagus nerve, anatomy of, in
        superior laryngeal block, 204f
Inferior hypogastric plexus, anatomy of, 350
Inferior lateral brachial cutaneous nerve, anatomy of,
        in pronated arm, 34f
Inferior vena cava, anatomy of
    in celiac plexus block, 340, 341f-342f, 344f
    in lumbar somatic block, 234f
    in superior hypogastric plexus block, 351f
Infraclavicular block, 59-66
    anatomy for, 39, 39f, 60-64, 61f-63f
    continuous catheter technique for, 66

Infraclavicular block (Continued)
    local anesthetics for, 60
    needle puncture for, 64, 64f
    nonstimulating catheter technique for, 18-20, 19f
    patient selection for, 60
    position for, 64
    problems with, 64
    stimulating catheter technique for, 18, 20, 21f-23f
    ultrasonography-guided, 65-66, 65f
Infraorbital fissure, anatomy of, in maxillary block,
        160f
Infraorbital nerve, anatomy of, 142f-143f, 143-144,
        146f
    in distal trigeminal block, 169f-170f
Inguinal block, 239-243
    anatomy for, 240-241, 240f-242f
    hematoma with, 243
    local anesthetics for, 240
    needle puncture for, 241, 242f-243f
    patient selection for, 240
    position for, 241
    problems with, 243
Inguinal herniorrhaphy
    inguinal block for, 240
    lumbar somatic block for, 232
Inguinal ligament
    anatomy of, in femoral block, 113f, 115f
    femoral nerve anatomy at, 114f
Inguinal perivascular block, 98-99, 98f
Innominate artery, anatomy of, in airway block, 194f
Intercostal block, 221-225
    anatomy for, 222, 223f
    breast block via, 218, 219f-220f
    lateral approach to, 225, 225f
    local anesthetics for, 222
    needle puncture for, 222-225, 223f-225f
    patient selection for, 222
    pneumothorax with, 225
    position for, 222, 223f
    problems with, 225
    sedation for, 222, 225
Intercostal muscle, anatomy of, 216f
Intercostal nerve, anatomy of, 216f, 219f
    in intercostal block, 222, 223f
    in interpleural block, 228f
Intercostobrachial cutaneous nerve, anatomy of
    in pronated arm, 34f
    in supinated arm, 34f
Intermediate supraclavicular nerve, anatomy of, in
        cervical plexus block, 178f
Intermesenteric aortic plexus, anatomy of, in lumbar
        sympathetic block, 336f
Internal carotid artery, anatomy of, in
        glossopharyngeal block, 201f
Internal jugular vein, anatomy of
    in cervical plexus block, 180f
    in glossopharyngeal block, 199f, 201f
Internal laryngeal nerve, anatomy of, in airway block,
        192-193, 193f-194f
Internal oblique muscle, anatomy of
    in inguinal block, 242f
    in transversus abdominis plane block, 256,
        257f-260f
Interpleural anesthesia, 227-230, 228f-229f
Interscalene block, 41-48
    anatomy for, 42-43, 42f-44f, 47-48, 47f
    local anesthetics for, 42-43, 45
    needle puncture in, 43, 45, 45f-46f
    patient selection for, 42
    phrenic nerve block with, 45
    position for, 43, 44f
    problems with, 43
    ulnar nerve block with, 45
    ultrasonography-guided, 45-48, 46f-47f
Interscalene groove, identification of, 43, 43f

Interspinous ligament, anatomy of, 264-266, 266f
in epidural block, 287f
in spinal block, 273f, 280f
Intervertebral foramen, anatomy of, in superior hypogastric plexus block, 356f
Intervertebral space, identification of, for spinal block, 276-280, 279f
Intracranial anatomy, 143-144, 144f
Intrathecal drug delivery. *See* Spinal drug delivery system.
Intravascular injection
with superior hypogastric plexus block, 356, 356f
with transforaminal injection, 360-361, 363
Intravenous regional block, 81-86
anatomy for, 82-85
distal IV site for, 82-85, 83f
early Bier block technique for, 82, 82f
equipment for, 83f
local anesthetics for, 82
mechanisms of action of, 85-86, 85f
needle puncture for, 82-85, 83f-84f
patient selection for, 82
position for, 82, 83f
tourniquet inflation pressure for, 82-85
venous exsanguination techniques in, 82-85, 84f
Intubation
glossopharyngeal block for, 198
superior laryngeal block for, 204
translaryngeal block for, 208
Ischial spine, anatomy of, in sacroiliac block, 330f-331f
Ischial tuberosity
anatomy of, in sciatic block, 104f, 106f-107f, 110f
cross section of, 96f

J

Jugular vein, anatomy of
in cervical plexus block, 180f
in glossopharyngeal block, 199f, 201f
in interscalene block, 42-43, 42f-43f
in supraclavicular block, 51f

K

Kidney, anatomy of, in celiac plexus block, 340, 344f
Knee surgery, femoral block in, 112-117
Kulenkampff supraclavicular block
needle puncture for, 50, 52f
position for, 50

L

Lacrimal artery, anatomy of, in retrobulbar (peribulbar) block, 172f
Lamina, anatomy of, 264, 265f
Laryngeal nerve, anatomy of
in airway block, 192-193, 193f-195f
in stellate block, 185f
in superior laryngeal block, 204-205, 204f
Lateral brachial cutaneous nerve, anatomy of, in pronated arm, 34f
Lateral decubitus position
for epidural block, 287
for spinal block, 273, 273f
Lateral femoral cutaneous block, 121-124
anatomy for, 94f, 122-123, 122f-123f
local anesthetics for, 122, 124
needle puncture for, 123-124, 124f
patient selection for, 122
position for, 123
Lateral femoral cutaneous nerve, anatomy of, 90f-94f, 92
in femoral block, 114f-115f
in inguinal block, 240f-241f

Lateral femoral cutaneous nerve, anatomy of (*Continued*)
in lateral femoral cutaneous block, 122-123, 122f-123f
in lumbar plexus block, 98f
in sciatic block, 103f-105f
Lateral malleolus, cross section of, 96f
Lateral pterygoid muscle, anatomy of, in trigeminal (gasserian) ganglion block, 153f-154f
Lateral pterygoid plate, anatomy of, 143-144, 145f
in mandibular block, 162f-163f, 164, 165f
in maxillary block, 159f-160f
in trigeminal (gasserian) ganglion block, 153f
Lateral rectus muscle, anatomy of, in retrobulbar (peribulbar) block, 172f, 174f, 176f
Lateral supraclavicular nerve, anatomy of, in cervical plexus block, 178f
Latissimus dorsi muscle, anatomy of, 216f
in transversus abdominis plane block, 257f, 259f-260f
Lead complications, with spinal cord stimulator implantation, 383
Leg. *See* Lower extremity.
Leg splints, during continuous nerve block, 27
Lesser occipital nerve, anatomy of, 142-143, 142f-143f, 146f
in cervical plexus block, 178f-179f, 179, 181f
in occipital block, 148f
Lesser splanchnic nerve, anatomy of, in interpleural block, 228f
Levator scapulae muscle, anatomy of
in cervical paravertebral block, 246f, 248f
in stellate block, 185f
Levobupivacaine, 6
for cervical paravertebral block, 247
Lidocaine, 4f, 5-6, 6f
for ankle block, 136
for axillary block, 68
for breast block, 218
for celiac plexus block, 340
for cervical nerve root block, 360
for cervical plexus block, 178
for elbow nerve block, 74
for epidural block, 286
for facet block, 316
for glossopharyngeal block, 198
for infraclavicular block, 60
for inguinal block, 240
for intercostal block, 222
for interscalene block, 42-43, 45
for intravenous regional block, 82, 85
for lateral femoral cutaneous block, 124
for lumbar nerve root block, 361
for obturator block, 127
for popliteal block, 130
for sacroiliac block, 328-330
for sciatic block, 102
for spinal block, 272
subarachnoid, 5-6
for superior hypogastric plexus block, 350
for superior laryngeal block, 204
for supraclavicular block, 50
for translaryngeal block, 208
Ligamentum flavum, anatomy of, 264-266, 266f-269f
in epidural block, 287, 287f-289f, 291f-293f, 295f-296f
in spinal block, 273f, 280f
Lingual nerve, anatomy of, in mandibular block, 164
Lithotomy position, lower extremity anatomy in, 94f
Liver, anatomy of, in celiac plexus block, 344f
Local anesthetics, 4-7, 5f
amino amide, 5-6, 6f
amino ester, 4-5, 4f-5f
for continuous nerve block, 20
structure of, 4, 5f

Local anesthetics (*Continued*)
timeline of, 4, 4f
toxicity of
with axillary block, 71
with epidural block, 297, 297f
vasoconstrictors with, 6-7, 6f-7f
Long ciliary nerve, anatomy of, in retrobulbar (peribulbar) block, 172-173, 176f
Long thoracic nerve, anatomy of, 33f
Longissimus capitis muscle, anatomy of, in stellate block, 185f
Longus capitis muscle, anatomy of, in stellate block, 185f
Longus colli muscle, anatomy of, in stellate block, 186f-187f
LORA syringe, in cervical paravertebral block, 246f
Loss-of-resistance technique
in lumbar epidural block, 287, 290f
in thoracic epidural block, 291-294, 294f
Low back pain
sacroiliac block for, 328
spinal cord stimulation for, 376
Lower extremity
anatomy of, 89-93, 90f-96f
in lithotomy position, 94f
on magnetic resonance imaging, 96f
dermatomes of, 94f
osteotomes of, 95f
Lower extremity block, anatomy for, 89-93, 90f-96f
Lower extremity pain, diagnosis of, obturator block for, 126, 128
Lower extremity procedures, obturator block for, 126
Lumbar artery, anatomy of, 267f, 269f
Lumbar cistern, intrathecal catheter placement within, 367, 368f-371f
Lumbar epidural block
anatomy for, 266-269, 267f-269f, 286-287
needle puncture for, 287-291, 290f
Lumbar facet block, needle puncture for, 321, 323f
Lumbar facet joints, anatomy of, 316, 317f-319f
Lumbar facet pain syndrome, 316
Lumbar lordosis, in spinal block, 276, 277f
Lumbar nerves, anatomy of, 233f, 237f
Lumbar paravertebral block (psoas compartment block), 99, 253, 253f-254f
Lumbar plexus, anatomy of, 90-92, 91f, 98f
in lumbar somatic block, 234f
in lumbar sympathetic block, 336f
Lumbar plexus block, 97-99
inguinal perivascular, 98-99, 98f
psoas compartment, 99, 253, 253f-254f
Lumbar roots, anatomy of, 267f
Lumbar somatic block, 231-237
anatomy for, 232, 233f-235f
local anesthetics for, 232
patient selection for, 232
position for, 232-237, 236f-237f
problems with, 237
skin markings for, 232, 236f
sympathetic block with, 237
Lumbar somatic nerve, third, anatomy of, in neuraxial block, 269f
Lumbar surgery, spinal cord stimulation after, 376
Lumbar sympathetic block, 335-338
anatomy for, 336-338, 336f
aorta puncture with, 338, 338f
dural puncture with, 338
local anesthetics for, 336
with lumbar somatic block, 237
needle puncture for, 336-338, 337f-338f
patient selection for, 336
position for, 336
problems with, 338, 338f
Lumbar transforaminal injection, 361-363, 362f
Lumbar vertebrae, anatomy of, 265f

Lumbosacral (Taylor's) approach, to spinal block, 280, 283f
Lumbosacral plexus, anatomy of, 90f-91f, 93
Lung, anatomy of
  in infraclavicular block, 62f
  in interpleural block, 228f
  in stellate block, 185f
  in supraclavicular block, 51f, 54f
Luschka, sinuvertebral nerve of, anatomy of, in facet block, 316, 319f-320f

M

Magnetic resonance imaging
  in celiac plexus block, 344f
  lower extremity anatomy on, 96f
  in superior hypogastric plexus block, 356f
  in supraclavicular block, 54f
Malleolus, cross section of, 96f
Mandible, anatomy of
  in airway block, 196f
  in mandibular block, 162f-163f, 165f
  in maxillary block, 159f
  in stellate block, 185f
  in trigeminal (gasserian) ganglion block, 154f
Mandibular angle, in glossopharyngeal block, 201f
Mandibular block, 161-165
  anatomy for, 162-164, 162f-164f
  hematoma with, 165
  local anesthetics for, 162
  needle puncture for, 164, 165f
  patient selection for, 162
  position for, 164
  problems with, 165
Mandibular nerve
  anatomy of, 142-143, 142f
    in mandibular block, 162-164, 162f-165f
    in maxillary block, 159f
    in trigeminal (gasserian) ganglion block, 152, 152f, 155f-156f
  pterygoid relationships of, 143-144, 145f
Mandibular notch
  plane of, 153f
  in trigeminal (gasserian) ganglion block, 153f
Mandibular ramus, anatomy of, in glossopharyngeal block, 199f
Mastoid, anatomy of
  in cervical plexus block, 181f
  in glossopharyngeal block, 201f
Maxilla, anatomy of, in glossopharyngeal block, 199f
Maxillary block, 157-160
  anatomy for, 158-160, 159f
  local anesthetics for, 158
  needle puncture for, 158-160, 160f
  patient selection for, 158
  position for, 158
  problems with, 160
Maxillary nerve
  anatomy of, 142-143, 142f
    in mandibular block, 163f
    in maxillary block, 158-160, 159f
    in trigeminal (gasserian) ganglion block, 152, 152f, 155f
  cutaneous innervation of, 158, 158f
  pterygoid relationships of, 143-144, 145f
Meckel's cave, anatomy of, in trigeminal (gasserian) ganglion block, 152, 153f-154f
Medial brachial cutaneous nerve, anatomy of
  in pronated arm, 34f
  in supinated arm, 34f
Medial malleolus, cross section of, 96f
Medial patellar retinaculum, anatomy of, in popliteal block, 132f
Medial plantar nerve, anatomy of, 93f-94f

Medial supraclavicular nerve, anatomy of, in cervical plexus block, 178f
Median antebrachial cutaneous nerve, anatomy of
  in pronated arm, 34f
  in supinated arm, 34f
Median cutaneous nerve, anatomy of, 33f
Median nerve
  anatomy of, 32, 33f
    in axillary block, 68-72, 69f-72f
    at elbow, 74-75, 74f-75f
    in infraclavicular block, 60-64, 62f-63f
    in pronated arm, 34f
    in supinated arm, 34f
    at wrist, 77, 77f-78f
  short-axis and long-axis imaging of, 13f
Median nerve block
  at elbow, 74-78, 74f-75f
  at wrist, 77, 77f-78f
Median sacral crest, anatomy of, in neuraxial block, 270f
Mental nerve, anatomy of, 142f-143f, 143-144, 146f
  in distal trigeminal block, 170f
Mepivacaine, 4f, 6, 6f
  for ankle block, 136
  for axillary block, 68
  for breast block, 218
  for cervical plexus block, 178
  for elbow nerve block, 74
  for epidural block, 286
  for infraclavicular block, 60
  for inguinal block, 240
  for intercostal block, 222
  for interscalene block, 42-43, 45
  for lateral femoral cutaneous block, 124
  for obturator block, 127
  for popliteal block, 130
  for sciatic block, 102
  for supraclavicular block, 50
Mesenteric artery, anatomy of, in celiac plexus block, 342f-343f
Mesenteric ganglion, anatomy of, in celiac plexus block, 341f-343f
Methylprednisolone, for sacroiliac block, 328-330
Middle cervical ganglion, anatomy of, in stellate block, 184f-185f, 185-186
Middle sacral artery, anatomy of, in superior hypogastric plexus block, 351f
Middle scalene muscle, anatomy of
  in cervical paravertebral block, 248f
  in infraclavicular block, 61f, 63f
  in interscalene block, 42f-44f, 46f
  in stellate block, 185f-187f
  in supraclavicular block, 37f, 51f, 53f, 55f
Midline approach
  to lumbar epidural block, 287
  to spinal block, 276-280, 279f-281f
M&Ms are tops mnemonic, 72
Morphine, for spinal pain therapy, 366
Multifidus muscle, anatomy of, 269f
Musculocutaneous nerve
  anatomy of, 32, 33f
    in axillary block, 68-72, 69f-72f
    in infraclavicular block, 60-64, 62f-63f
    in pronated arm, 34f
    in supinated arm, 34f
  block of, 68-70, 70f
  ultrasonography of, 72, 72f
Myalgia paresthetica, diagnosis of, lateral femoral cutaneous block for, 122

N

Neck and head block. *See* Head and neck block.
Needles, 7-8, 7f-8f
Nerve protection, during continuous nerve block, 27

Nerve root injection, selective. *See* Transforaminal injection.
Nerve stimulators, 9-10, 9f
Neuraxial anatomy, 263-270
  bony, 264, 265f
  ligamentous relationships in, 264-266, 266f
  lumbar, 266-269, 267f-269f
  sacral, 269-270, 270f
  surface relationships in, 264, 264f, 289f
  vertebral column relationships in, 264, 265f
Neuraxial block
  anatomy for, 263-270
    bony, 264, 265f
    ligamentous, 264-266, 266f
  caudal, 301-307
  epidural, 285-298
  spinal, 271-284
Neurologic injury
  with axillary block, 71
  with celiac plexus block, 348
  with epidural block, 297
  with spinal block, 284
Neurolysis
  of celiac plexus, 340
  of superior hypogastric plexus, 350

O

Oblique muscle, anatomy of
  in inguinal block, 242f
  in retrobulbar (peribulbar) block, 176f
  in transversus abdominis plane block, 256, 257f-260f
Obturator block, 125-128
  anatomy for, 126f-127f, 127
  local anesthetics for, 127
  needle puncture for, 127
  patient selection for, 126
  position for, 127
  problems with, 128
Obturator canal, anatomy of, in obturator block, 127
Obturator foramen, anatomy of, in obturator block, 126f-127f
Obturator internus muscle, anatomy of, in obturator block, 127
Obturator nerve, anatomy of, 90f-91f, 92-93, 93f-94f
  in femoral block, 115f
  in lumbar plexus block, 98f
  in obturator block, 126f-127f, 127
  in sciatic block, 103f-105f
Occipital artery, anatomy of, 143f
  in occipital block, 148, 148f
Occipital block, 147-149, 148f
Occipital nerve, anatomy of, 142-143, 142f-143f, 146f
  in cervical plexus block, 178f-179f, 179, 181f
  in occipital block, 148, 148f
Occipital protuberance, anatomy of, in occipital block, 148f
Olecranon, anatomy of, in elbow nerve block, 74f
Olecranon process, anatomy of, in ulnar nerve block, 76f
Omohyoid muscle, anatomy of, in stellate block, 185f
Ophthalmic artery, anatomy of, in retrobulbar (peribulbar) block, 172-173, 172f, 174f, 176f
Ophthalmic nerve, anatomy of, 142-143, 142f
  in trigeminal (gasserian) ganglion block, 155f
Opioids, for spinal pain therapy, 366
Optic nerve, anatomy of, in retrobulbar (peribulbar) block, 172f, 174f, 176f
Orbicularis oculi muscle, Van Lint's block of, 174, 175f
Orbit, anatomy of, 172-173, 172f, 176f
Osteotomes
  of lower extremity, 95f
  of upper extremity, 35f
Ovarian artery, anatomy of, in celiac plexus block, 341f

P

Pain, chronic
celiac plexus block for, 339-348
cervical paravertebral block for, 247
cervical transforaminal injection for, 358-361, 359f-360f
facet block for, 315-326
lumbar sympathetic block for, 335-338
lumbar transforaminal injection for, 361-363, 362f
nerve blocks for, 311-313, 312f. *See also specific nerve blocks.*
sacroiliac block for, 327-334
spinal cord stimulation for, 376
spinal drug delivery system for, 365-373
superior hypogastric plexus block for, 349-356
Palantine tonsil, anatomy of, in glossopharyngeal block, 200f
Palmar digital nerve, anatomy of, in digital nerve block, 79f
Palmaris longus tendon, anatomy of, in wrist nerve block, 77f-78f
Paramedian approach
to spinal block, 280, 282f
to thoracic epidural block, 288f, 291-294, 293f
Paraplegia, after celiac plexus block, 348
Paraspinous muscle
anatomy of, 216f
in lumbar somatic block, 233f-234f
in lumbar sympathetic block, 336f
spasm of, with superior hypogastric plexus block, 356, 356f
Paravertebral block, 245-254
breast block via, 218
cervical, continuous, 246-250, 246f, 248f-249f
lumbar (psoas compartment block), 99, 253, 253f-254f
lumbar somatic, 231-237, 233f-237f
thoracic, 250-253, 251f-252f
Paravertebral space, anatomy of, in thoracic paravertebral block, 251f
Parotid, anatomy of, in trigeminal (gasserian) ganglion block, 154f
Patellar ligament, anatomy of, in popliteal block, 132f
Patellar retinaculum, anatomy of, in popliteal block, 132f
Pectoralis major muscle, anatomy of, in infraclavicular block, 39f, 62f
Pectoralis minor muscle, anatomy of, in infraclavicular block, 39f, 62f-63f
Pediatric position, for caudal block, 303-304, 304f
Pelvic cancer pain, superior hypogastric plexus neurolysis for, 350
Peribulbar block. *See* Retrobulbar (peribulbar) block.
Peroneal nerve, anatomy of, 91f, 93f-94f
in ankle block, 136-137, 136f
in popliteal block, 130-131, 130f-131f, 133, 134f
Peroneal nerve block, at ankle, 137f, 138
Peroneus brevis tendon, cross section of, 96f
Peroneus longus tendon, cross section of, 96f
Pharyngeal nerve, anatomy of, in airway block, 192, 193f
Phenol, for superior hypogastric plexus neurolysis, 350
Phenylephrine, 7, 7f
for spinal block, 272
Phrenic nerve, anatomy of
in cervical plexus block, 179, 179f
in interscalene block, 43f
in stellate block, 185f
in supraclavicular block, 37f, 38, 51f
Phrenic nerve block
with cervical paravertebral block, 249
with interscalene block, 45
with stellate block, 188
with supraclavicular block, 55

Pia mater, anatomy of, 266-269, 267f-268f
Piriformis muscle, anatomy of, in sciatic block, 104f-105f, 107f
Plantar nerve, anatomy of, 93f-94f
in ankle block, 136f
Pleura, anatomy of
in interscalene block, 44f
in thoracic paravertebral block, 251f
Pleural space, anatomy of, in interpleural block, 228-230, 228f
Plumb bob supraclavicular block
needle puncture for, 53-55, 53f-55f
position for, 53
Pneumothorax
with breast block, 220
with intercostal block, 225
with supraclavicular block, 55-56
Popliteal artery, anatomy of, in popliteal block, 134f
Popliteal block, 129-134
anatomy for, 130-131, 130f-131f
local anesthetics for, 130
needle puncture for, 131, 132f
patient selection for, 130
position for, 131
ultrasonography-guided, 133-134, 133f-134f
Popliteal fossa, anatomy of, 130-131, 130f-131f
Popliteal neurovascular bundle, cross section of, 96f
Posterior brachial cutaneous nerve, anatomy of, in pronated arm, 34f
Posterior cutaneous nerve, anatomy of, in sciatic block, 104f
Posterior femoral cutaneous nerve, anatomy of, 93f-94f
Posterior sacrococcygeal ligament, anatomy of, in caudal block, 269-270
Posterior scalene muscle, anatomy of
in interscalene block, 46f
in stellate block, 185f
Posterior spinal artery, anatomy of, 267f
Posterior superior iliac spine, anatomy of
in caudal block, 302-303, 302f-303f
in epidural block, 289f
in sacroiliac block, 330f-331f
in sciatic block, 106f-107f
Posterior tibial nerve block, at ankle, 137-138, 137f
Posterior vagal trunk, anatomy of, in celiac plexus block, 342f-343f
Prevertebral fascia, in brachial plexus, 32
Prilocaine, 6, 6f
for intravenous regional block, 82
Procaine, 4-5, 4f
Prone jackknife position
for epidural block, 287
for spinal block, 273, 276f
Prone position
for caudal block, 303-304, 304f
for facet block, 316-321, 321f-322f
Proper palmar digital nerve, anatomy of, in digital nerve block, 79f
Provocative testing, of sacroiliac joint, 328, 328f-329f
Psoas compartment block (lumbar paravertebral block), 99, 253, 253f-254f
Psoas major muscle, anatomy of
in celiac plexus block, 341f
in superior hypogastric plexus block, 351f
Psoas minor muscle, anatomy of, in celiac plexus block, 341f
Psoas muscle, anatomy of
in femoral block, 113f
in inguinal block, 241f-242f
in lateral femoral cutaneous block, 122f
in lumbar paravertebral block, 253f
in lumbar plexus block, 98f
in lumbar sympathetic block, 336f
in obturator block, 126

Pterygoid muscle, anatomy of, in trigeminal (gasserian) ganglion block, 153f-154f
Pterygoid plate, anatomy of, 143-144, 145f
in mandibular block, 162f-163f, 164, 165f
in maxillary block, 159f-160f
in trigeminal (gasserian) ganglion block, 152f
Pterygopalatine fossa, anatomy of, in maxillary block, 159f
Pubic tubercle, anatomy of
in femoral block, 114f-115f
in obturator block, 126f-127f, 127
in sciatic block, 108f
Pudendal nerve, anatomy of, 92f
in inguinal block, 240f
Pump migration, with spinal drug delivery system, 373
"Push, pull, pinch, pinch" mnemonic, in brachial plexus block, 36

Q

Quadratus femoris muscle, cross section of, 96f
Quadratus lumborum muscle, anatomy of
in celiac plexus block, 341f
in femoral block, 113f
in inguinal block, 241f
in lateral femoral cutaneous block, 122f
in lumbar paravertebral block, 253f
in lumbar plexus block, 98f
in lumbar somatic block, 234f
in lumbar sympathetic block, 336f
in superior hypogastric plexus block, 351f
Quadriceps muscle, continuous block involving, leg splints during, 27
Quincke-Babcock needle, for spinal block, 276
Quincke needle, 8f

R

Radial nerve, anatomy of, 32, 33f
in axillary block, 68-71, 69f-72f
at elbow, 74-75, 74f-75f
in infraclavicular block, 60-64, 62f-63f
in pronated arm, 34f
in supinated arm, 34f
at wrist, 77
Radial nerve block
at elbow, 74-78, 74f-75f
at wrist, 77, 77f-78f
Radial prominence, distal, anatomy of, in wrist nerve block, 78f
Radicular artery
anatomy of
in cervical transforaminal injection, 358, 359f-360f
in lumbar transforaminal injection, 361
injection of, with cervical transforaminal injection, 360-361
Radiocontrast agent
for cervical transforaminal injection, 360
for facet block, 316, 321, 323f-325f, 326
for lumbar transforaminal injection, 361
for sacroiliac block, 328-330
for superior hypogastric plexus block, 350, 354
Radiography, in spinal cord stimulation, 383
Radius, anatomy of, in wrist nerve block, 77f
Rami communicantes, anatomy of, 216f, 222, 223f
in celiac plexus block, 343f
in lumbar sympathetic block, 336
in neuraxial block, 269f
Ramus(i)
dorsal, 222, 223f
in neuraxial block, 269f
in truncal block, 214, 216f
posterior, in facet block, 316, 319f-320f
primary, anterior and posterior, 142f

Ramus(i) (Continued)
  ventral
    in cervical plexus block, 178-179, 179f
    in intercostal block, 222, 223f
    in truncal block, 214, 216f
Rectum, anatomy of, in superior hypogastric plexus
  block, 351f
Rectus abdominis muscle, anatomy of, in inguinal
  block, 242f
Rectus muscle, anatomy of, in retrobulbar
  (peribulbar) block, 172f, 174f, 176f
Recurrent laryngeal nerve, anatomy of
  in airway block, 192-193, 193f-195f
  in stellate block, 185f
Recurrent laryngeal nerve block, with stellate block,
  188
Red triangle, for superior hypogastric plexus block,
  350, 352f, 355f
Regional anesthesia
  catheters for, 8, 8f
  drugs for, 4-7. See also Local anesthetics.
  needles for, 7-8, 7f-8f
  nerve stimulators in, 9-10, 9f
  ultrasonography-guided. See Ultrasonography.
  vasoconstrictors in, 6-7, 6f-7f
Retrobulbar (peribulbar) block, 171-176
  anatomy for, 172-174, 172f
  hematoma with, 176
  local anesthetics for, 172
  needle puncture for, 173-174, 174f-175f
  patient selection for, 172
  position for, 173, 173f
  problems with, 176
  Van Lint method for, 174, 175f
Retrocrural needle puncture, for celiac plexus block,
  340-346, 345f-347f
Rib
  anatomy of
    in interpleural block, 228f
    in thoracic paravertebral block, 251f
  first
    anatomy of
      in infraclavicular block, 61f-63f
      in interscalene block, 43f
      in stellate block, 185f
      in supraclavicular block, 37f-38f, 51f,
        53f-55f
    brachial plexus anatomy at, 38-39
  second, anatomy of, in stellate block, 185f
  twelfth, anatomy of, in celiac plexus block, 341f
Ropivacaine, 4f, 6, 6f
  for ankle block, 136
  for axillary block, 68
  for breast block, 218
  for celiac plexus block, 340
  for cervical paravertebral block, 247
  for cervical plexus block, 178
  for elbow nerve block, 74
  for epidural block, 286
  for facet block, 316
  for femoral block, 112
  for infraclavicular block, 60
  for inguinal block, 240
  for intercostal block, 222
  for interpleural block, 228
  for interscalene block, 42-43, 45
  for lateral femoral cutaneous block, 124
  for obturator block, 127
  for popliteal block, 130
  for sacroiliac block, 328-330
  for sciatic block, 102
  for stellate block, 185
  for superior hypogastric plexus block, 350
  for supraclavicular block, 50
  for transversus abdominis plane block, 256

S

Sacral anatomy, 268f
  in sacroiliac block, 330f-331f
  sex of patient and, 302-303, 303f
  in superior hypogastric plexus block, 352f
Sacral canal, anatomy of, in caudal block, 269-270,
  270f, 305f
Sacral cornu, anatomy of, in caudal block, 269-270,
  270f, 304f-305f
Sacral hiatus, anatomy of
  in caudal block, 269-270, 270f, 302-303, 302f-303f,
    305f
  in sciatic block, 107f
Sacral nerves, anatomy of, 233f
Sacral roots, anatomy of, 267f
Sacrococcygeal ligament, anatomy of, in caudal
  block, 269-270
Sacroiliac block, 327-334
  anatomy for, 330, 330f-331f
  fluoroscopy in, 332-334, 334f
  groin pain relief after, 334
  needle puncture for, 332-334, 332f-334f
  patient selection for, 328, 328f-329f
  pharmacologic agents for, 328-330
  position for, 330f-333f, 332
  problems with, 334
Sacroiliac joint
  anatomy of, 330, 330f-333f
  provocative testing of, 328, 328f-329f
Sacroiliac ligament, anatomy of, in sacroiliac block,
  330, 330f-331f
Sacrospinalis muscle, anatomy of, 269f
Sacrospinous ligament, anatomy of, in sacroiliac
  block, 330f-331f
Sacrotuberous ligament, anatomy of, in sacroiliac
  block, 330f-331f
Saline solution, in interpleural block, 228-230
Saphenous block
  anesthetic volume in, 134
  needle puncture for, 131, 132f
  with popliteal block, 130
Saphenous nerve, anatomy of, 91f, 93f-94f, 132f
  in ankle block, 136-137, 136f
  in popliteal block, 132f
Saphenous nerve block, at ankle, 137f, 138
Saphenous vein, cross section of, 96f
Sartorius muscle
  anatomy of, in popliteal block, 132f
  cross section of, 96f
Scalene muscle, anatomy of
  in cervical paravertebral block, 248f
  in infraclavicular block, 61f-63f
  in interscalene block, 42f-44f, 43, 46f-47f
  in stellate block, 185f-187f
  in supraclavicular block, 37f-38f, 51f, 53f-55f
Scapula, anatomy of, in epidural block, 289f
Sciatic block, 101-110
  anatomy for, 102, 103f-105f
  anterior approach to
    needle puncture for, 108, 108f-109f
    position for, 108
  classic approach to, 102
    needle puncture for, 102, 106f-107f
    position for, 102, 106f
  local anesthetics for, 102
  patient selection for, 102
  problems with, 109
  subgluteal approach to, 109-110, 110f
  ultrasonography-guided, 109-110, 110f
Sciatic nerve
  anatomy of, 102, 103f-105f
  on magnetic resonance imaging, 109f
Sedation, for intercostal block, 222, 225
Selective nerve root injection. See Transforaminal
  injection.

Semimembranosus muscle and tendon
  anatomy of, in popliteal block, 130f, 132f
  cross section of, 96f
Semitendinosus muscle and tendon
  anatomy of, in popliteal block, 130f, 132f
  cross section of, 96f
Seroma formation
  with spinal cord stimulator implantation, 383
  with spinal drug delivery system, 373
Serratus anterior muscle, anatomy of, 216f
  in infraclavicular block, 60-64, 61f
Short ciliary nerve, anatomy of, in retrobulbar
  (peribulbar) block, 172-173, 176f
Shoulder surgery
  cervical paravertebral block for, 247
  interscalene block for, 43, 45
Side-port device, during catheter placement for
  infraclavicular block, 18-20, 19f
Sinuvertebral nerve of Luschka, anatomy of, in facet
  block, 316, 319f-320f
Sitting position
  for epidural block, 287
  for spinal block, 273-276, 274f-275f
Skin bridge, catheter tunneling with, 20, 24f-25f
SnapLock device, in continuous nerve stimulation,
  20-26, 26f
Solar plexus. See Celiac plexus.
Soleus muscle, cross section of, 96f
Somatic nerve, anatomy of
  in celiac plexus block, 343f
  in lumbar somatic block, 234f, 237f
Spinal artery, anatomy of, 267f
Spinal block, 271-284
  anatomy for, 272, 273f
  backache with, 284
  cerebrospinal fluid aspiration in, 280, 281f
  combined spinal-epidural technique in, 284
  continuous, 284
  fentanyl in, 284
  headache with, 272, 276, 284
  high, dyspnea with, 284
  hyperbaric, 272
  hypobaric, 272
  local anesthetics for, 272
  lumbosacral (Taylor's) approach to, 280, 283f
  midline approach to, 276-280, 279f-281f
  needle puncture for, 276-280, 279f-283f
  neurologic injury with, 284
  paramedian approach to, 280, 282f
  patient selection for, 272
  position for, 273-276, 273f-277f
  problems with, 284
  vasoconstrictors for, 272
Spinal canal, anatomy of, in spinal block,
  277f-278f
Spinal cord injury, with spinal drug delivery system,
  373
Spinal cord stimulation, 375-383
  anatomy for, 377
  antibiotics with, 383
  battery failure and, 383
  bleeding with, 382
  dural puncture with, 382-383
  equipment placement for, 377-382, 378f-381f
  infection with, 382
  lead complications with, 383
  patient selection for, 376
  pocket for, 377, 378f-381f, 382
  position for, 377, 378f-381f
  problems with, 382-383
  radiography in, 383
  seroma formation with, 383
  trial of, 376-377
  tunneling device for, 378f-381f, 382
  wound dehiscence with, 383

Spinal drug delivery system, 365-373
  abdominal wall pocket for, 367, 368f-371f
  anatomy for, 366
  antibiotics with, 373
  bleeding with, 373
  catheter placement for
    intrathecal, 367, 368f-371f
    permanent epidural, 367-373, 372f
  infection with, 373
  patient selection for, 366
  position for, 366-367, 368f-371f
  problems with, 373
  pump migration with, 373
  seroma formation with, 373
  spinal cord injury with, 373
  subcutaneous port for, 367-372, 372f
  sutures for, 367, 368f-371f
  tunneling device for, 367, 368f-372f, 372-373
  wound dehiscence with, 373
Spinal fluid injection, in epidural block, 297, 297f
Spinal ganglion, anatomy of, 216f
Spinal needles, 8, 8f
  for glossopharyngeal block, 201
Spinal nerve, anatomy of
  in epidural block, 288f, 292f
  in facet block, 319f
Spinal nerve root injection. See Transforaminal
    injection.
Spinous process, anatomy of, 264, 265f
  in epidural block, 292f
Splanchnic nerve, anatomy of
  in celiac plexus block, 340, 341f-344f
  in interpleural block, 228f
Splanchnic plexus. See Celiac plexus.
Splenic artery, anatomy of, in celiac plexus block, 343f
Sprotte needle, 8f
  for spinal block, 276
Stellate block, 183-188
  anatomy for, 184f-185f, 185-186
  local anesthetics for, 185
  needle puncture for, 186, 187f
  patient selection for, 184
  position for, 186, 186f
  problems with, 188
Stellate ganglion, anatomy of, in stellate block,
    185-186, 185f
Sternocleidomastoid muscle, anatomy of, 143f
  in cervical plexus block, 180f-181f
  in infraclavicular block, 62f-63f
  in interscalene block, 43f-44f, 46f
  in stellate block, 185f-187f
  in supraclavicular block, 37f-38f, 51f, 53f-55f
Sternohyoid muscle, anatomy of, in stellate block, 185f
Sternum, anatomy of, in infraclavicular block, 62f
Stimulating catheter technique, for continuous nerve
    block, 18, 20, 21f-23f
Styloid process, anatomy of, in glossopharyngeal
    block, 199f, 201f
Subarachnoid anesthesia
  with caudal block, 306
  with lumbar somatic block, 237
  with transforaminal injection, 361, 363
  with trigeminal (gasserian) ganglion block, 156
Subarachnoid space, 266-269
  anatomy of
    in epidural block, 287f-288f
    in superior hypogastric plexus block, 356f
Subclavian artery, anatomy of
  in infraclavicular block, 63f
  in interscalene block, 43f
  in stellate block, 185f
  in supraclavicular block, 38, 38f, 51f, 53f-57f, 56
Subclavian vein
  anatomy of
    in infraclavicular block, 62f

Subclavian vein, anatomy of (Continued)
    in interscalene block, 43f
    in supraclavicular block, 51f, 53f-55f
  puncture of, during supraclavicular block, 55
Subcostal nerve, anatomy of, 92f
  in inguinal block, 240f, 242f
  in lumbar somatic block, 233f
Subdural injection, in epidural block, 297, 297f
Subdural space, 266-269
  anatomy of, in epidural block, 287f
Subgluteal approach, to ultrasonography-guided
    sciatic block, 109-110, 110f
Subscapular nerve, anatomy of, 33f
Superficial cervical plexus, anatomy of, 142-143, 143f
Superficial cervical plexus block, 180-182, 181f
Superficial peroneal nerve, anatomy of, 91f, 93f-94f
  in ankle block, 136-137, 136f
Superficial peroneal nerve block, at ankle, 137f, 138
Superior articular process, anatomy of, in epidural
    block, 292f
Superior cervical ganglion, anatomy of, in stellate
    block, 184f-185f, 185-186
Superior gemmelus muscle, anatomy of, in sciatic
    block, 110f
Superior hypogastric plexus
  anatomy of, 350, 351f-354f
  neurolysis of, 350
Superior hypogastric plexus block, 349-356
  anatomy for, 350, 351f-354f
  fluoroscopy in, 350-354, 356
  intravascular injection with, 356, 356f
  magnetic resonance imaging in, 356f
  needle puncture for, 350-354, 353f-355f
  paraspinous muscle spasm with, 356, 356f
  patient selection for, 350
  pharmacologic agents for, 350
  position for, 350, 352f
  problems with, 356, 356f
  red triangle for, 350, 352f, 355f
  skin markings for, 354f
Superior laryngeal block, 203-205, 204f-205f
Superior laryngeal nerve, anatomy of
  in airway block, 192-193, 193f-195f
  in superior laryngeal block, 204-205, 204f
Superior mesenteric artery, anatomy of, in celiac
    plexus block, 342f-343f
Superior mesenteric ganglion, anatomy of, in celiac
    plexus block, 341f-343f
Superior nuchal line, anatomy of, in occipital block,
    148f
Superior oblique muscle, anatomy of, in retrobulbar
    (peribulbar) block, 176f
Superior orbital fissure, anatomy of, 143-144, 144f
Superior rectus muscle, anatomy of, in retrobulbar
    (peribulbar) block, 172f, 174f, 176f
Supraclavicular block, 49-57
  anatomy for, 37-39, 37f-38f, 50, 51f
  AXIS block versus, 56
  classic (Kulenkampff) approach to
    needle puncture for, 50, 52f
    position for, 50
  local anesthetics for, 50
  patient selection for, 50
  pneumothorax with, 55-56
  problems with, 55
  ultrasonography-guided, 56-57, 56f-57f
  vertical (plumb bob) approach to
    needle puncture for, 53-55, 53f-55f
    position for, 53
Supraclavicular nerve, anatomy of, 142f-143f, 146f
  in cervical plexus block, 178f-179f, 179, 181f
  in pronated arm, 34f
  in supinated arm, 34f
Supraorbital nerve, anatomy of, 142f-143f, 143-144, 146f
  in distal trigeminal block, 169f-170f

Suprarenal plexus, anatomy of, in celiac plexus block,
    341f
Suprascapular nerve, anatomy of, 33f
Supraspinous ligament, anatomy of, 264-266, 266f,
    269f
  in epidural block, 287f
  in sacroiliac block, 330f-331f
  in spinal block, 273f, 280f
Supratrochlear nerve, anatomy of, 142f-143f, 146f
  in distal trigeminal block, 169f
Sural nerve
  anatomy of, 93f-94f
    in ankle block, 136-137, 136f
  cross section of, 96f
Sural nerve block, at ankle, 137-138, 137f
Sutures, for spinal drug delivery system, 367, 368f-371f
Sympathetic nervous system, plexuses of, 340
Sympathetic trunk, anatomy of, 216f
  in celiac plexus block, 341f-342f
  in glossopharyngeal block, 199f, 201f
  in lumbar somatic block, 234f, 237f
  in lumbar sympathetic block, 336, 336f
  in neuraxial block, 269f
  in stellate block, 186f-187f
  in superior hypogastric plexus block, 351f
Syringe technique, for cerebrospinal fluid aspiration,
    280, 281f

T

TAP block. See Transversus abdominis plane (TAP)
    block.
Taylor's (lumbosacral) approach, to spinal block,
    280, 283f
Temporalis muscle, anatomy of, in trigeminal
    (gasserian) ganglion block, 154f
Testicular artery, anatomy of, in celiac plexus block,
    341f
Tetracaine, 4f-5f, 5
  for spinal block, 272
Thoracic epidural block
  anatomy of, 286-287, 288f
  needle puncture for, 291-294, 291f-294f
Thoracic facet joints, anatomy of, 316, 317f
Thoracic paravertebral block, 250-253, 251f-252f
Thoracic sympathetic ganglion, first, anatomy of, in
    stellate block, 184f
Thoracic vertebrae, anatomy of, 288f
Thoracodorsal nerve, anatomy of, 33f
Three-in-one block, 98-99, 98f
Thyroepiglottic ligament, anatomy of, in airway
    block, 195f
Thyrohyoid membrane, anatomy of
  in airway block, 195f
  in superior laryngeal block, 205f
  in translaryngeal block, 208f-209f
Thyroid cartilage, anatomy of
  in airway block, 194f-196f
  in interscalene block, 43f
  in superior laryngeal block, 204f-205f
  in supraclavicular block, 51f
  in translaryngeal block, 208f-209f
Thyroid gland, anatomy of, in stellate block, 187f
Tibial collateral ligament, anatomy of, in popliteal
    block, 132f
Tibial nerve
  anatomy of, 91f
    in ankle block, 136f
    in popliteal block, 130-131, 130f-131f, 134f
    in sciatic block, 103f
  cross section of, 96f
Tibial nerve block, at ankle, 137-138, 137f
Tibial tuberosity, anatomy of, in popliteal block, 132f
Tibialis anterior tendon, cross section of, 96f
Tibialis posterior tendon, cross section of, 96f

Tongue, anatomy of, in airway block, 196f
Tonsillar nerve, anatomy of, in airway block, 192
Tourniquet inflation pressure, for intravenous
    regional block, 82-85
Trachea, anatomy of
  in airway block, 195f
  in translaryngeal block, 208f-209f
Tracheal intubation
  glossopharyngeal block for, 198
  superior laryngeal block for, 204
  translaryngeal block for, 208
Transforaminal injection, 357-363
  cervical, 358-361, 359f-360f
  coaxial technique for, 363
  lumbar, 361-363, 362f
Translaryngeal block, 207-209, 208f-209f
Transverse cervical nerve, anatomy of, 142f, 146f
  in cervical plexus block, 178f-179f, 179, 181f
Transverse process, anatomy of, 264-266, 266f
Transversus abdominis muscle, anatomy of
  in celiac plexus block, 341f
  in inguinal block, 242f
  in transversus abdominis plane block, 256,
    257f-260f
Transversus abdominis plane (TAP) block, 255-260
  anatomy for, 256, 257f
  local anesthetics for, 256
  needle puncture for, 258, 258f
  patient selection for, 256
  problems with, 260
  triangle of Petit approach to, 258-259, 260f
  ultrasonography-guided, 258, 259f
Trapezius muscle, anatomy of
  in cervical paravertebral block, 246f, 248f
  in infraclavicular block, 62f
  in interscalene block, 46f
Triamcinolone
  for cervical nerve root block, 360
  for lumbar nerve root block, 361
Triangle of Petit, in transversus abdominis plane
    block, 257f, 258-259, 260f
Trigeminal block, distal, 167-168, 169f-170f
Trigeminal ganglion, anatomy of, 152, 152f-156f
  in mandibular block, 163f
Trigeminal (gasserian) ganglion block, 151-156
  anatomy for, 152, 152f-154f
  local anesthetics for, 152
  needle puncture for, 154-156, 156f
  patient selection for, 152
  position for, 154, 155f
  problems with, 156
  subarachnoid injection with, 156
Trigeminal nerve
  anatomy of, 143-144, 144f
    in airway block, 192, 192f, 196f
    in trigeminal (gasserian) ganglion block, 152,
      152f-154f
  distal, anatomy of, 168, 169f
Trigeminal nerve block, distal, 167-168, 169f-170f
Truncal anatomy, 213-214, 215f-216f
  cross-section of, 216f
  dermatomes in, 215f
Truncal block
  anatomy for, 213-214, 215f-216f
  breast, 217-220, 219f-220f
  intercostal, 221-225, 223f-225f
  interpleural, 227-230, 228f-229f
Tuffier's line, 264
  in lumbar paravertebral block, 254, 254f
Tunneling device
  with spinal cord stimulator implantation,
    378f-381f, 382
  for spinal drug delivery system, 367, 368f-372f,
    372-373

Tuohy needle, 8f
  for lumbar epidural block, 287
  for spinal block, 276

U

Ulna, anatomy of
  in ulnar nerve block, 76f
  in wrist nerve block, 77f
Ulnar artery, anatomy of, in wrist nerve block,
    77f
Ulnar groove, palpation of, 76f
Ulnar nerve, anatomy of, 32, 33f
  in axillary block, 68-71, 69f-72f
  at elbow, 74-75, 74f, 76f
  in infraclavicular block, 60-64, 62f-63f
  in pronated arm, 34f
  in supinated arm, 34f
  at wrist, 77, 77f-78f
Ulnar nerve block
  at elbow, 74-78, 74f, 76f
  interscalene approach to, 45
  at wrist, 77, 77f-78f
Ulnar styloid process, anatomy of, in wrist nerve
    block, 78f
Ultrasonography, 10-14
  for axillary block, 71-72, 72f
  beam focus in, 12, 13f
  color Doppler, 12-13
    for interscalene block, 48
  for femoral block, 117-119, 118f
  gain and time gain compensation in, 12
  "imaging" needle in, 7f
  for infraclavicular block, 65-66, 65f
  for interscalene block, 45-48, 46f-47f
  physics of, clinical issues related to, 12, 12f-13f
  for popliteal block, 133-134, 133f-134f
  for regional anesthesia
    ASRA recommendations for, 10b
    hydrodissection and doughnut sign formation
      in, 18-20
    in-plane and out-of-plane needle approaches in,
      14, 14f-15f
    PART maneuvers in, 14, 16f
    principles of, 13-14
    short-axis and long-axis views in, 13, 13f
  resolution in, 12, 12f
  for sciatic block, 109-110, 110f
  for supraclavicular block, 56-57, 56f-57f
  for transversus abdominis plane (TAP) block, 258,
    259f
  ultrasound generation in, 10-12, 11f
  wave properties in, 10, 11f
Umbilicus, anatomy of, in inguinal block, 243f
Upper extremity
  dermatomes of, 34f-35f
  osteotomes of, 35f
Upper extremity block. See also Brachial plexus
    block.
  anatomy for, 31-39. See also Brachial plexus,
    anatomy of.
  distal, 73-79
    at digits, 78-79, 79f
    at elbow, 74-78, 74f-76f
    problems with, 77
    at wrist, 77, 77f-78f
  intravenous regional, 81-86. See also Intravenous
    regional block.
  ipsilateral, with stellate block, 188

V

Vagal trunk, anatomy of, in celiac plexus block,
    341f-343f

Vagus nerve
  anatomy of
    in airway block, 192-193, 192f-194f, 196f
    in glossopharyngeal block, 199f, 201f
    inferior ganglion of, anatomy of, in superior
      laryngeal block, 204f
Van Lint's block, of orbicularis oculi muscle, 174,
    175f
Vancomycin
  with spinal cord stimulator implantation, 383
  with spinal drug delivery system, 373
Vasoconstrictors, 6-7, 6f-7f
  for spinal block, 272
Vastus lateralis muscle, cross section of, 96f
Vastus medialis muscle
  anatomy of, in popliteal block, 132f
  cross section of, 96f
Vena cava, inferior. See Inferior vena cava.
Venous exsanguination techniques, in intravenous
    regional block, 82-85, 84f
Ventricle, anatomy of
  in airway block, 195f
  in translaryngeal block, 208f
Vertebrae
  anatomy of, 264, 265f
  lumbar, anatomy of, 265f
  thoracic, anatomy of, 288f
Vertebral artery
  anatomy of
    in cervical plexus block, 180f
    in cervical transforaminal injection, 359f-360f
    in interscalene block, 43, 44f
    in stellate block, 184f, 186f
    in supraclavicular block, 37-38, 37f, 51f
  injection of
    with cervical transforaminal injection, 360-361
    in stellate block, 188
Vertebral body
  cervical, sixth, anatomy of, in cervical
    paravertebral block, 248f
  pedicle of, in thoracic paravertebral block, 251f
Vertebral column, 264, 265f
Vertebral ganglia, anatomy of, in stellate block,
    184f
Vertebral ligaments, lumbar, 266f
Vertebral notch, anatomy of, in epidural block, 292f
Vertebral prominence, 264
Vertebral tubercle, cervical, sixth, palpation of, in
    stellate block, 186, 186f, 188
Vestibular fold, anatomy of
  in airway block, 195f
  in translaryngeal block, 208f
Visceral pain, celiac plexus block for, 340
Vocal ligament, anatomy of
  in airway block, 195f
  in translaryngeal block, 208f

W

Whitacre needle, 8f
  for spinal block, 276
Wound dehiscence
  with spinal cord stimulator implantation, 383
  with spinal drug delivery system, 373
Wrist nerve block, 77, 77f-78f
Wrist surgery, cervical paravertebral block for, 247

Z

Zygoma
  anatomy of
    in maxillary block, 159f
    in trigeminal (gasserian) ganglion block, 154f
  plane of, 153f